The Collected Works of MHE Milton H. Erickson

Volume 10

Hypnotic Realities

Editors:
Ernest Lawrence Rossi
Roxanna Erickson-Klein
Kathryn Lane Rossi

Forward by Jeffrey Zeig

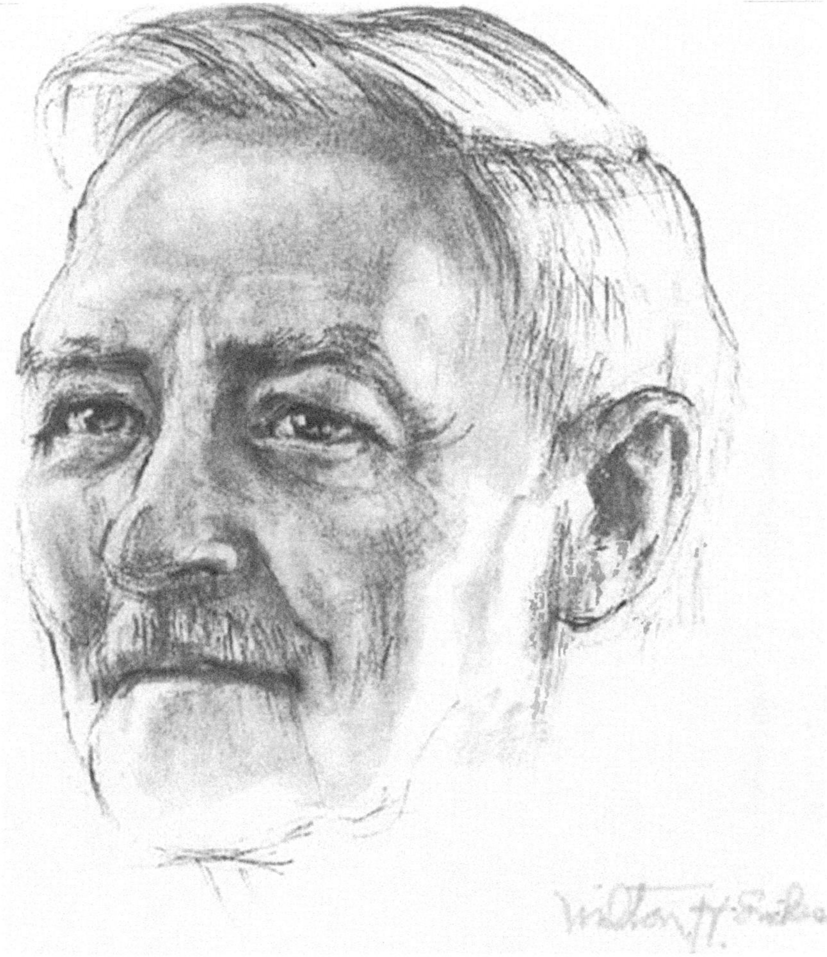

Milton H. Erickson, MD 1901 - 1980
Artist: Ida Libby Dengrove, 4 July 1976

Library of Congress Cataloging-in-Publication Data

ISBN: 978-1-7351114-7-6

Editors:
Rossi, Ernest Lawrence.
Erickson-Klein, Roxanna.
Rossi, Kathryn Lane.

The Collected Works of Milton H. Erickon. MD, Volume 10: Hypnotic Realities

1. Indirect Suggestion
2. Hypnosis
3. Induction
4. Conversational
5. Handshake
6. Therapeutic
7. Suggestion

Further Information:
Erickson-Milton.com
Erickson-Rossi.com
ErnestRossi.com

About the 2021 Digital Series

We hold an ambitious vision: To gather as many of the original works of Milton H. Erickson as within our capacity and publish in a format that reaches as many interested students as possible. Each of these volumes were originally published in printed books. This series of 16 digital volumes represents the editor's ongoing efforts to keep classic materials current and available to readers. Over the decades we three editors, Ernest and Kathryn Rossi and Roxanna Erickson-Klein, have worked together and individually on various stages of this series. We are guided by a shared commitment to bring these classic works to the students of today and tomorrow. Our friendship has been a pillar of strength on the path to publication in this format that has endured many challenges. When one of us was tired or bereft, another picked up and carried on.

Each of these volumes was originally published in printed book form. The last 15 years has brought a new age of digitization and broadened possibilities of access to these seminal works. Our vision is one of integration that allows students to explore with a depth that was not previously possible. We are working on the development of a search engine that spans across the all of the volumes for comprehensive information for individual readers interests. We hope our commitment to continue the work begun here will extend its wisdom to an ever-broadening audience and encourage ongoing exploration of infinite healing possibilities.

Many of these materials have been previously published in book form. The earlier publications included ***Advanced Techniques of Hypnosis and Therapy*** Edited by Jay Hayley and a 4-volume set of ***The Collected Papers of Milton H. Erickson,*** 1980 Edited by Ernest Rossi. The titles of the 4-volume set are:

The Nature of Hypnosis and Suggestion

Hypnotic Alteration of Sensory, Perceptual and Psychophysical Processes

Hypnotic Investigation of Psychodynamic Processes

Innovative Hypnotherapy

All of the papers from these five books are now included in Volumes 1-8 of the 2021 Digital Series along with additional new materials.

Volume 9, ***The February Man*** (2009) was published as an individual volume. Volumes 10, 11, and 12 were written as an experiential trilogy and are published in the 2021 Digital Series with the original titles:

Hypnotic Realities (2010)

Hypnotherapy, An Exploratory Casebook (2014)

Experiencing Hypnosis: Therapeutic Approaches to Altered States (2014)

Volumes 13-16 were published as a 4-volume set with the same titles as appears in the 2021 Digital Series.

Healing in Hypnosis:
The Seminars, Workshops and Lectures part one (2014)

Life Reframing in Hypnosis:
The Seminars, Workshops and Lectures, part two (2014)

Mind Body Communication in Hypnosis:
The Seminars, Workshops and Lectures part three (2015)

Creative Choice in Hypnosis:
The Seminars, Workshops and Lectures, part four (2014)

What you will find within these works are the words of Milton Erickson as he wrote, conversed and spoke. You will also see how he interacted, explained, and failed to explain, with patients and colleagues. The harmony of voices shows how conscious explanations leave off as unconscious processes begin. Erickson valued what emerged as his own ideas developed over the years. Through our forewords, we include voices of colleagues who carry Erickson's work onward. It is an ongoing treasure to investigate and advance techniques, ideas and approaches, exploring the healing legacy left by Milton H. Erickson.

Ernest Rossi, PhD & Kathryn Rossi PhD,
Los Osos, California

Roxanna Erickson-Klein PhD,
Dallas, Texas

2021 Message to Our Readers

This is a momentous and joyous time for us, the editors: Ernest and Kathryn Rossi, and Roxanna Erickson-Klein. The release of this digital volume represents reaching the peak of a mountainous journey through time.

As we gaze out to the horizon, we release the first volume of 16 volumes of the Collected works of Milton H. Erickson in the digital integrated format. While this collection has been previously published in hardback and paperback books through the non-profit Milton H. Erickson Foundation Archives, our current efforts represent the construction an integrated search capability that extends through all 16 volumes.

Milton H. Erickson, MD, began his professional writing a century ago. He dedicated his career to the dream of bringing clinical hypnosis from the dappled shadows of history to blaze a trail in science and medicine. Ernest Rossi, a colleague mentored by Erickson in the use of hypnosis, began his studies with Erickson half a century ago. The two of them, Ernest Rossi and Milton Erickson, sought to identify the hypnosis and rehabilitation understandings Erickson had developed and to decipher techniques to further advance the work and knowledge in written form.

By the time Erickson died in 1980, he and Ernest Rossi had co-authored twelve books, signed contracts with publishers and enjoyed a sense of progress in their shared endeavor. At the time, the Erickson family felt a depth of gratitude to Ernest Rossi and to the other colleagues who had contributed and made their own efforts to compile and preserve the ideas of Milton H. Erickson, the great thinker, who had accomplished ambitious goals undertaken early in his lifetime. Within a few years, both Rossi and the Erickson family became aware that the works were not as available to readers as had been promised in the contracts.

Over the next several decades, the three of us: Ernest and Kathryn Rossi along with Roxanna as a representative of the Erickson family, joined forces to work through the legal, business, financial and practical concerns associated with this process of making these important contributions available. We three committed ourselves to make the primary works of Milton Erickson available to scholars, clinicians, historians, and explorers of the future. It was an arduous journey, but one in which the Rossi's and Roxanna reinforced working alliances as we deepened our rewarding friendship.

At the time this journey began, the concept of the effects of psychotherapy on the physiology of genes was merely a whisper not yet scientifically understood. The idea of digitizing reading materials was beyond the scope of day to day audiences. Yet, while we have traveled this journey, science has advanced and digitization has claimed the right of way for publications. Thus, our initial goals of making these primary works available shifted to address these relevant changes. Ernest Rossi has annotated the originals to discuss the interface of what is now understood from a neuroscience and genomic perspective. What we now offer is the original works that illustrate how the words and works of Milton Erickson invite healthy change in the context of today's understandings.

Now that the pragmatics of bringing this all together have been mapped out, the remaining volumes with search capabilities will soon follow. Eventually, we hope to expand beyond the first 16 volumes to include as many of the primary works of Erickson as possible, some of which have yet to be published for the first time. Our work is not complete, but this step shows the sunrise on the far side of the mountainous path.

Ernest Rossi, PhD & Kathryn Rossi PhD
Los Osos, California

Roxanna Erickson-Klein PhD
Dallas, Texas

The Structure of This Volume

Hypnotic Realities is a the first of a trilogy wherein Milton Erickson experientially trains Ernest Rossi in clinical hypnosis. The two additional volumes of this trilogy are ***Hypnotherapy: An Exploratory Casebook*** (published first in 1979, now Volume 11 of this Collected works series) and ***Experiencing Hypnosis*** (1981, now Volume 12). Taken together, these three volumes present a deepening view of what hypnosis is and the ways in which a creative process of hypnotherapy can be achieved. The material in these volumes touches ultimately on the nature of human consciousness and suggests a variety of open-ended approaches to facilitate its exploration in hypnotherapy as well as in more formal research situations.

Our object in this series of trancework, has been to learn as much as possible about Erickson's approaches so that other clinicians and research workers could study, test, and utilize our findings. Because Erickson's approaches presuppose a certain amount of clinical skill, a major goal of this volume has been to carefully delineate exactly how Erickson goes about his work, the observations and inferences he makes, and the hypotheses he tests. Any fair evaluation of his approaches requires that the clinician and researcher acquire some of Erickson's hypnotherapeutic skills. To facilitate this process of skill acquisition, we have outlined the types of study and exercises that other workers might well pursue to further their clinical practice and research in hypnosis.

This volume is the record of a series of training sessions in which both Dr. S (a professional who serves as the primary hypnotic subject) and Ernest Rossi (the student / colleague) were experientially learning hypnosis. The sessions were carefully recorded on audio cassettes and later reviewed by the authors. At this time, Erickson was 72 years of age, and Rossi looked up to him as the senior contributor to the material, thus refers to Erickson as the senior author and himself as the junior author. In the discussions, which took place both during the hypnotic sessions and afterwards, Rossi's inquisitive mind stimulated a lot of why, how and what questions. Erickson answered in his own unique manner - usually to use the inquiry as a jump off point for the next demonstration session with Dr. S.

Within this book are the transcripts of hypnotic inductions done while Rossi observed and participated in a variety of roles. The chapters are divided into carefully transcribed records of Erickson's induction of clinical hypnosis and his work with a subject along with commentary to elucidate his procedures. In these records there is some repetition of the procedures utilized, the questions asked, the issues discussed and nonverbal behavior is described. This repetition came about naturally because Erickson was engaged in training Rossi in hypnotherapy. Rossi in turn, frequently had to ask the same questions over and over to be sure he understood what Erickson was trying to convey. The repetition of similar themes in different contexts allows the reader to explore the significant features of Erickson's work and how he utilizes them in the contingencies of daily practice.

The transcript of the trancework is bolded so that readers are able to identify what was actually spoken to the subject. During the sessions, there are a multitude of comments between Erickson and Rossi as the subject sits quietly in trance state. These questions and comments are included as they took place in the context of the trancework, differentiated with bold type.

After a session, the recording was then transcribed for further discussion. In the follow-up discussions techniques, intentions, strategies, meanings and responses were further discussed. These commentaries are likewise positioned so they can assist readers in a fuller understanding of the nature of the trancework.

To make this book more useful as a training text, Rossi added information and exercises for readers to skill build. While these elements were largely Rossi's contributions, Erickson reviewed and approved all of the material that is contained herein. For clarity, we have separated the transcripts of the trance sessions from the conceptual discussions and summaries of information.

Because both Rossi and Dr. S were both relative beginners in the study of hypnosis, Erickson introduced and demonstrated basic principles in a manner that makes this volume suitable as an introductory text. In studying this volume readers may do best by first reading the induction sections that are the "purest" indications of Erickson's work.

Readers can then draw their own conclusions and ask their own questions about the work before progressing to the commentary sections. They can then determine for themselves the adequacy of the explications of the inductions. Readers may then write their own analyses of the relevant variables and perhaps test them, adding to the general knowledge. At the end of each chapter or section where new material has been introduced, a number of graduated exercises are offered as a guide to aid hypnotherapists in developing their own skills in the clinical arts of observation, hypnotic induction, and the formulation of indirect suggestions. Many of these exercises will be of value to the general psychotherapist with or without the formal induction of clinical hypnosis.

1976 Foreword by André Weitzenhoffer

An Encounter with Milton H. Erickson

For the many who never had the opportunity and never will have the opportunity to attend workshops led by Milton Erickson, this work will serve as an invaluable surrogate. Psychotherapists, in general, as well as hypnotherapists, will find the work rewarding reading and study, for Erickson is above all a psychotherapist, and his ***modus operandi*** transcends clinical hypnotism. As for academicians and researchers, I believe they will find enough food for thought and research here, to keep them busy for some time to come.

My first encounter with Milton H. Erickson was in 1954 or 1955 at a meeting of the Society for Clinical and Experimental Hypnosis in Chicago. When I met him he was engaged in conversation with a small group of colleagues in a hotel lobby. I had never seen the man or even a photograph of him. Yet, in a strange way, as it then seemed to me, as I saw him from some distance out of hearing range, I knew this was Milton Erickson. I have thought back to this incident a number of times. Conceivably, I had heard somewhere that he had had polio and the fact he leaned on a cane might have been the clue to his identity. I cannot be sure, but I am inclined to believe the clues were more subtle. In a way, I had encountered Milton a number of times previously—through his writings which I had studied exhaustively. Through these, I had begun to appreciate the uniqueness of his person. I believe that some of the qualities which have made him the individual he is, were communicated to me through these writings, and that I experienced them more directly as they were manifesting themselves as he interacted with others.

In the years which followed, I was to have other occasions, by far too few to suit me, to meet with him, watch him demonstrate, watch him doing therapy, and listen to him talk about hypnotism as well as other matters. More particularly, I had the opportunity to see why, as the years have gone by, he has grown into a quasi-legendary figure to whom the title of "Mr. Hypnosis" was once given. I have also had the opportunity to see in action such famed stage hypnotists of the forties and fifties as: Ralph Slater, Franz Polgar, and others, many of whom billed themselves as "America's Foremost Hypnotist," the "World's Fastest Hypnotist," etc., and who extolled their fantastic prowess ***ad nauseam***. Good entertainers, yes. As hypnotists, however, they came up poor seconds to Milton Erickson, and yet, there never was a more quiet, unassuming man.

It is not surprising then that many professionals have tried to emulate him. None thus far have ever truly succeeded, although a few have managed to become a fair approximation. Some of the reasons for this become clear on reading this work. Some of these will still remain unclear. If the authors have failed to deal with them to the extent that their importance calls for, it is only because they are not exactly the kind of things one can adequately teach merely through the written word. Perhaps, it is also because they are not teachable and, I suspect, there is some unwillingness on their part to admit this to themselves and the reader.

As the work makes it most clear, not only what one says to the patient or subject, how one says it, when one says it, and where one says it are all extremely important factors in the effective use of hypnotism, particularly in a clinical, therapeutic setting. It also becomes clear that one must view the hypnotherapeutic interaction in its totality and not piecemeal, and go even a step further by viewing it within the totality of its utilization. This takes the use of suggestion, and more broadly, of hypnotism out of the domain of the use of simple magic formulas and places it within the framework of the science of interactional and communication networks.

Erickson, however, is not just a master of verbal communication as the work makes evident. He is equally adept at nonverbal communication, which is one of the aspects to which the work does not and can not really do justice. This is unfortunate, but unavoidable and certainly not an oversight on the part of the authors. One of the more memorable demonstrations of his skill at nonverbal communication that he has given in his career was in Mexico City in 1959 when he hypnotized and demonstrated various hypnotic phenomena with a subject with whom verbal communication was impossible. He spoke no Spanish and the subject spoke no English. From beginning to end, communication was carried entirely nonverbally through pantomime.

I can personally attest to the effectiveness of his nonverbal communications, through an experience I had with Milton Erickson some 15 or 16 years ago. Here I think I should make it clear that, to my knowledge, I have never been hypnotized by him, at least formally. A group of us had met in Philadelphia with Milton, in a special seminar aimed at gaining some understanding of his ***modus operandi.*** One morning, I was alone with him sitting at the breakfast table, facing him somewhat obliquely toward his left. As I recall, I was doing most of the talking. As I talked, partially absorbed in my thoughts, I became vaguely aware, peripherally, of Milton making peculiar repetitious gestures with one of his hands. Momentarily I made nothing of this, then with my awareness increasing, two things happened in very close sequence. My right hand moved out, spontaneous-like, to pick up the coffee pot which was on the table and begin to lift it. With this, the realization dawned on me that Milton wanted coffee. At that point, to use the terminology of this work, my "conscious mind" took over the action and I completed the act, while realizing now, that Milton's gesturing had, indeed, clearly spelled out a nonverbal request to have coffee poured into his cup. This sort of thing, as I learned in time, is one of his favorite ways of teaching or answering a question about a related matter. It is also his way of subtly testing an individual's suggestibility or hypnotizability. It is also his way of keeping himself in shape, so to speak. I said, toward the beginning of this paragraph, that I had never been "formally" hypnotized by Milton Erickson. True, if by "formal induction," we mean the use of any of the usual classical and semi-classical techniques described over and over in various texts on hypnotism. For reasons that will become clear presently, and certainly after reading the present work, I am sure that the authors would say that I had indeed been hypnotized by Milton at least on that particular occasion.

There is, of course, much more to effective verbal communication than saying words according to appropriate syntactical and other linguistic rules, or the introduction of appropriate nonverbal elements at the correct time and place. In my experiences with Milton Erickson, I have found that his control of such features as intonation and voice modulation, to mention only these two aspects, forms an intrinsic part of his approach to hypnotism. One has to hear and watch him to get the full flavor of his manner of speech. To say that he speaks gently, yet incisively, slowly, calmly, softly, enunciating clearly and carefully each word, sometimes each syllable, the whole with certain cadence, can only give but a sketchy flavor of the process. There is, unfortunately, no way for a book to convey to the reader the kinds of information that would allow him to duplicate these features. However, attention can be called to this matter so that after studying the book, if the reader finds himself somewhat less effective than Erickson in spite of his efforts to do everything just so, he will not draw the wrong conclusions.

Another element which I believe enters into Milton's effectiveness and which, in my opinion, this work does not sufficiently bring out, is the quiet confidence, and strangely enough in view of his permissive approach, the authority too, that he exudes. There is a conviction expressed by his voice and his actions that everything is, or will be, as he says. Perhaps part of this exuded conviction has its roots in another feature of Erickson's interaction with his subjects and patients. As one watches him, one becomes very much aware of his ability to communicate to the subject and patient that he is participating in some of his experiences and sharing these with him. This is particularly evident when he elicits hallucinatory phenomena. As one witnesses Milton Erickson tell a subject about a skier "out there" on a distant snow covered hill which he describes in some detail, or about a rabbit "right down there at your feet and what color is it?" one often has the eerie feeling that he too sees the skier, the hill, the snow, and the rabbit. How then, can the subject indeed fail to see them too? Whether or not Milton actually shares in the subject's subjective experiences, the impression is verbally and nonverbally communicated to the latter that he does. In my opinion this is an extremely powerful adjunct in his elicitation of the desired responses.

This is to say then, as a warning to readers who might expect much more than is reasonable from this work, that I believe there are important elements Milton Erickson brings to bear in his production and utilization of hypnosis which are not given as much attention as they deserve. This is not being written in a judgmental manner, an action hardly appropriate to a foreword. That aspect of the induction and utilization of hypnosis upon which the authors have chosen to focus is sufficiently complex and central as to justify certain omissions, particularly of material extremely difficult to deal with in writing.

Indeed, as every modern educator knows, the three major modes of communication, audio, visual, and written, each contributes in a unique and noninterchangeable way to the total process of education. What I have just stated merely reflects this fact. As written communication goes, the present work does a superlative job in elucidating the complexities of Erickson's approaches to clinical hypnotism. Indeed it accomplishes admirably that which can only best be done by the written word.

All of this leads me to one last point I would make for all those readers who would aspire to become another Milton Erickson. The book will teach them some of Milton's "secrets," which actually were never secrets at all. It is simply that what he did, and still does, was so obvious and natural to him that he assumed everyone knew what was going on. Whether knowing the secrets will be enough is a moot question. Milton did not become "Mr. Hypnosis" overnight. Many events and experiences have preceded his 50 years and more of experience with hypnotism. Many other events have also filled these fifty years. Which ones have materially contributed to make the man, the hypnotist, and the clinician that he is? No one can really tell, even Milton himself. Some can be specified. Of these, some could be duplicated, some could not, and there are some which one would hardly want to duplicate. A wide experience with the phenomenology of hypnotism, especially in a naturalistic setting, extensive and long experience teaching, applying, demonstrating, and experimenting with hypnotism, all of these must be seen as undoubtedly having played an essential part in Milton Erickson's spectacular success. These are duplicable. Potentially duplicable by deliberate inoculation, but hardly the kind of experience anyone would readily undergo, is being stricken twice with poliomyelitis as Milton Erickson was. Certainly not duplicable is being born tone deaf and color blind. Erickson attributes much of his heightened sensitivity to kinesthetic cues, body dynamics, and altered modes of sensory perceptual functioning to his lifelong struggle with his innate and acquired infirmities. In his study and effort to mitigate these problems he acquired a personal awareness of altered patterns of functioning that was channeled into his lifework as healer. Additionally, Erickson has brought to his lifework a remarkable imagination and creativity, a high degree of sensitivity and intuition, a keen observing power, a prodigious memory for facts and events, and a particular ability for organizing what he experiences on a moment to moment basis. There is little here that can be duplicated on demand.

If one is not likely to ever be another Milton Erickson, one can at least learn something about his ***modus operandi*** and utilize it as completely as possible within one's own limitations and in terms of one's own personal assets. If this work does nothing more than help the reader accomplish this, it will have attained its purpose.

In approaching this work the reader should keep in mind that it is the product of pragmatists, and that it is specifically about therapeutic or clinical hypnotism, and neither about theoretical or experimental hypnotism. The reader might as well know from the outset that he will not find in this book any well defined and worked out theory, nor any solid scientific documentation of many stated facts. Quite clearly, the authors espouse a certain theoretical position with regard to the nature of hypnosis, of hypnotic phenomena, of suggestion, and of suggested behavior. One may or may not agree with them, and many alternative explanations will come to the reader's mind as he follows the authors' explanations of what takes place when Erickson makes a certain intervention or takes a certain step. However, to get the most out of this work, one needs to keep in mind that its focus is not so much upon developing a scientific theory as it is upon elucidating how Milton Erickson obtains the kinds of results that he does; results which most would agree involve behavior which may be labeled as being "suggested" and/or being "hypnotic." From a practical, pragmatic standpoint it is relatively immaterial whether these elicited behaviors are "veridical," "roleplaying," "a product of cognitive restructuring," involve some sort of "dissociative process," or are the consequences of a "shaping" process, and so on. Eventually, the "true" scientist wants to know what is what. This the authors have well recognized, often pointing out areas for investigation and suggesting experiments which could be made. But for the busy clinician and for the long suffering patient it is results, and quick ones at that, which count. Efficacity is the issue. For this reason effective hypnotherapists, which the three authors are, do not limit themselves to hypnotic procedures per se. On the contrary, as is evident from this book, and even more so from other writings of Erickson and of Rossi, effective hypnotherapy constantly interweaves the utilization of hypnotic and nonhypnotic behavioral processes. To take just one tiny example, the use of the "D*ouble Bind*," be it as understood by Bateson, or in the special sense that the authors use it, is not a hypnotic technique or approach per se, nor does it involve a hypnotic or suggestion process, but it can be used as a specific tool to induce hypnosis and/or as a tool to elicit further behaviors from a hypnotized individual.

Although theory is neither the strength nor the focus of this book, a very definite theoretical position is reflected by Erickson's modus operandi, or at least guides it. It has been traditional, and this is still widely done, to view hypnotic behavior as behavior elicited by "suggestions" given while the subject is in a state of "hypnosis." However, even prior to Bernheim, and earlier, it has also been widely recognized that suggestions leading to the sort of behaviors exhibited by hypnotized individuals can also be effectively used in the absence of any induction of hypnosis. That is, they can be effective with persons who have presumably not been hypnotized. One interpretation of this observation, to which a small number of modern investigators have ascribed, is that hypnosis is not only unnecessary for the production of hypnotic behavior, but is also actually an unnecessary concept. This interpretation leads to the position there is no hypnosis as a state. However, one alternative to this position, and this is the one taken by the authors, is that all ***bonafide*** responses to suggestions are associated, ***ipso facto***, with a hypnotic or trance state. From this standpoint there is no longer any distinction between "waking" and "hypnotic" suggestions, or if one prefers, between extra and intrahypnotic suggestions. To respond adequately to a suggestion is to be hypnotized. To put it a little differently, according to the authors, one cannot respond adequately to a suggestion without first, or at the same time, developing a hypnotic trance. This particular view of the situation comes about in a two-fold way: for the authors, if a response is to be an adequate response to a suggestion, it must be mediated by a different aspect of the mind than so-called conscious behavior. Thus they distinguish between behavior executed by the subject's unconscious and conscious mind. Normally, the conscious dominates the unconscious. The traditional inductions of hypnosis are nothing more or less than a freeing of the unconscious from conscious dominance, which is what they see as also momentarily existing any time an individual responds adequately to a suggestion. For them to function completely at the unconscious level is to be in a trance or hypnotic state, too. Any shift from conscious to unconscious functioning is a passage from a non-trance to a trance state ("waking" to "hypnotic state"). Although this will most likely be clear to many readers, it may be well to make the point here that the authors' conception of the "unconscious" is definitely not the one held by Freud. Morton Prince's "subconscious" is perhaps the closest to it. In any case it is an intelligent, complex level of mental functioning which appears to retain certain ego functions possessed by the conscious mind, while relinquishing, or not being affected by, some of the other functions usually associated with the ego.

One consequence of the above view of suggestion and hypnotism is that the notion of hypnosis as a state of hyper-suggestibility becomes meaningless. To be suggestible is to be hypnotized. These are merely alternative ways of speaking of the same thing. It follows from this then, that it is also meaningless to speak of testing an individual's waking or non-hypnotic suggestibility, as a predictor of his hypnotizability. Finally, a formal induction of hypnosis, when it is successful, might be viewed in this framework as nothing more than an obtrusive technique which brings about a shift in degree of increased unconscious participation in a steplike fashion. The real impact of viewing hypnotic and suggested behavior as the authors do, however, is to be found in the central topic of this work. How to facilitate, activate, cultivate, and, to some extent, utilize unconscious levels of functioning. This is what this book is about.

I have spoken at great length about Milton Erickson, and justifiably so, since this is a book about his approach to the therapeutic utilization of hypnotism. Still, this work is a joint effort and, had it not been for another of the authors, in particular, Ernest L. Rossi, it would never have seen the light of day. Rossi has done much more than record and report that which Erickson does and says. He has spent an enormous amount of time and effort getting him to explicate what has been so clear to Milton, but so obscure to everyone else. Having done so, Rossi has proceeded to unravel, sift, analyze, translate, organize, and finally integrate what must at first have seemed to him to be a bewildering collection of data. This has been no small task, as I can attest to from my own unsuccessful past efforts to do something similar on a much smaller scale. Furthermore, Rossi has succeeded, I believe, in giving us an opportunity to see in a unique way, what Erickson does through the latter's very own eyes. Ernest Rossi's particular contribution does not stop there, however, and is to be further found in his compilation of interesting, useful, and thought provoking exercises, questions, commentaries and suggestions for research.

Finally, I believe that students of Erickson will find in this book answers to questions they wish they could have asked of him, but never did or could, and even more so, answers they sought but never got.

André M. Weitzenhoffer, PhD
Oklahoma City, Oklahoma

2022 Foreword by Jeffrey K. Zeig

Hypnotic Realities Visited 40 Years Later

Ernest Rossi, Kathryn Rossi and Roxanna Erickson-Klein graciously asked me to write the foreword for the volume of my choice for the eBook version of ***The Collected Works of Milton H. Erickson, MD***, and I chose Volume 10, ***Hypnotic Realities***. I had wanted to reread this volume first published in 1976, and this honor gave me that opportunity. It is a pleasure to revisit Erickson's work as a seasoned professional now more expert in the methods developed by my mentor. There is a lot to learn from Erickson and in reading ***Hypnotic Realities*** and I discovered more – even 40 years after his death.

Although ***Hypnotic Realities*** is not the first volume in ***The Collected Works***, it well could be, because it is the most important book in introducing Erickson's hypnotic methods. Even those who have advanced their practice of hypnotherapy will benefit from reading and re-reading it.

And there is another reason why I chose Volume 10. It conjures up a pleasant memory. It was gifted to me by Milton Erickson who inscribed in my copy, "Just another book to curl your hair." Let me explain: When I first visited Erickson in 1973 it was at the end of my counterculture days, and my curly hair was so long it could be pulled down to my waist. I had my hair styled before my next visit with him. I wore more professional clothing. Those changes represented a life transition.

These musings aside, Bernhard Trenkle, a dear friend and expert in hypnosis and the therapeutic use of humor, once told me a joke, which goes like this:

> A man named John, a serious stutterer, confidently strides into an employment office and declares that he wants a job selling Bibles. The employment officer cannot help but notice John's speech defect, so he suggests John consider another line of work. John is recalcitrant and insists that he can sell Bibles.
>
> For nearly a half hour, John argues his case, and eventually the employment officer acquiesces and gives John a Bible saying, "Obviously you need to see for yourself that you cannot sell Bibles because you stutter. Now go out and try to sell a copy."
>
> This leads to another long argument because John insists on getting a box of Bibles, not just one. Finally, the employment officer reluctantly hands John a box of Bibles and tells him he should come back at the end of the day having learned that sales is not for him.
>
> To the surprise of the employment officer, John returns in an hour with an empty box. He sold the entire box of Bibles. Since no one had ever sold a box of Bibles in an hour, the employment officer quizzed John about his method. It seems that John confidently declared to homeowners, "D-d-do you wa-wa-want to b-b-buy a B-B-Bible, or sh-sh-should I re-re-read it to you?"

Jokes can elicit humor. They are evocative forms of communication. We laugh because we have an experience, not because we have learned information. If I give you reasons why you should laugh, it will not prompt a smile. Humor is something that must be experienced.

In rereading ***Hypnotic Realties***, I am reminded of the essential nature of hypnosis as something that must be experienced. Once elicited it can be a foundation for subsequent therapy through which the client can have adaptive realizations.

Hypnotic Realities elicits in me the sense of once again being with Milton Erickson, watching his precision; watching as he strategically targets a conceptual goal using the lens of his uncommon perceptiveness. Erickson explored the possibilities inherent in evocative communication. He was a conceptual communicator who oriented people toward a realization by using evocative communication. Erickson's inductions and therapy were evocative, because like humor, evocative communication is required to prompt a realization.

Erickson was wise in selecting Ernest Rossi to be his Boswell. Many brilliant and accomplished therapists studied with Erickson, but Rossi was a superlative and dedicated student and collaborator – and a great writer. And he continued exploring and teaching what he learned from Erickson until his death in 2020.

Ernest Rossi was new to hypnosis when he visited Erickson in the early 1970s. Much of the book is dedicated to hypnotic induction. In it the author provides a roadmap of learning from the master. The transcripts and annotations in ***Hypnotic Realities*** pop off the page, bringing the spirit of Erickson to life. When the practice of hypnosis began in the medical field, inductions were scripted. Erickson expanded the world of hypnosis. Rather than using rote procedures, he improvised for each patient, tailoring both the induction and subsequent therapy

Hypnotic Realities codifies some of Erickson's methods. This revised version benefits from being cast in a contemporary neuroscience framework.

The only issue I have with Volume 10 is that some terms Rossi uses reflect earlier understandings. For example, "confusion" may be better seen as "destabilization," which is a milder and more accurate term. Also, "indirection" may be more appropriately described as "eliciting" or "orienting toward." When someone tells a joke, it orients the recipient toward the realization of humor, in the same way an induction may orient someone toward trance. Jokes also have destabilizing elements that prompt humor in the same way that effective hypnotherapy has destabilizing elements that prompt realizations.

Reading ***Hypnotic Realities*** is a journey worth embarking on because it will orient you toward realizations about hypnosis and its induction and the masterful work of Milton H. Erickson.

I am honored to write this foreword, but also recommend carefully studying the foreword of my esteemed predecessor, André Weitzenhoffer.

And finally, I thank and congratulate Ernest and Kathryn Rossi and Roxanna Erickson-Klein for their dedicated efforts in making this work available as an eBook.

Jeffrey K. Zeig, PhD
Founder and Director, The Milton H. Erickson Foundation
www.erickson-foundation.org
Phoenix, Arizona

2024 Editors' Preface

Eliciting Creative Change

Hypnotic Realities was the first work done collaboratively by Ernest Rossi and Milton H. Erickson. The cooperative way in which the two explored the territory of hypnotic trance, consciousness and the multitude of phenomena related to these ideas radiates a sense of trust, appreciation and joie de vivre. Roxanna remembers those treasured years when Ernest came to stay at the Erickson family home. The two of them would focus their attention as long as Erickson's stamina would carry him. As they quieted down for the evening, they would continue to talk about ideas for the morning.

This volume includes the original 1976 Foreword by André Weitzenhoffer as well as recent 2021 Foreword by Jeffrey Zeig. Each of these contributions reflects a deep appreciation for the uniqueness of the work of Milton Erickson. Over the many years of Erickson's professional exploration, we have been enriched by the collegial relationships, the similarities of perspectives and the differences, agreements and disagreements, the intense discussions and the mutual collaboration in a quest for understandings. With each of these individuals, as will the multitudes of other clinicians, researchers. And students of art who seek a more holistic understanding of the nature of consciousness we see this work as a piece of a much larger collective of wisdom.

Erickson demonstrates a myriad of approaches by which psychotherapists of all persuasions can facilitate psychological development with or without the formal induction of trance. Erickson teaches that trance itself is a different experience for every person; indeed, clinical trance may be understood as a freedom in which individuality can flourish. From this point of view one comes to understand Erickson's work as an active approach to the basic endeavor of all psychotherapy: helping individuals outgrow learned limitations so that inner potentials can be realized in service of therapeutic goals.

It will be seen on the following pages that clinical hypnosis and therapeutic trance (using these terms synonymously) are carefully planned extensions of some everyday processes of normal living. Without quite realizing it, we all experience the ***Common Everyday Trance*** wherein we are absorbed in a moment of inner reverie or preoccupation. During such periods we go about our daily routine somewhat automatically; much of our attention is actually focused inward as we experience ourselves a bit more deeply and possibly gain a fresh perspective or even solve a problem. Similarly, in the clinical utilization of trance we can be more receptive to our own inner experience and unrealized potentials in ways that are most surprising. With the help of a therapist's guidance, these potentials may be explored and further developed.

Most people are startled to learn how Art, Beauty, and Truth turn on gene expression and brain growth during creative activity. It is profound to realize that our highest and most inspired states of consciousness can facilitate optimal gene expression and brain plasticity while negative stress can distort and suppress it. Mind-gene communication engages the transformational alchemy of mind, body, and spirit, which generates our health and well-being as well as personal illness and the clash of cultures. These are the important insights that eventually emerged from publication of Erickson & Rossi's Hypnotic Realities in 1976.

"What is a Suggestion?" added in 2010,tells the story of how neuroscience research on activity or experience-dependent gene expression and brain plasticity builds a bridge over the Cartesian gap between body and mind. The new world of neuroscience is entirely consistent with our emerging view that the function of consciousness in general, and the focus of attention and expectancy in therapeutic hypnosis in particular, are to turn on activity and experience-dependent gene expression and brain plasticity for creative adaptation, problem solving, and healing. This is the deep secret that generations have searched for since the beginning of mesmerism and hypnosis more than two centuries ago. This is the science of what is behind many of the purported "mysteries of the human mind," the ever-popular myths of everything that seems strange or mysterious, and so-called "fascinating powers of stage hypnosis." Activity or experience-dependent gene expression and its attendant brain plasticity is the basic psychobiological mechanism for understanding the changes and transformations evident in therapeutic hypnosis, psychotherapy, and the creative insights of human consciousness in art, science, and culture. This is how we can "talk to our genes" and change the neural networks of our own brain and mind.

This new neuroscience framework was not available to us when we published the first edition of ***Hypnotic Realities*** in 1976. Yet, as can be seen when we read this volume today, every chapter and line anticipates our new neuroscience perspective to a remarkable degree. The subtitle of the original ***Hypnotic Realities: the Induction of Clinical Hypnosis andForms of Indirect Suggestion,*** which emphasized Erickson's use of "indirect suggestion", is being re-framed today with the more apt concept of "implicit processing heuristics." "Implicit" is the current neuroscience term, for the "unconscious." "Heuristics" are hints we give each other for priming and prompting a new activity, thought, emotion or experience of consciousness. Implicit processing heuristics are linguistic tools psychotherapists use to turn on experience-dependent gene expression and brain plasticity for creative change and healing. This leads to propose that "implicit processing heuristics" provides a more general neuroscience framework for understanding the subtlety of Erickson's indirect forms of suggestion in therapeutic hypnosis and psychotherapy. In common parlance "indirect suggestion" has the unfortunate connotation of being tricky or sneaky. This was certainly not Erickson's intention. Rather, implicit processing heuristics are the open questions and linguistic tools we use to creatively activate genc expression, brain plasticity, and Milton H. Erickson's use of neuropsychophysiology for facilitating mind-body healing and the so-called "spiritual transformations" of consciousness. Each reader will have to ponder these issues as they seek to integrate the creative edge of Erickson's contributions with their own evolving understanding and efficacy in the therapeutic arts.

Hypnotherapists share many views in common with other well-trained psychotherapists: an understanding of the dynamics of unconscious processes in behavior; an appreciation of the significance of emotional and experiential learning as well as intellectual knowing; a high regard for the unique life experience of each individual; and so on. Hypnotherapists are distinct in practice, however, in that they are more specialized in the deliberate utilization of these processes within individuals to help them achieve their own, individual, therapeutic goals in their own unique ways.

This volume can thus serve as a heuristic, stimulating practicing psychotherapists to improve their own education and training. It also provides researchers with a clinical source of hypothesis about hypnotic phenomena and hypnotherapy that can be tested in a more controlled experimental fashion. Erickson was a creative innovator, and even the most basic of his demonstrations contain a depth of sophistication making this material of great interest to all psychotherapists, regardless of their level of training or area of specialization.

Hypnotic Realities remains an original source for understanding Milton H. Erickson's essential contribution to therapeutic hypnosis, psychotherapy, and current consciousness studies. We editors take great pleasure in bringing forth this digital volume ***of Hypnotic Realities***, as part of our ongoing efforts to make the works of Ernest Rossi and Milton Erickson more widely available. Thank you for your interest.

Ernest Rossi, PhD & Kathryn Rossi, PhD
Los Osos, California

Roxanna Erickson-Klein, PhD
Dallas, Texas

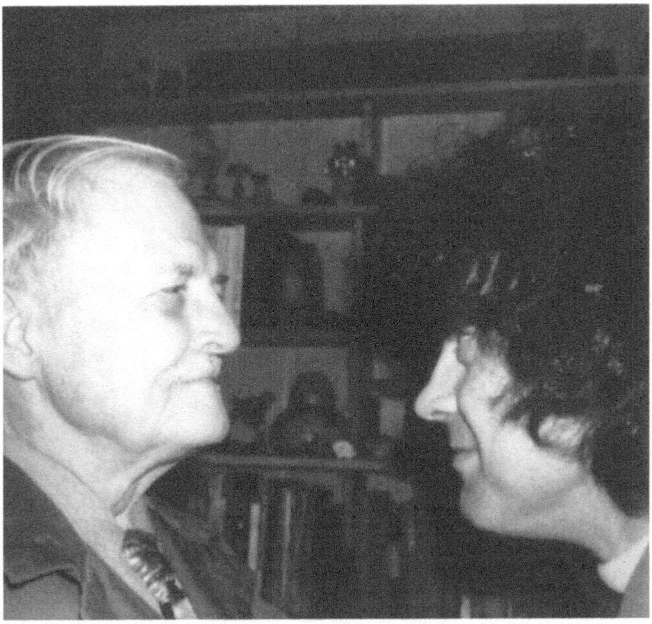

**1973. Phoenix, Arizona. 1201 E. Hayward.
Milton Erickson & Ernest Rossi.
Taking on a new student.**

Table of Contents

Legend	**The Four-digit Code Listed in the Captions Refers to:**
10.0.P.0	Volume
10.**0**.P.0	Location: Frontmatter, Chapter or References
10.0.**P**.0	What is displayed: Table, Figure or Photo
10.0.P.**0**	Number of Table, Figure or Photo within this chapter

Chapter One

A Conversational Induction

Dr. S is a psychologist and mother who was available to cooperate in a unique demonstration to ascertain if it was possible to train a professional person to become a hypnotherapist by having her learn by experiencing hypnosis personally. Dr. S had no experience with hypnosis apart from one demonstration where she experienced a short induction. This served to arouse her interest in the field, and she agreed to being tape recorded in return for the free training she would receive.

Erickson initiates the process in this first session with what we may call the "Early Learning Set" induction. He simply requests that Dr. S focuses on a spot while he talks with her. His approach is casual, gentle, warm, and friendly. Erickson simply talks about kindergarten and learning, imagery and comfort, the abilities of the unconscious and some alterations of the blink reflex. This is an example of conversational induction so innocuous and indirect that it is often difficult to recognize that trance is being induced.

The impatient novice waits in vain for him to begin the hypnosis. Where are the mysterious manipulations that will take possession of the subject's mind and body? Where are the frenzy, prostration, stupor, and bizarre gesticulations that ancient medical lithographs have illustrated as possession and trance?

Modern hypnotherapy is quite different from the popular conception of hypnosis as a mysterious drama. Therapists are not showmen. They are, however, highly skilled in observation and can recognize even minor variations in behavior that provide important clues to the patient's interests and abilities. These clues are then utilized to help guide the patient into those interesting states of altered awareness that are generally called "trance." Therapy then proceeds by "taking the learnings that the person already has and applying them in other ways." Erickson is wary about suggesting or adding anything new to the patient; he would rather facilitate the patient's ability to creatively utilize and develop what he already has.

In this first session, Erickson introduces a number of themes that will be repeated in ever-widening contexts in the later sessions: focusing the patient inward, freeing unconscious (autonomous) processes from the limitations of a patient's conscious sets, some principles and forms of indirect suggestion, and the ethics of trance and hypnotherapy. The beginning student in hypnotherapy often wants to learn everything all at once. That approach cannot really succeed. An understanding of the material develops naturally over time as Erickson goes over the fundamentals again and again in successive sessions. Frequently, the significance of the material in the early sessions is not entirely understood until later. Because of this, serious students may find themselves returning to restudy each session many times before it will be well understood.

Session 1: Erickson's Initial Trance with Dr. S & Rossi

> **MHE: Look at the far upper corner of that picture.**
> **[to ER] Now, you watch her face.**
> **The far upper corner of that picture.**
> **Now, I'm going to talk to you. [Pause]**

MHE: So often the therapist does not even look at the patient's face. Yet, changes in facial expression, muscle tonus throughout the body, and the breathing tell you how much of the patient's attention has been directed to the problem at hand. No sense in trying to work with a patient who's making restless movements.

ER: The quieter the patient, the more he's directing energy to what is being said.

MHE: Yes! And you also notice whether the patient can be distracted from the therapy. Can the patient be disturbed by a bus outside or a siren? The less disturbed they are by such outer distractions, the more focused is their energy on therapy. You can only tell these things by carefully watching the patient.

> **MHE: When you first went to kindergarten, grade school,**
> **this matter of learning letters and numerals**
> **seemed to be a big insurmountable task.**

MHE: Now here you are merely taking the learnings that the person already has and applying them in other ways. But you're not creating anything new.

ER: You're utilizing a learning set that already exists in the patient. It is a learning set that you're evoking by this particular induction.

MHE: Yes.

> **MHE: To recognize the letter A**
> **to tell a Q from an O was very, very difficult.**
> **And then too, script and print were so different.**
> **But you learned to form a mental image of some kind.**
> **You didn't know it at the time,**

but it was a permanent mental image.

ER: You are using a series of very obvious truths, truisms, as suggestions here. As you speak of these early experiences, your words tend to evoke early memories and may facilitate an actual age regression in some subjects.

MHE: Yes, suggestions are always given in a form that the patient can accept easily. Suggestions are statements that the patient cannot possibly argue with.

MHE: And later on in grammar school
you formed other mental images of words
or pictures of sentences.
You developed more and more mental images without knowing
you were developing mental images.
And you can recall all those images. [Pause]

MHE: The average hypnotherapist says, "Look at this spot," and tries to focus the patient's attention to the spot. But it is easier to deal with the images the person has in his mind. There's a large variety of images in his mind, and he can slip easily from one to another without leaving the situation.

ER: So internal imagery is therefore much more effective in holding attention.

MHE: Some external thing has no real value to them, but the images they have within are of value. Furthermore, you're only talking about what did occur in their past. It is their past and I'm not forcing anything on them. They did learn the alphabet, their numerals. They did learn many, many images. They can be pleased and select any image they want.

ER: Far from arousing resistance, you're actually on their side in sympathy with them. You sympathize with their difficulty in learning, so you align yourself with the patient's difficulties.

MHE: That's right. And you know from your own experience it was hard.

ER: With all that early accomplishment you're tapping, you also arouse their motivation for their current work in hypnosis.

> **MHE: Now you can go anywhere you wish, and transport yourself to any situation.**
> **You can feel water**
> **you may want to swim in it.**
> **[Pause]**
> **You can do anything you want.**

MHE: This sounds like a great deal of freedom, but note, I have given the suggestion to "transport" your consciousness to another situation. It can be any place you wish. It will probably be associated with water and you can do anything you want, but your consciousness need not be focused here in the therapy room.

> **MHE: You don't even have to listen to my voice**
> **because your unconscious will hear it.**
> **Your unconscious can try anything it wishes.**
> **But your conscious mind isn't going to do anything of importance.**

MHE: The patient is not paying attention to me with her conscious mind, but the unconscious ***will*** pick up what I'm saying.

ER: So, your method gets directly to the unconscious without the intervention and distortion of consciousness.

MHE: Sometimes patients will later say, "I wish you had let me stay in the water or the garden longer."

ER: So, being in an "inner garden" is a way you have of holding their conscious attention. You're having their conscious attention focused on an internal image just as watching a spot focuses their attention on an outer image. But being absorbed in an internal image is much more effective for focusing attention.

MHE: Much more effective!

ER: And while they are so absorbed, their consciousness is distracted, so you can make suggestions directly to their unconscious.

MHE: They are far more interested in the conscious things. They are not paying attention to what I say consciously. They are paying attention unconsciously, so there is no interference from consciousness.

ER: That's the important use of images: they bind a person's conscious attention while you make other (e.g., therapeutic) suggestions directly to their unconscious.

MHE: And it is very important for a person to know their unconscious is smarter than they are. There is a greater wealth of stored material in the unconscious. We know the unconscious can do things, and it's important to assure your patient that it can. They have to be willing to let their unconscious do things and not depend so much on their conscious mind. This is a great aid to their functioning. So, you build your technique around instructions that allow their conscious mind to withdraw from the task and leave it all up to the unconscious.

ER: You don't want them to have conscious control but to allow their unconscious to function smoothly by itself.

MHE: And then the results of that unconscious functioning can become conscious. But first they have to get beyond their conscious understanding of what is possible.

> **MHE: You will notice that your conscious mind is somewhat concerned since it keeps fluttering your eyelids.**

MHE: Here, I limited the fluttering to the eyelids rather than letting her generalize it into believing her whole system was fluttering or uncertain.

ER: That slight, rapid, vibratory flutter of the eyelids during the initial phase of an induction is frequently taken as an indication of beginning trance.

> **MHE: But you altered your rate of breathing.**
> **You've altered your pulse.**
> **You've altered your blood pressure.**
> **And without knowing it, you're demonstrating the immobility that a hypnotic subject can show.**

MHE: They don't know, but when you tell them they have altered their functioning, they can become aware of it. Their functioning is already altered, so they cannot resist or deny it. They have their inner proof.

ER: They have proof of an altered state. You inform the patient of these things to prove the hypnotic state rather than using a challenge.

MHE: That's right. I don't like to use the lack of the swallow reflex as a challenge because they tend to test that one. I'd rather use things they cannot test.

ER: Because patients tend to swallow less during trance, some therapists have used it as a test of trance depth. They will challenge patients by telling them they cannot swallow. During the initial stages of trance training, however, such a challenge might actually arouse some patients.

> **MHE: There is nothing really important**
> **except the activity of your unconscious mind,**

MHE: That downgrades traffic sounds or any other outside distractions without emphasizing that there are outside distractions. They can then apply this downgrading to whatever irrelevant stimuli that might be intruding.

ER: You don't project your distractions on the patient and you don't even suggest there are distractions. But if there are distractions this phrase helps the person to downgrade them.

> **MHE: and that can be whatever your unconscious mind desires.**

MHE: This is an example of what Kubie calls "illusory freedom." The person has a very great subjective feeling of freedom of choice, but actually, I hold my subject to the task at hand through subtle directives and implications. For example, in the above I did say, "You can go anywhere you wish," but then I did define a place: Water.

ER: So, the art of giving suggestions is to give careful direction, but you let the person have a certain illusion of freedom within the framework you have constructed.

MHE: When I earlier said, "Your unconscious can try anything it wishes," it sounds as if I were giving freedom, but actually that word "try" implies the opposite. The word "try" implies a block. You use the word "try" for your own purpose when you want to imply a block.

ER: Use of the word "try" at that point actually blocked or tied up the unconscious until it received further directives from you.

MHE: Then when I say, "Your conscious isn't going to do anything of importance," it implies that your unconscious will do something of importance.

ER: And the unconscious cannot do anything it wishes because you have already tied it up. In sum, this implies that the unconscious is going to do something important, and it's going to be what you suggest.

> **MHE: Now physical comfort exists,**
> **but you don't even need to pay attention**
> **to your relaxation and comfort.**

MHE: Notice how I emphasize, "You don't even need." Patients drag along too much, so you emphasize all they don't need so energy can be focused on the task at hand.

ER: This reinforces your earlier remark, "You don't even have to listen to my voice." It facilitates trance induction when the patient does not have to know or do anything.

> **MHE: I can tell your unconscious mind**

that you are an excellent hypnotic subject,
and whenever you need to or want to,
your unconscious mind will allow you to use it.

MHE: "I can tell your unconscious" implies I don't have to convince your conscious.

ER: In other words, *every sentence has implications, and it is in these implications that the important message is given.*

MHE: Yes!

MHE: And it can take time, its own time
letting you go into a trance
helping you to understand anything reasonable

MHE: You can take your time, but you are going to do it. That's the important implication. And they don't know how much time, so they have to rely on you.

MHE: I can speak to you or anyone else I choose,
but only when I speak to you is it necessary for you to listen.
I can direct my voice elsewhere
and you will know I am not speaking to you
so you will not need to pay any attention.

MHE: Here I'm setting up a lot of freedom for myself in future work.

ER: You are also giving suggestions for rapport wherein she will pay attention only when you are addressing her.

MHE: Dr. Rossi, I think you see a lot of behavior of great interest.
The alteration of the blink reflex.
The alteration in facial muscles, the total immobility.

ER: The slowing of the blink reflex before the final closing of the eyes and the relaxation of the facial muscles so the face has a smoother or "ironed out" expression are typical indications of trance.

ER: Would you like to go on now and demonstrate more phenomena?

MHE: I might like to, but I did not discuss it with her consciously. Therefore, if I go on I must first wake her up and ask her permission. The unconscious always protects the conscious.
Would you like to awaken now?

MHE: I cannot ask for permission to do something in trance while she is in trance. Asking for permission belongs to the normal state of awareness, and we must therefore ask while she is awake. You must be careful to protect the integrity of the personality and not exploit the trance state.

ER: That would break trust and only arouse the so-called resistance.

[Dr. S opens her eyes and stretches a bit.]

MHE: Notice the body reorientation when she came back.
Now, is there anything you want to tell us?

ER: This reorientation to the body at the termination is another cue the therapist can use to recognize the patient has been in a trance. The stretching, blinking, shifting of body posture, yawning, wetting of lips, smoothing of hair, touching various parts of the body, etc., are all indications that the patient is reorienting from the trance to the awake state.

Dr. S: Oh I enjoyed it; it was very peaceful. I was watching the point up there and it got foggy.

ER: I see, a perceptual alteration.

ER: This report of a fogging of the visual field is another fairly common indication of trance development. Others may report blurring, tunnel vision, alterations in the color of the background or the size and shape of things, etc.

Dr. S: I tried to listen in the beginning but then I went off onto my own thing. It would have been tedious to listen to you Dr. Erickson. I just felt like relaxing.

[After the tape recorder was turned off and the session had formally ended, Dr. S mentions her experience of "drifting" in the early stages of trance induction.]

ER: Her relaxation and inner absorption to the point where she no longer made an effort to listen to you are further indications of trance. She was also following your earlier suggestion that she need not listen to your voice consciously because her unconscious could pick up what you were saying. She obviously was responding on an unconscious level since she did end her inner absorption when you told her to awaken.

Chapter Two

Observation and Erickson's Basic Approach

Observation is the most important aspect of the early training of the hypnotherapist. For Erickson, this training began in youth and has continued through his life. Observation of the invariants and correlations in human behavior is the sine qua non, the stock-in-trade, of the creative hypnotherapist. The anecdotes and stories that Erickson tells on the following pages reveal him to be an acute observer of the regularities of human behavior. Erickson enjoys humor, and all of his original jokes are based on a sound knowledge of what people would do in a given situation.

As a child walking through the Wisconsin snow to school, for example, he delighted in leaving home early in the morning, so he could set a crooked path on the straight roads of the flat plains and later observe how everyone who came after him followed his exact footsteps. People did not follow the straight road they knew was there; they apparently found it easier to follow the crooked path he made until he began to straighten it by cutting out some of the crooked loops on his later walks to school.

It is the regularities of behavior that are of great significance. These regularities are tools he uses to shape hypnotic phenomenon and behavior. Given a certain stimulus, it is useful for him to know that a certain response will follow. Or, if he can evoke one piece of behavior, it is important for him to know that another piece of behavior is closely related to it and is likely to occur. Thus, he can use one stimulus to evoke a certain response and then use that response to evoke, by association, another specific response.

The situation is subjectively experienced as hypnotic when these responses appear to take place without conscious intention because patients are not aware of these predictable associations within themselves. Patients do not know all of the possibilities within their own behavioral repertory. Consequently, when they experience something that they could not have predicted (although the therapist can, because of his knowledge of the patients' behavioral associations), they assume the hypnotherapist somehow caused it. The hypnotherapist did arrange the behavioral situation so that a certain response by the patient would naturally follow. But the hypnotherapist was able to cause the response only by knowing how to ***Utilize*** preexisting structures within the patient's behavioral matrix.

From this it follows that the more therapists know about the lawfulness of behavior, the more adequately will they be able to evoke desired responses in any specific situation. The more therapists are able to observe about the specific regularities of the individual patients, the more will they be able to facilitate therapeutic responses in those individuals.

Exercises in Observation

1. Look for and carefully study regularities in patients' behavior. These regularities can range from the mannerisms and rituals of saying "Hello" and adjusting themselves in the first minute or two to the therapy session to the habitual patterns in their associative structure when they talk about problems. To what degree can you observe how a patient's problem is defined by a closed circuit of associations, a habitual and invariant pattern of associations that the patient does not know how to break out of. What intervention can you make to help the patient break out? (Rossi, 1968, 1972a, 1973a)

2. Observe to what degree various patients are open and available to change and capable of following you and to what degree they are fixed, closed, unavailable for change—and actually expect you to follow them. Erickson looks for response attentiveness (the degree to which a person is absorbed in what another is saying) in assessing the degree to which a person would be a capable hypnotic subject. The more response attentiveness, the better the subject. We might therefore assume that the more a patient is open to therapist direction and the greater his capacity to be absorbed in what the therapist is saying; the greater his capacity as a hypnotic subject.

This requires that therapists focus on the process aspect as well as the content, of their relation to their patients' behavior. Therapists who would become adept in hypnotherapy train themselves to observe the dynamics of availability and following in the transference-countertransference relation. The greater the openness and availability, the greater the following and capacity for hypnotic response. What helps a particular patient become more open and available to therapists? What can therapists do to make themselves more open and available to each patient?

We note that availability and following comprise a two-way street. The more sensitively therapists are capable of responding to patients' needs, emotions, and world view, the more will patients learn to be open and available to following the therapeutic suggestions. The more adequately therapists relate to their patients in the I-Thou experience, the more relevant and therefore acceptable will their understanding and suggestions be.

3. The practical art of trance induction requires that therapists learn to observe behavior and tie suggestions to it. What changes are occurring in facial behavior? Does one observe a preliminary quiver of the eyelids? If so, then it can be suggested that the patient will soon blink his eyes. Is the blink reflex slowing? If so, the therapist can note it and suggest it will soon get slower until the lids finally close. When it is observed that the patient has just exhaled, that is the precise moment to suggest he take a deep

breath. When it is observed that body movements are slowing, it can be suggested that the patient is becoming immobile and will soon be completely quiet and comfortable. Therapists can become so conversant with suggestions that they can automatically associate the patient's manifest behavior with further suggestions. They gradually develop a flow of language that permits them to speak and reflect while carefully studying the patient's behavior to determine what is to be suggested next. One can practice such careful observation in many situations of everyday life. People in audiences and fellow passengers on a bus, plane, or train will be in a range of states from tenseness and alertness to trance. Learn to recognize the behavioral correlates of such states. In early practice inductions, one can learn the art of observing behavior, commenting on it, and adding suggestions that will anticipate and further develop the behavior. In the sections that follow, we will gradually introduce the various forms of indirect hypnotic suggestion that can be learned as one gains more experience.

The Conscious and Unconscious in Clinical Hypnosis

Erickson emphasizes certain aspects of the relations between the conscious and unconscious and the many ways of utilizing them for therapeutic purposes in his work with clinical hypnosis. This is a major theme that is introduced in this first commentary and will be discussed further in practically all the following sessions. We believe that consciousness, programmed by the typical attitudes and beliefs of modern rationalistic man, is grievously limited. It has been estimated that, at best, most people do not utilize more than 10 percent of their mental capacity. Most of us simply do not know how to utilize our individual capacities. Our educational system has taught us how to measure up to certain external criteria of learning only. We learn our A B C's, how to read and write, and similar skills. The adequacy of our learning is measured by our scores on standardized achievement tests rather than the degree to which we utilize our own unique neural circuits for our individual goals. Our educational system, as yet, has little or no means of training and measuring the individual's ability to utilize his own unique behavioral matrix and associative processes, even though this internal ability is of the essence in creativity and personality development.

Consciousness is thus programmed to meet outer consensual standards of achievement, while all that is unique within the individual remains in abeyance. That is, most of our individuality remains unconscious and unknown. Erickson can say, "It is very important for people to know their unconscious is smarter than they are. There is a greater wealth of stored material in the unconscious."

Patients have problems because their conscious programming has too severely limited their capacities. The solution is to help them break through the limitations of their conscious attitudes to free their unconscious potential for problem solving.

Again and again, we will find that Erickson's approaches to inducing trance and problem solving are usually directed toward circumventing the rigid and learned limitations of the patient's conscious and habitual attitudes. We will later demonstrate and discuss means of "depotentiating conscious sets," "coping with consciousness," and the like. All these phrases denote the same effort to free individuals from their learned limitations. As Erickson so clearly states, "You build your technique around instructions that allow their conscious mind to withdraw from the task, and leave it all up to the unconscious."

To implement this goal of freeing unconscious potentials from the limitations of consciousness, Erickson has pioneered the ***indirect*** approaches to hypnotic suggestion. These approaches are in marked contrast to most previous and current work in hypnosis, where ***direct*** suggestions are still considered to be the major therapeutic modality. The following sessions and commentaries will be a gradual introduction to these indirect approaches. So multifaceted and vast are the possibilities of these indirect approaches that Erickson has never been able to organize them into a comprehensive system; in fact, he does not always understand why and how they work. Indirect approaches are thus still a virgin field, a terra incognita, that some readers will hopefully explore and extend further in their own research and therapeutic practice.

The *Utilization Theory* of Hypnotic Suggestion

We recently outlined the ***Utilization Theory of Hypnotic Suggestion***as follows (Erickson and Rossi, 1975):

> Trance is a special state that intensifies the therapeutic relationship and focuses the patient's attention on a few inner realities; trance does not insure the acceptance of suggestions. Erickson depends upon certain communication devices . . . to evoke, mobilize and move a patient's associative processes and mental skills in certain directions to sometimes achieve certain therapeutic goals. He believes that hypnotic suggestion is actually this process of evoking and utilizing a patient's own mental processes in ways that are outside his usual range of intentional or voluntary control.

The effective hypnotherapist learns to use words, intonations, gestures, and other things that evoke the patient's own mental mechanisms and behavioral processes. Hypnotic suggestion is not a kind of verbal magic that can be imposed on patients to make them do anything. Hypnotic suggestions are effective only to the degree that they can activate, block, or alter the functioning of natural mental mechanisms and associations already existing within the patient. Erickson likes to emphasize that hypnotic suggestion can evoke and ***Utilize*** potentials that already exist within patients, but it cannot impose something totally alien. Hyper-suggestibility is not necessarily a characteristic of therapeutic trance as he uses it.

In his first published paper on hypnosis (1932), Erickson found that "hyper-suggestibility was not noticed" as a necessary characteristic of trance. His work with 300 subjects involved in several thousand trances led him to this conclusion:

> Far from making them hyper-suggestible, it was found necessary to deal very gingerly with them to keep from losing their cooperation and it was often felt that they developed a compensatory negativism toward the hypnotist to offset any increased suggestibility. Subjects trained to go into a deep trance instantly at the snap of a finger would successfully resist when unwilling or more interested in other projects. In brief, it seems probable that if there is a development of increased suggestibility, it is negligible in extent.

Erickson was not alone in this finding. In his review of the history of hypnosis, Weitzenhoffer (1961, 1963, 1971) has pointed out that the earliest investigators, (such as Bertrand, Despine, and Braid,) did not view suggestibility as the essential feature of trance. It was Liebeault, and especially Bernheim (1895), who paved the way for viewing hyper-suggestibility as a necessary condition for speaking of hypnosis or trance. This may have been accepted by modern experimentally oriented investigators (Hull, 1933; Hilgard, 1965) because it lent itself easily to the development of "hypnotic susceptibility scales," which were thought necessary for the quantitative study of hypnotic phenomena. Weitzenhoffer, however, has maintained the necessity of exploring the concepts of ***trance*** and ***suggestibility*** as separate issues.

For Erickson, trance and hypnotic suggestion are separate phenomena that may or may not be associated in any given individual at any given moment. Because of this Erickson (1952) has emphasized the difference between "trance induction versus trance utilization." In his early work, he found it necessary to spend "four to eight or even more hours in inducing trances and in training the subjects to function adequately, before attempting hypnotic experimentation or therapy." The eight sessions of Erickson's work with Dr. S in this volume are thus a typical example of training a subject to experience trance. It will be seen that trance is a highly individualized process that can be experienced very differently even by the same person on separate occasions. For the therapeutic purposes of clinical hypnosis, however, we will focus our interest on exploring and facilitating only one particular aspect of trance. ***We are interested in the therapeutic aspect of trance wherein the limitations of one's usual conscious sets and belief systems are temporarily altered, so that one can be receptive to an experience of other patterns of association and modes of mental functioning.***

Erickson views the separate issue of hypnotic suggestion as a problem in communication and ***Utilization***. To facilitate suggestion, one must learn how to communicate more effectively. A major objective of this volume is to isolate the hypnotic forms of communication Erickson uses to facilitate suggestion. ***These hypnotic forms are communication devices that facilitate the evocation and Utilization of the patient's own associations, potentials and natural mental mechanisms in ways that are usually experienced as involuntary by the patient.*** Ordinary, everyday, nonhypnotic suggestions are acted upon because we have evaluated them with our usual conscious attitudes and found them to be an acceptable guide for our behavior, and we carry them out in a voluntary manner. Hypnotic suggestion, by contrast, is different in that the patient is surprised to find that experience and behavior are altered in a seemingly autonomous manner; experience seems to be outside one's usual sense of control and self-direction. ***A successful clinical hypnotic experience, then, is one in which trance alters habitual attitudes and modes of functioning so that carefully formulated hypnotic suggestions can evoke and Utilize other patterns of associations and potentials within the patient to implement certain therapeutic goals.***

The ***Utilization Approach*** to trance induction (Erickson, 1958, 1959) and the ***Utilization*** of the patient's presenting behavior and symptoms as an integral part of therapy (Erickson, 1955, 1965b) are among Erickson's original contributions to the field of clinical hypnosis. This ***Utilization Approach***, wherein each patient's individuality is carefully studied, facilitated, and ***Utilized***, is one of the ways clinical hypnosis is different from the standardized approaches of experimental and research hypnosis as it is usually conducted in the laboratory. It is in the clinician's ability to evaluate and ***Utilize*** patients' uniqueness together with the exigencies of their ever-changing real life situation that the most striking hypnotic and therapeutic results are often achieved. The ***Utilization Approaches*** achieve their results precisely because they activate and further develop what is already within the patient rather than attempting to impose something from the outside that might be unsuitable for the patient's individuality.

Most of the indirect forms of hypnotic suggestion that were pioneered by Erickson to facilitate his ***Utilization Approach*** were developed in clinical practice and field experiments without the benefit of detailed analysis or controlled experimental validation. In this volume, therefore, we will begin the process of analyzing a number of these indirect hypnotic suggestion, first to achieve some understanding of their clinical application, and second, to propose research that will be needed to further explore their nature and use. In this chapter, we will discuss "truisms" and "not doing, not knowing" as two of the most basic forms of indirect hypnotic suggestion.

Truisms Utilizing Mental Mechanisms

The simplest form of suggestion is a truism—a simple statement of fact about behavior that the patient has experienced so often that it cannot be denied. Erickson frequently talks about such psychological processes as if he were simply describing objective facts to the patient. Actually, these verbal descriptions can function as indirect forms of hypnotic suggestion when they trip off associated ideomotor and ideosensory processes that already exist within the subject (Weitzenhoffer, 1957); the truism can evoke and ***Utilize*** the patient's own repository of life experience, associations, and mental mechanisms. The Generalized Reality Orientation (Shor, 1959) usually maintains these subjective associations and mental mechanisms in appropriate check when we are talking in ordinary conversation. When attention is fixed and focused in trance, however, the following truisms may actually trip off a literal and concrete experience of the suggested behavior.

1. You already know how to experience pleasant sensations like the warmth of the sun on your skin.
2. Everyone has had the experience of nodding their head "Yes" or shaking it for "No" even without quite realizing it.
3. We know when you are asleep your unconscious can dream.
4. You can easily forget that dream when you awaken.

Practical experience demonstrates that evoking a subject's personal experience by way of a concrete image, as illustrated in Example 1, is an effective approach for evoking ideosensory experience. The idea of warmth and the image of the sun on the skin evoke personal associations from previous experiences that generate an actual sensation of warmth on the skin. In a similar manner, talking about a common life experience, like nodding a head "Yes" in Example 2, is an idea that tends to evoke the actual motor response of head nodding. Such ideomotor and ideosensory processes were early recognized as the basis of many hypnotic phenomena (Bernheim, 1895), and they can be easily measured today with psycho-physiological instruments. Many forms of biofeedback (Brown, 1974), for example, can be understood as ideosensory and ideomotor responses that are amplified and reinforced by electronic instrumentation. More cognitive processes, like dreaming and forgetting, can be facilitated when suggested by truisms that the average subject usually cannot deny, as in Examples 3 and 4. This, then, is a basic mechanism of hypnotic suggestion: we offer simple truths that automatically evoke conditioned associations in a particularly vivid way. Suggestion is a process of evoking and ***Utilizing*** potentials and life experiences that are already present in subjects, but perhaps outside their usual range of control. Therapeutic suggestion helps patients gain access to their own associations and abilities to solve their own problem.

Truisms Utilizing Time

One particularly important form of truism is that which incorporates time. When Erickson makes a request for a definite behavioral response, he usually tempers it with time. He would never say, "Your headache is gone," because it might not be, and the patient would, with some justice, begin to experience a loss of belief. Instead, Erickson turns the direct suggestion into a truism by saying, "The headache is going to leave shortly." It could be a few seconds, minutes, hours, or even days. In a similar vein, the following suggestions all become truisms because the time factor allows patients to ***Utilize*** their own associations and experience to make them true.

Sooner or later, your hand is going to lift [eyes close, etc.]

Your headache [or whatever problem] will disappear as soon as your system is ready for it to leave.

It probably will happen just as soon as you are ready. We will

allow the unconscious to take as much time as it needs to let that happen.

Exercises with Truisms

1. Plan how truisms Utilizing mental mechanisms and time can be used to facilitate trance induction and an experience of any of the classical hypnotic phenomena.
2. Do the same for any psychological function (e.g., memory, learning ability, time sense, emotional processes) your patient is interested in exploring for therapeutic purposes.
3. Make up verbal suggestions that can be used to alter body temperature, digestion, respiration, or any other psychophysiological function you have been trained to deal with in your professional work. It might be well first to write down these suggestions in a direct form and then convert them into truisms Utilizing time and common everyday descriptions of natural psychological and physiological processes.
4. Plan how truisms Utilizing mental mechanisms and time can be used to help you cope with typical clinical problems you have been trained to deal with.

Not Doing, Not Knowing

A basic aspect of trance experience is allowing mental processes to take place by themselves. We ask the subject to "relax and let things happen." Not doing is thus a basic form of indirect hypnotic suggestion that is of particular value in inducing trance. Most people do not know that most mental processes are autonomous. They believe they think by driving and directing their own associative processes. And to a certain extent they do. But it comes as a pleasant surprise when they relax and find that associations, sensations, perceptions, movements, and mental mechanisms can proceed quite on their own. This autonomous flow of undirected experience is a simple way of defining trance. Hypnotic suggestion comes into play when the therapist's directives have a significant influence in facilitating the expression of that autonomous flow in one direction or another.

When one is relaxed, the parasympathetic system is predominant, and one is physiologically predisposed ***not to do*** rather than to make any active effort of doing. Because of this it is very easy to accept the following suggestions for not doing during the initial stages of trance induction.

You don't have to talk or move or make any sort of effort.

You don't even have to hold your eyes open.

You don't have to bother trying to listen to me because your unconscious can do that and respond all by itself.

People can sleep and not know they are asleep.

They can dream and not remember that dream.

Not doing is a precondition for most hypnotic experience. Most hypnotic phenomena can be experienced by relaxing to the point where we simply give up our habitual patterns of control and self-direction. This is the opposite of the usual situation of everyday life, where we make concentrated efforts to remember. In trance, we are congratulated for forgetting (hypnotic amnesia). In normal living, we are enjoined to pay attention; in trance, we are applauded for allowing the mind to wander (reverie, hypnotic dreaming). In daily affairs, we are forced to act our age; in trance, we achieve success simply by allowing a comfortable age regression to take place. In normal life, we continuously expend strenuous effort to achieve veridical perceptions; in trance, we allow sensory and perceptual distortions to take place and can even indulge ourselves in hallucinations. From this point of view, we can understand how it is indeed much easier and enjoyable to experience trance than the extensive effort that is required to stay normally awake!

Thus, Erickson's initial direction in trance training is to help the subject have a comfortable experience in ***not doing***. Frequently, this can be experienced as momentarily losing abilities that are usually performed in an automatic and unthinking manner. Subjects can lose the ability to stand up or to keep a hand on the thigh. They can lose the ability to focus their eyes and see clearly; they can lose the ability to speak. How often in everyday life do we say, "I stood there like an idiot, unable to say anything or even think in that situation." That is an example of the common everyday trance where for a moment we were lost in not doing.

Closely related to not doing is ***not knowing***. In everyday life, we must continuously expend energy and effort to know. How pleasant, then, to find a situation where we can relax and do not need to know. What a relief! Most subjects can look forward to trance experience as a newfound freedom from the demands of the world. They really don't have to know or do anything; their unconscious can handle it all by itself.

To help subjects realize this, Erickson frequently gives a preinduction talk about the conscious and unconscious—or the "front" and "back" part of the mind. He emphasizes how the unconscious is usually capable of regulating the body (breathing, heartbeat, all the physiological processes) and the mind all by itself. Indeed, people frequently have problems because their conscious mind is trying to do something that the unconscious can do better. He talks about infancy and childhood when one was natural and happy and ***did not know***. At one time one did not know how to walk or talk or even make sense of visual and auditory impressions. One did not know that one's hand belonged to oneself, as when infants are observed to reach for their right hand with their right hand.

Erickson frequently introduces puzzles and beguiling tasks to prove how amusing it can be when one does not know. He will ask if a person knows whether he is right or left thumbed. Few people do. He then asks people to put their hands behind their head and then fold their fingers together. The subjects then bring their folded hands to their lap to learn whether their left or right thumb is on top; that is the dominant thumb. Erickson then emphasizes how the patients' unconscious, their body, knew this all their life even though their conscious mind did not. With many anecdotes, stories, and interesting bits of behavior he carefully lays the groundwork to help patients realize and value the fact that the unconscious knows more and that the conscious can help best simply by relying upon the unconscious to do things. This permits subjects to adopt a receptive and ***Acceptance Set*** wherein they become more acutely sensitive to their own inner processes as well as the suggestions of the therapist.

Exercises with Not Doing and Not Knowing

1. Practice changing direct, positive suggestions into indirect suggestions of the "You don't have to" form. For example, instead of "Remain quietly seated with your eyes closed," one may say "You don't have to move or even bother keeping your eyes open," or "You can just remain comfortable and quiet and not bother with anything."
2. Formulate suggestions for not doing and not knowing that are appropriate for the induction and maintenance of trance.
3. Formulate suggestions for "Not doing" that will achieve interesting (a) hypnotic phenomena (catalepsy, anesthesia, age regression, etc.) and (b) psychotherapeutic goals (coping with phobias, compulsions, habits such as nail biting, smoking, overeating; self-understanding, etc.)

Chapter Three

Indirect Induction by Recapitulation

The indirect approach is a basic theme in Erickson's work and the source of a great deal of his originality. In this session, he reveals his beliefs about how a patient learns to experience trance and illustrates many of his indirect approaches to suggestion. The therapist helps the patient learn to experience trance by depotentiating conscious sets and by creating a definite demarcation or dissociation between the trance state and the ordinary awake state. One of the major controversies in the past few decades of research in hypnosis has been between the traditional clinical view of trance as an altered state that is different and discontinuous from being awake, versus the theories of trance as a special form of roleplaying (Sarbin & Coe, 1972), goal-directed imagining (Barber & De Moor, 1972), or communication (Haley, 1963). There can be no doubt that Erickson maintains the traditional view of trance as a special state (Erickson & Rossi, 1974/2021), but it is in his indirect approaches to suggestion that he is most innovative and nontraditional.

In this session, Erickson illustrates with simplicity and seeming casualness a few cornerstones of the indirect approach: the ***Yes Set***, implication, the ***Double Bind***, and the use of truisms to align a patient's associative processes for creative trance work. He also illustrates indirect approaches for discharging resistance, ***Utilizing*** personal motivation, and facilitating new learning and individuality. He takes some initial steps toward training Dr. S for the experience of dissociation, ideomotor signaling, hallucination, amnesia, posthypnotic suggestion, and the separation of conscious and unconscious processes. We witness a simple secret of the effectiveness of his approach: he offers suggestions in an open-ended manner that admits many possibilities of response as acceptable. Suggestions are offered in such a manner that any response the patient makes can be accepted as a valid hypnotic phenomenon. These open-ended suggestions are also a means of exploring the patient's response tendencies (the response hierarchy of learning theory and behavior therapy). The therapist can ***Utilize*** these response tendencies to effect therapeutic goals.

Erickson begins this session with an indirect induction by recapitulation. He does not begin by directly asking the subject, Dr. S, to recall and recapitulate experiences on the first session. Such a direct request would only evoke a plaintive, "But I don't know how." Instead, in the first sentence he ***Utilizes*** her motivation for learning and then immediately touches gently, but completely, on many associations that will automatically evoke memories of her previous session and therefore tend to reinduce that trance. Dr. Rossi (ER) was present in the room while Dr. Erickson (MHE) worked with the subject: Dr. S. Near the conclusion of the trancework, Dr. Rossi addressed his questions directly to the subject. This transcript of an audiotape ***Utilizes*** bold to indicate words and actions that took place during the session, followed by later discussion. This begins with body orientation in preparation for the trance.

Session 2: Body Orientation for Trance with Dr. S

MHE: Both feet on the floor and your hands on your thighs, elbows at your sides.
Pick a spot here on this paper weight.

MHE: Here we exactly reproduce the previous hypnotherapeutic position. She went into a trance the first time with this position, so the position will help her to do the same now.

MHE: Now the thing for you to do,
actually for your own education,
your own training,
your own experiences,
is to look at a spot there,
anywhere you wish,
and try to recall
what I said to you
and keep on
thinking,
trying to recall
the formation of mental images,
of letters, numbers
the unimportance of keeping your eyes open
and then permitting Dr. Rossi and me to talk
while you listen
and then beginning to drift away.
[Pause]

ER: This is a fantastic sentence; it completely recapitulates the first hypnotherapeutic situation. You touch upon many associations to her previously successful hypnotic work and thereby facilitate your current hypnotic induction. You also deftly utilize her professional motivation by touching upon "for your own education." Instead of suggesting eye closure directly at this point, you prepare for it indirectly simply by mentioning "the unimportance of keeping your eyes open." I notice you use the word "drift" here, which she introduced at the very end last time to describe her subjective experience of entering a trance.

MHE: You always use the patient's own words and experience as much as possible for trance induction and suggestion. (Direct suggestion for inevitable behavior.)

MHE: Your eyes can now close,

ER: This direct suggestion for eye closure was now more appropriate since she had that fixed, glassy stare at this point. You only give direct suggestions when you're absolutely certain the patient is ready to accept them. (Direct suggestion for inevitable behavior.)

MHE: It is always safe to suggest behavior that is inevitable in the natural course of things.

MHE: And you will note
that the drifting can occur
more rapidly.
That there is less and less importance
to be attached to my voice
and that you can experience
progressively
[Pause]
any kind of sensations you wish.

MHE: By emphasizing "more rapidly," you imply that drifting will occur.

ER: Implication is thus a safe way of evoking and talking about behavior that may or may not be present. If you simply said, "You will now drift," that could arouse resistance. (Implication.)

MHE: For example, if I say, "I don't know what chair you are going to sit in . . ."

ER: That implies you will sit down; you are structuring their behavior, but so subtly that it's not likely to arouse resistance.

MHE: Another example: "Will you pay by cash or by check?"

ER: By using the word "progressively," you throw the statement "you can experience" into an implication, and then you pause to let it take place and the burden for it taking place rests with the patient.

MHE: And I pause with confidence that it will.

ER: Further, it is a very safe statement to make because they are certainly experiencing some sensations. You give them permission to experience whatever they are experiencing, and then take credit for evoking it.

MHE: That's right.

> **MHE: Bear in mind that when you first formed**
> **an image of the letter A**
> **it was difficult.**
> **But as you continued in school**
> **you learned to form**
> **mental images of letters and words and pictures**
> **with increasing ease**
> **until finally all you had to do**
> **was to take a look.**
> **[Pause]**

ER: You're evoking the early learning set again just as you did in the first session.

MHE: You imply that just as you overcame difficulties in the past, so you will now.

MHE: In the matter of experiencing other sensations,
you learn to recognize cold
warm
muscle tension.

MHE: All these things are taking place in her body, so I am limiting her attention to herself and downgrading all outside distractions. By mentioning her "experiencing," I am referring to her own history. I am now evoking her personal history, and she knows it and cannot dispute it.

MHE: In your sleep at night, you can dream.
In those dreams, you can hear
you see, you move
you have any number of experiences.

ER: These are truisms about dreams. Your mention of "dream" tends to evoke partial aspects of the dream state as contributions to the current trance experience. I notice you frequently state obvious truths as if to evoke a *Yes Set.*

MHE: That's right!

[Erickson here recounts how in his earliest experiences with hypnosis he discovered that he could ask subjects a dozen or so casual questions and make remarks that required an obvious "Yes" answer so that positive momentum was gradually built up until they would finally also agree to enter a trance and then succeed in doing it.]

MHE: You also develop a *Yes Set* by saying, "You wouldn't do such and such," and they answer, "Yes, I wouldn't."

ER: For a person who is negatively inclined, you would emphasize all the things they wouldn't do.

MHE: And thereby evoke a "Yes."

ER: This is like mental judo. Actually, it is a U***tilization Technique:*** you are ***Utilizing*** the person's characteristic attitudes.

MHE: That's right.

> **MHE: And as a part of that experience**
> **is forgetting that dream after you awaken.**
> **An experience of forgetting in itself**
> **is an experience**
> **that is not alien to anybody.**
> **[Pause]**

MHE: The mention of "forgetting" tends to evoke posthypnotic amnesia without direct suggestion.

ER: The verbal naming or description of a neuropsychological mechanism such as forgetting tends to evoke it. This seems to be a fundamental method of modern hypnosis.

> **MHE: Now with your background**
> **you'll have many questions about many things.**
> **You really don't know what those questions are.**
> **You won't know what some of those questions are until they are half answered.**

MHE: "You'll have many questions" implies: you will want to learn all you can and therefore you will participate fully.

ER: You're evoking a learning set again.

MHE: And very forcefully.

ER: By mentioning her background as a professional psychologist you evoke her professional pride and personal motivation.

MHE: That's right! And without boldly identifying what you're doing.

ER: Yes. You did not say, "Because you are a psychologist you are going to be interested in this." You simply said, "with your background," and thereby evoked the best of her personal pride in herself as a professional.

> **MHE: And sometimes the answers**
> **seem to be one thing**
> **and turn out to be another.**

ER: The implication here is that new learning will take place: new answers to change the mental sets or mental habits that may be the source of a personal problem. You are structuring a learning set for therapeutic change, using an indirect evocation of new learning.

MHE: Yes, new and different learnings for psychotherapeutic change. Without saying, "Now I'm going to cram down your throat some new understanding."

MHE: The word April is a child's name —
it means a month.
[Pause]
But it can also mean April fool.
And so in your experiences be aware of the fact
that you really don't know where you are going to go,
but you are going to go.

ER: Now, you do a charming thing. You know that Dr. S has a young daughter named April and you talk about her here. Why?

MHE: She can say, "Let's not drag my child into this." Now notice my emphasis on "April *fool*." All her rejection has to go on that one word.

ER: I see. You've picked up her rejection with that one word "fool?" You've crystallized and discharged her resistance.

MHE: Discharged it!

ER: "April fool" discharged rebelliousness of the situation. So, if resistance was building up, you've discharged it here. You've discharged it indirectly with a pun. so, you were indirectly discharging her resistance.

MHE: Yes, and "April fool" also has pleasant associations. But this does imply that you *are* going someplace.

MHE: It all belongs to you.

MHE: If it all belongs to you, you want to take charge of it, don't you?

ER: The burden is placed on her for carrying out the experience; she is to be the source of her own experience. You engaged her motivation in a way that was meaningful to her.

MHE: And because it belongs to her she ***wants*** it.

ER: So, you're again engaging her personal pride and motivating her.

MHE: That's right.

> **MHE: And it can be shared in any way that you decide.**

MHE: You can't share a thing unless you've got it.

ER: And with these hidden directives, you imply there will be something to share. You again give the illusion of freedom when you say, "And it can be shared in any way you decide," but the hidden directives are (1) there will be something to share and (2) she will share it

> **MHE: And one of the nicest things about hypnosis is**
> **that in the trance state you can dare to look at**
> **and think and see and feel things**
> **that you wouldn't dare in the ordinary waking state.**

MHE: I'm telling her that she has a lot more courage than she knows, and there will be more to become aware of than she knows.

ER: Which of course is a scientific truism again: there is much more in our memory banks and associative structures than we are usually aware of in the normal conscious state. You use this truism here to evoke both courage and a set for self-exploration.

MHE: And it is hard for any person to think
that he can be afraid of his own thoughts.
But you can know that in this hypnotic state
you have all the protection of your own unconscious,
which has been protecting you in your dreams,
permitting you to dream what you wish,
when you wish,
and keeping that dream
as long as your unconscious thought necessary,
or as long as your conscious mind
thought would be desirable.

MHE: She has all the control.

ER: She has all the protection she needs. She need not fear, her unconscious mind will take care of her. Is that right?

MHE: Right!

ER: You're again verbally describing a scientific truism or natural mental mechanism that will by association tend to set that mechanism into operation. You earlier evoked "forgetting" in this way and now self-protection as a means of deeply reassuring her. The truisms are evoking mental mechanisms of protection and flow from the unconscious.

MHE: But your conscious mind will keep it only with the consent of your unconscious mind.

ER: Is this again putting the conscious mind under the control or protection of the unconscious? Is this a way of depotentiating consciousness?

MHE: Yes and it emphasizes that the unconscious can give to the conscious.

ER: Again, opening up a set for self-exploration, for things to flow into consciousness. I'm seeing this more and more: you're again *Utilizing* a natural psychological mechanism, in this case the unconscious giving to the conscious, for therapeutic purposes here and now.

MHE: Now the important achievement
for you
is to realize
that everybody
does not know
his capacities.
[Pause]

MHE: Who is important? She is! When you stop to think about it, nobody does know his capacities.

ER: So again, you're *Utilizing* a scientific truism; in this case you're setting her up to enhance her latent potentials in any possible way.

MHE: That's right.

MHE: And you have to discover these capacities in whatever slow way you wish.

MHE: In other words, you don't have to feel you must do it instantly.

ER: This is an important principle in administering suggestions. When you don't know whether her unconscious is ready to carry out a particular suggestion, you allow her an indefinite time period to carry it out. Allowing indefinite time for suggestions is thus a fail-safe device. If the suggestion is not carried out immediately, it's not registered as a failure. The suggestion remains in a latent condition until it can be responded to. You must always allow enough time for the subject to respond in their own way.

[Erickson now tells a case history wherein a patient called him up 16 years after the termination of therapy to tell him of a new development in her life that was directly related to something he had told her in trance.]

MHE: And one of the things I want you to discover is you don't need to listen to me.

ER: Again, dismissing the conscious mind in favor of the unconscious.

MHE: And I'm also saying, "I'm not the important person; you are."

ER: I see, again emphasizing the central role of the patient. The patient tends to think the therapist is the important person.

MHE: He isn't!

ER: Patients keep pulling at the therapist for the cure, the magic, the change, rather than looking at themselves as the change agent. The patient has a central role. You are continually putting the responsibility for change back on the patient.

MHE: On to them always!

> **MHE: Your unconscious mind can listen**
> **to me without**
> **your knowledge**
> **and also deal with something else at the same time.**
> **[Pause]**

MHE: A scientific truism, just as you step up and down from a curb without thinking about it.

ER: You actually are evoking this psychological mechanism of listening on an unconscious level simply by describing it verbally. It is words evoking mental mechanisms. This is rather profound when you stop to think of it: you are using words to describe certain psychological mechanisms that you want to happen. Your verbal description evokes the psychological mechanism described.

MHE: It does.

> **MHE: A person seeking therapy**
> **comes in and tells you one story that is believed fully at the conscious level**
> **and in nonverbal language, can give you a story that is entirely different.**
> **And the unconscious mind has had little opportunity**
> **to give recognition to its own ways of understanding.**

ER: Again, a therapeutic truism, but why are you presenting it?

MHE: I'm telling them, "You really don't know what's wrong with you." You tell them that so they won't think, "I know everything about my problem, my illness."

ER: You're developing a learning set again for something new to come in, facilitating change and development. You're trying to open up their horizon, their experience. That's what the cure is going to be. You say the unconscious is going to have a new opportunity for expressing itself.

MHE: Too often the conscious behavior keeps you too busy so you deprive the unconscious of an opportunity to express itself. It's another scientific truism.

ER: And so stated here it opens up the way for change and inner development.

> **MHE: We learned to nod our heads for "Yes"**
> **to shake our heads for "No."**
> **[Pause]**

MHE: That is a fact and you pause to let them reflect on the factual nature of that statement. They have a chance to recognize that you are really speaking the truth.

ER: This is actually your way of introducing her to ideomotor signaling. You don't tell her to nod and shake her head for "Yes" and "No." You simply mention the possibility of nonverbal communication and let her own individuality decide how and when.

> **MHE: But that is not necessarily true of all people.**
> **A cave people of the South Seas**
> **recently discovered have their own ways**
> **of nonverbal communication**
> **where the cues are much slighter than we have.**
> **Yes. Now each of us is an individual.**

ER: I see, that is the implication in describing these cave people with their own ways of communication. You are implying there is a place for her individuality, and you're evoking it thereby, you are facilitating her individuality.

MHE: Yes, evoking it thereby.

ER: Because that in fact is the problem with patients: many of their symptoms and so-called mental problems are due to a suppression of their individuality. The cure is to let that individuality come out and flower in all its particular genius.

MHE: That's right. That's what you need to do, and that is why they are seeing you.

> **MHE: And your willingness to rely**
> **upon your unconscious mind**
> **to do anything**
> **that can be of interest**
> **or value to you**
> **is most important.**
>
> **[Dr. S begins to nod her head very slowly.]**

MHE: Emphasizing *she* is going to do something.

ER: The fact that she does begin the ***very slow, repetitive*** head nodding characteristic of an autonomous ideomotor response indicate that she is accepting your suggestion to rely on her unconscious mind.

MHE: Not only are you to learn positive things
but you need to learn negative things.
[Pause]
One of the negative things
you need to learn is that of forgetting.
Consciously, you can say to yourself,
"This, I will remember."
To forget something seems very hard for some people.
And yet if they would look into their history,
they can forget as easily.
In teaching students in medical school,
you tell them most impressively,
"The examination will be held
in such and such a room
at such and such a time
and in Building C
and will begin at 2:00."
And they will all listen
with great interest,
and you turn to leave the classroom
and you will see
the students lean toward each other
and say,
"What day?"
What hour?
Building?
You know they heard it,
and they forgot it immediately.

ER: Here you again talk about forgetting and give common examples of forgetting in everyday life to facilitate the possibility of evoking forgetting in the form of posthypnotic amnesia. Your suggestions are open ended and of forgetting and recall while your subject continues her very slow, slight, and repetitive head nodding throughout your words here. Does that mean she is accepting your ideas and will act upon them? In this case, will she forget and experience an amnesia?

MHE: At some level, she is responding with recognition or acceptance of what I am saying. But I don't know how she will act on it yet.

ER: You can offer this loosely structured network of associations about forgetting, and it may or may not actually trip off forgetting mechanisms in her own mind. You do not impose suggestions or commands, you simply *offer* verbal associations that her individuality may or may not ***Utilize***. Trance does not ensure the acceptance of suggestions (Erickson & Rossi, 1975); it is simply a modality wherein the patient's mental processes have an opportunity to interact in a more spontaneous and autonomous manner with the therapist. At this early stage of trance training, you are simply exploring how her individuality will respond to suggestions you offer in an open-ended manner.

MHE: That is a facility in behaving
that serves many good purposes.
And you should enjoy learning
to forget not only ideas,
but nonverbal performances.
Purposely forgetting
that you know a certain name,
doing as you did as a child
when you decided you liked a different name
and perhaps for a half day
you entertained that your name was Darlene
or Ann Margaret

[Dr. S appears to renew her slow head nodding at this point in apparent recognition or acceptance of what is being said.]

MHE: This is a very common game among children and it reminds her of a forgotten game.

ER: Giving her yet another example of a forgotten experience. This is a way of proving you can forget.

MHE: But they will ***recall*** the forgotten memory of their experience with the game.

ER: They will do the opposite of forgetting when they recall; they then prove they have forgotten.

MHE: And at the same time, they are verifying the validity of what I have been saying.

ER: And it is possible you may have elicited a forgotten memory. So, you have done two things that are the opposite of one another. You have facilitated forgetting and you have facilitated recall. You are juxtaposing mental mechanisms that are usually very delicately balanced: forgetting and recall. They are delicately balanced in our neurophysiology, and you delicately balance them here for therapeutic purposes. We will call this the apposition of opposites wherein you attempt to balance opponent mental processes. This careful balance is another means by which you give her individuality a chance to express itself.

> **MHE: It's a very remarkable thing**
> **to discover**
> **that you can lose an arm,**
> **a leg,**
> **an entire moment.**
> **You can forget where you are.**
> **[Pause]**

ER: Another set of examples of how forgetting can take place by dissociation.

MHE: And everybody has that experience.

ER: Yes. You would never take a chance and say something that everyone doesn't always have. You speak in truisms for complete acceptance. People have to accept what you say because it is all true. You then pause to let them assimilate your message.

MHE: And I'm evoking memories

MHE: Now there are some
different ways
in which the mind can function
in which the unconscious can join
with the conscious,
many different ways
in which the unconscious can avoid
the conscious mind
without the conscious mind
knowing that it is
just received a gift.
[Pause]

ER: A series of truisms about the relations between conscious and unconscious here. You continually use these truisms to:

(1) Establish that you are a reliable source of the truth
(2) To evoke certain mental mechanisms and modes of functioning.

When these truisms do trip off the described psychological mechanisms (for example, the unconscious releasing a forgotten memory to the conscious), you also thereby establish the validity and value of trance in a very safe way. In therapeutic work, you never use direct challenges to prove the trance.

MHE: That's right.

ER: This is a much more effective and interesting way of establishing the validity of trance, and you are less likely to arouse resistance.

> **MHE: The very complexity of mental functioning**
> **you can go into a trance to find out**
> **a whole lot of things that you can do.**
> **And they are so many more than you dreamed of.**
> **[Pause]**

MHE: This implies: ***You*** do have an important purpose in going into a trance. It is not what I can do but what ***you***, the patient, can do. You emphasize all the things the patient can do.

ER: You are using implication to initiate a process of inner exploration that may facilitate the recognition of potentials she did not know she had.

> **MHE: You can dream of yourself as a small child,**
> **wondering who that child is.**
> **[Pause]**

ER: This may be evoking early memories or an age regression, but with the safe distancing device of "wondering who that child is." You do not precipitate the patient into an actual experience of reliving the past since that might be traumatic at this early stage of therapy.

MHE: You do not elicit the common response, "But I can't be a child." But they ***can*** wonder who the child is. While they wonder they can say, "I can be that child."

ER: You speak of it in the context of, "You can dream of yourself as a small child." Is that actually evoking mechanisms of dream formation?

MHE: Yes, and using them in another way.

ER: So again you are ***Utilizing*** a natural neuropsychological mechanism by evoking it verbally.

MHE: And when you say, "You ***can*** dream," it implies you can also do it any other way you want to.

ER: You did not say, "You will dream of yourself." That would be limiting it to dreams only. You say, "You ***can*** dream" and imply, "But you could fantasize it, talk to yourself about it, or whatever."

MHE: You can do it any way you wish, but you will do it.

> **MHE: And you can watch that child grow older,**
> **week by week,**
> **month by month,**
> **year by year.**
> **Until finally**
> **you are able to recognize**
> **who that child is**
> **who is growing up.**
>
> **[Dr. S's head appears to nod very slightly.]**

ER: You are now ratifying the regression by having her watch herself grow up.

MHE: Yes, if she watches herself grow up, that implies and ratifies the fact that she experienced herself as a child.

MHE: Every person has abilities
not known to the self,
abilities discredited by the self.
If there is an ability
that the unconscious wants to disown,
it can examine that ability,
examine it very fully,
very completely,
and when it desires,
obliterate that ability,
but doing so with an adequate understanding
of the fact that an obliteration
has been effected.

[The discussion between MHE and ER diverts for approximately 15 minutes while MHE discusses a fairly complex clinical example of how the unconscious can obliterate a memory.]

MHE: Everyone does this; a truism again.

ER: By discussing this disowning of abilities, you are actually setting the stage for facilitating processes of dissociation?

MHE: You only obliterate when there is that ability. By actively illustrating it, you prove it is there. Since it is there we will use it.

ER: So while you ratify the age regression through dissociation, you are also evoking the obliteration mechanism in the unconscious?

MHE: Yes, but only temporarily to let her know it is there.

ER: Oh, are you implying that the unconscious has obliterated a lot of things but it can also bring them forward when it wants to?

MHE: Yes.

ER: So you are setting her up for possible memory recall of anything the unconscious has obliterated.

MHE: That's right. Only she does not know what you are doing.

ER: You are speaking directly to her unconscious here.

MHE: And using her own growth and experience, that's all your talking about.

MHE: Now, I am trying to map out some things you can learn.

ER: You make such a direct statement here. I'm shocked.

MHE: "I am trying," and since you feel kindly toward me this implies: you will help me. [You refers to the subject]

ER: Indirectly placing the essential burden on her again. So even when you make a direct statement, you may be implying other things, and the really important suggestion is contained in that implication.

> **MHE: Now in hallucinating visually**
> **sometimes you want to start it**
> **by keeping your eyes closed**
> **and knowing they are closed.**
> **[Pause]**
> **There is no set time**
> **for you to learn**
> **to remain in trances**
> **with your eyes wide open.**
> **[Pause]**

MHE: Here she is beginning to realize that a hallucination is not just a psychotic thing. She can see it in her mind's eye.

ER: You are redefining hallucination as something that can be seen in the mind's eye with one's eyes closed. You're making it a safe and easy thing they can do.

MHE: It may look like a challenge, but it isn't one. You may "start it by keeping your eyes closed," implies that it doesn't make a damn bit of difference whether your eyes are open or shut.

ER: Then you throw in the safety phrase, "There is no set time." It can happen now or next week. She is hallucinating her own training.

MHE: In the final pause, you exude confidence.

> **MHE: You have already had**
> **some experiences of**

being in a trance
with your eyes wide open.
[Pause]

MHE: Anyone absentmindedly looking out the window during a lecture is experiencing trance with eyes wide open. You are oblivious to the external lecture and your surroundings as you tune into inner realities. Everyone has had that experience.

ER: You are defining trance in this way: not paying attention to your immediate surroundings, being off someplace else mentally.

MHE: Trance is a common experience. A football fan watching a game on TV is awake to the game, but is not awake to his body sitting in the chair, or his wife calling him to dinner.

MHE: Now, we'll shift over
to another part of your learning.
You can awaken
from the trance at will,
awaken by counting back
from 20 to 1.

ER: You seemed fairly tentative as you gave these awakening instructions. You thus gave her a creative option to awaken at this time. But if she was absorbed in interesting and important work at that moment, there was an implication that she could continue for a while yet. This ensures that awakening will be a pleasant experience rather than a rude interruption.

MHE: You can as a person awaken,
but you do not need
to awaken as a body.
[Pause]

ER: With the following sentence, this forms a ***Double Dissociation Double Bind.***

MHE: Yes. You are making it possible for the subject to comprehend the idea of a dissociation between the mind and the body.

> **MHE: You can waken**
> **when your body awakes,**
> **but without**
> **a recognition of your body.**
> **[Pause]**

MHE: Here, I'm giving the possibility of posthypnotic suggestion.

ER: Now, this is a very important aspect of your technique. You give possibilities for posthypnotic behavior and you wonder yourself which of these will be fulfilled. You have no way of knowing which will be realized, but when they are, you can take credit for them.

MHE: You take credit only when you are given credit.

ER: You just smile when they fulfill a posthypnotic suggestion, and they know you've had a hand in it, which you have.

MHE: But not to the extent that they think.

ER: So, throughout the induction you may give many possibilities of posthypnotic behavior, but not in a bold way, as I once did in my early work when I told a subject that he would "casually touch the ashtray after the trance was terminated." When he awakened, he said he remembered my posthypnotic suggestion, but he "did not feel like carrying it out." He came back the next session saying he had been preoccupied all week with why he had not touched the ashtray.

Obviously, he was influenced by the suggestion, but I presented it so directly that it aroused resistance and actually precipitated a conflict between touching and not touching and the question "Why?" that bothered him all week. It may be dramatic for the purposes of the stage hypnotist to select subjects who will obey direct commands, but the hypnotherapist who must work with all patients must carefully study what natural tendencies the individual patient has that can be funneled into therapeutically useful posthypnotic behaviors.

MHE: Our understanding
of ourselves
is very complicated.
A child first learns,
I love me,
[Pause]
and then proceeds
one day,
I love my brother,
my father,
my sister,
but what the child
is saying—
I love the me
in you.
[Pause]
And that's all the child does love.
The me in you.
[Pause]
As the child progresses,
[Pause]
the child now learns
to love your beauty,
your grace,
intelligence,

but that is his perception of the you.
[Pause]

ER: Here, you are exploring identity formation. The focus is on the person's identity and how it developed?

MHE: You're evoking, "I am me, I am doing this, I'm going to keep on doing this."

ER: You're focusing on the work to be done by her in trance?

MHE: Yes.

ER: By this general description of identity formation, you are offering a series of truisms that may help keep her focused on her own individual inner work. You also may be helping her explore important facets of the development of her own identity.

MHE: In the final stage,
it is learning
in your happiness,
I will find
my happiness,
[Pause]
and that is the separation
of the identity
of one person
from the identity
of the other.

MHE: "In your happiness I will find my happiness." Everyone wants to give and find happiness. Their happiness right now in the trance will be some accomplishment.

ER: I see, you're actually motivating her to accomplish something for which she will be happy. You do everything you can to create an atmosphere of positive motivation and reward in trance experience. By interspersing this positive feeling within the general context of exploring her identity, you also may be associating a reward with the development and separation of personal identity. You are indirectly facilitating the growth of her identity.

[Dr. S spontaneously opens her eyes and reorients to her body.]

ER: You did not know she was going to open her eyes at this point?

MHE: No.

ER: Yet, you gave her the option earlier of counting from 20 to 1 to awaken. Your open-ended manner gave her the creative option of awakening when she felt ready to. You structured an awakening, yet you gave her the freedom of when even if it was inconvenient for you.

MHE: That's right. You give them the freedom to awaken at the wrong time for you. Then, they are in the mood to continue for you.

ER: There is a give and take in your relationship with patients.

MHE: Now, what's happened to you?

Dr. S: Me?

MHE: Yes, what happened to you?
[Pause]
You wait and don't discuss it because what you're going to do is separate your understandings and clarify those and individualize them.

At the present time, you have a partially conscious and partially unconscious understanding, and we don't know where to place the emphasis.
[Pause]

ER: Now that she's awakened, we enter that important period of ratifying the trance. Her question, "Me?" implies she is not completely oriented yet. It takes most people a moment or two to awaken from trance. That is another indicator of a genuine trance experience.

MHE: You will "separate your understandings" implies: You have got understandings of two varieties, conscious and unconscious.

ER: And you are going to do more work on them as time goes on.

MHE: That's right.

MHE: There is one thing in therapy that is so important.
[Pause]
When you touch upon another person's emotions,
[Pause]
you always touch tender places, and they don't know where those tender
places are.
[Pause]
You have had your first experience of a quick withdrawal.

[Pause]
Maybe you were trying to find why you were withdrawing, or what you were withdrawing from.

Dr. S: I didn't know I was.

ER: You say that you didn't know you were withdrawing from hypnosis?

Dr. S: Yes.

ER: Here, you soften any possible negative implications of her awakening by generalizing about tender places and emotions in therapy. You provide a frame of reference for talking about tender emotions. You avoid direct questioning about such tender spots since that tends to arouse resistance and at best, only elicits an answer that is hedged by all sorts of conscious inhibitions and limitations. By simply providing her with a gentle frame of reference, on the other hand, you're giving her an opportunity to say something that's important if she wants to; you're providing her with an opportunity for growth that is automatically appropriate for whatever level she is at, since she can choose to say whatever she wants within the frame you've provided. The frames of reference offer a shelter of safety for what she is experiencing.

MHE: I'm asking for what she may be thinking without being blunt and putting her on the spot.

ER: Yes, your statement about withdrawing provides a frame that may enable her to say something about whatever she might have experienced as negative. Her statement that she did not know she was withdrawing indicates she feels her awakening was a natural and satisfying termination rather than an abrupt withdrawal or escape from something unpleasant in trance.

> **MHE: By the way, what time do you think it is?**
>
> **Dr. S: I thought it was about 4:30.**
>
> **MHE: Does it feel a half-hour has passed?**

ER: Were you trying to distract us by throwing in that question?

MHE: Yes. It was a distraction. You don't want too much self-analysis immediately. A person freshly out of the trance is still lingering close to it, and unconscious knowledge is easily available. You don't know if that should be used yet. So, you distract them.

ER: You want to make a definite separation between trance and waking behavior. You don't want the in-between state that blurs the distinction.

MHE: You do not want to blur that distinction.

> **Dr. S: Well, it's kind of hard to judge because I was flashing back to when I was 16. I think the first time, I went ahead in time to about 40 years of age and we were visiting April's children. There were four kids that were climbing around a banyan tree.**
>
> **ER: You went into the future?**
>
> **Dr. S: Yes, I lived in the future. Well, I have thought about it, but I dreamed about it too.**
>
> **MHE: Where was April when you were thinking about her and her children?**
>
> **Dr. S: Where was she? I don't know where she was; it seemed as**

if she was off doing something. She was going to be there soon.

MHE: Where was that place? What was that place?

Dr. S: She just had these girls playing around a banyan tree. Just some time in the future.

MHE: The implication of this, of course, is that Dr. S did want to have four children herself (this was later verified as true), and she is now projecting it into a fantasy of the future when she can play with her daughter April's four children. But she does not know I know this, she does not know it herself. Her unconscious knows a lot she does not know. In not promptly analyzing this and telling her about it, I've also let her know it is safe to fantasize and project herself in this way.

ER: Yes. You've made the trance experience safe for her. You did not learn anything from her trance that is going to frighten or traumatize her life. You make the trance a safe and pleasant experience.

MHE: And she can trust me.

ER: So, we go on talking about the trance in an intellectual way that's safe.

[Erickson gives an example of a patient who once slapped him across the face because she was not yet ready to talk consciously about trance events she was still partly associated with in the first moments of awakening.]

MHE: Do you know what you just said?

Dr. S: No.

MHE: What is the approach some people make toward active

hallucination?

Dr. S: A while before, you said something about not having to pay attention to your voice, but your voice had already gotten pretty distant because I felt pretty relaxed. But you mentioned something about hallucinations. Just about then I saw a great heart, and it had different layers. I don't know if it had something to do with that (referring to the irregular green-tinted glass, an art object, she had used for an eye fixation point.) Well, when I first looked at it, it looked like seaweed, but I was imagining I was just swimming along in the ocean.
[Pause]
I guess I'm just skipping around now.

MHE: Yes. To get a real hallucination is an unreality, and what is more unreal than April's four children?

Dr. S: Well, it was like a dream in that respect. They were cute little girls climbing through the tree.

ER: Here, she gives an excellent description of some of the subjective experiences of trance. Especially noteworthy is her comment to the effect that when she was relaxed, your voice already became "pretty distant." In relaxation, then, we automatically diminish the subjective experience of all the sensory modalities.

This is the basis of using relaxation and hypnosis for pain and similar problems.

Her internal imagery with eyes closed was a symbolic approach toward experiencing visual hallucinations with eyes open. This was her first response to your earlier suggestions about hallucinating visually.

MHE: And a very effective one. She is very sophisticated with terminology—more so than she realized—and she betrayed that fact by seeing April's children.

ER: Seeing April's children is in the visual modality, the modality of visual hallucinations.

MHE: Yes.

> **ER: You saw all that? So this was your first approach to hallucinatory experience.**
>
> **MHE: And very, very real approach, and the approach of someone who is sophisticated without knowing that she is sophisticated.**

ER: And without knowing that she is approaching hallucinatory behavior.

MHE: At a completely sophisticated level.

ER: Let me ask what you mean by "sophisticated."

MHE: She knows what hallucination is. She accepted my abstract and sophisticated concept "hallucination" and used it to see an unreality projected into the future.

ER: I can see we were both very quick to reinforce her first step toward hallucinations with very supportive remarks here. It is also fascinating to see how she spontaneously oriented herself into the future without any suggestion from you. I suppose this is how most hypnotic phenomena were discovered. Someone does something interesting spontaneously, and then an alert investigator tries to evoke it in others.

Dr. S: Now, I'm trying to think better. It was kind of hard to think, flashing around in that state.
ER: In the trance, it's harder to think?

Dr. S: Yes
[Pause]
Another thing flashed into my mind when Dr. Erickson mentioned going back and assuming another identity. I used the name Amy for a while in high school because we were all using different names. When you mentioned Ann Margaret, that Amy identity flashed in my mind.

[Dr. S continues to recount other memories of her teen years that she touched upon in trance.]

MHE: How long had it been since you thought about Amy?

Dr. S: About 20 years. That's funny. Oh well, I think you said something about awakening by counting back from 20 or something and I did it, but then I didn't know if I was right in waking up.

ER: Such spontaneous comments as these about how hard it is to think in trance suggest that trance (at least as she experienced it) is an altered state characterized by less control over cognitive processes. Trance is a giving up of controls over internal processes as well as external behavior. Thus, processes of cognition, imagery, and emotion are experienced as flowing by themselves in an involuntary manner. Awakening is a process of reasserting control over thinking (as she expresses so well here) and behavior (body reorientation).

MHE: You were giving signs that I had hit on a definition of identity.

ER: What were the signs?

MHE: Movements in her muscles here and there, especially in the thighs.

ER: I see, that's why you were watching her hands resting on her thighs. You were watching those muscles. I also noticed her fingers were moving at a certain point. I'd like to have you say more about this, Dr. Erickson. About the signs you were picking up on her-- about the trance characteristic, and the relationship of movement to identity.

ER: You mentioned that when a patient's identity is touched, they show certain body movements. How would you suggest a beginning hypnotherapist train himself to deal with this? Would you wake up a patient when he begins showing such movements and ask about them or simply ask while the patient is in trance?

MHE: When you continue with one subject long enough, they will gradually tell you everything without your even asking.

ER: Sensing that Dr. S was caught up in her identity by observing the movements in her muscles and fingers—did that motivate you to suggest termination by counting backward from 20 to 1?

MHE: I knew she was going to wake up in a direct relationship to the identification with maturity.

> **MHE: Usually a patient in a trance remains immobile. When you see her move, you immediately try to connect the movement with the words you have been using.**
>
> **ER: When you see her finger move, you try to connect it with what you have been saying?**
>
> **MHE: Yes.**
>
> **ER: A more naive hypnotherapist, a beginner like myself, might think, "Oh she is just waking up." But her awakening**

> **has psychodynamic meaning. You saw those twitches starting to take place and you understood this as a show of recognition or identity with what you were saying.**
>
> **MHE: Yes.**

ER: After this session, Dr. S casually mentioned to me that she had recently witnessed a demonstration of finger signaling. She felt that even though you did ***not*** suggest the possibility of finger signaling to her, the finger movements I noticed were her initial efforts at finger signaling. She wanted to experience finger signaling because she was fascinated with it when she had previously witnessed it. She therefore used this trance as an opportunity to experience something she was interested in without even telling you about it. She said she was surprised and delighted when she noticed that her fingers moved all by themselves. It is a curious dissociation: she wanted to experience finger signaling and yet she did it in an entirely spontaneous and autonomous manner. Of course, her finger signaling could also be a generalization from your earlier suggestions for head signaling.

> **Dr. S: What did they mean, if I wasn't aware of them?**
>
> **MHE: You were having flashes of identity of yourself as a child, maybe flashes of your identity as you grew, flashes of your identity as an adolescent and then, a very strong identification of yourself as a woman.**

ER: So in this presentation, Dr. Erickson, you allowed her many possibilities. You used a buckshot approach which allowed her unconscious to select just what it wanted to experience. You offered suggestions in an open-ended manner.

MHE: Yes, you phrase your suggestions in such a manner that the patient's own unconscious can select just what experience is most appropriate at that time.

Chapter Four

The *Yes Set*

The Yes Set is another basic hypnotic form for coping with the limitations of a patient's rigid and negativistic conscious attitudes. Much initial effort in every trance induction is to evoke a set or framework of associations that will facilitate the work that is to be accomplished. In the first session, for example, he evoked the early learning set as an analog of the new learning situation that hypnosis represented for Dr. S. Just as she successfully learned her ABC's, so she would successfully learn to experience trance. Thus, the early learning set could itself be understood as a Yes Set serving as a framework to orient her to the trance work at hand.

One of Erickson's favorite anecdotes is about a beginning student who discovered the usefulness of the ***Yes Set*** in hypnotic induction. The student found himself confronted by a hostile subject who adamantly refused to accept the possibility that he could experience trance. The student, acting on a creative hunch, then simply proceeded to ask the resistant subject a series of 20 or 30 questions all of which would elicit an obvious answer of "Yes." All sorts of simple and boring questions such as the following could be used.

Are you living at x address?

Do you work at x?

Is today Tuesday?

Is it 10:00 AM?

Are you seated in that chair?

Without realizing, it the subject develops a ***Yes Set*** and also becomes a bit bored with the situation. At this point, the student finally asked again if the subject would like to experience trance. The subject then acquiesced simply because of the ***Yes Set*** and his desire to escape the dull circumstance of simply saying, "Yes," to obvious questions.

Exercises with the *Yes Set*

1. We believe the ***Yes Set*** is closely related to the concept of rapport, which has traditionally been regarded as a basic feature of the therapist-patient relationship in hypnosis. It is the essence of Erickson's approach to the resistant patient, who is usually unable to control his own antagonistic, defensive, and self-defeating behavior.

Erickson (1964/2022a) illustrates as follows:

Perhaps this can be illustrated by the somewhat extreme example of a new patient, whose opening statement as he entered the office characterized all psychiatrists as being best described by a commonly used vulgarity.

MHE: [Immediately] You undoubtedly have a damn good

reason for saying ***that and even more.***

The italicized words were not recognized by the patient as a direct intentional suggestion to be more communicative, but they were most effective. With much profanity and obscenity, with bitterness and resentment, and with contempt and hostility, the patient related his unfortunate, unsuccessful, repeated, and often prolonged futile efforts to secure psychotherapy.

MHE: [Commented simply, casually, during a pause] **Well, you must have had a hell of a good reason to seek therapy from me.** (This gave definition to the patient's visit unrecognized by him.)

Plan how you can learn to recognize, share, and ***Utilize*** a patient's own words and frames of reference to facilitate the transformation of "seemingly uncooperative forms of behavior into good rapport, a feeling of being understood, and an attitude of hopeful expectancy of successfully achieving the goals being sought."

Psychological Implication

An understanding of how Erickson uses implication will provide us with the clearest model of his indirect approach to hypnotic suggestion. Since his use of ***implication*** may involve something more than the typical dictionary definition of the term, we will assume that he may be developing a special form of ***psychological implication*** in his work. For Erickson, psychological implication is a key that automatically turns the tumblers of a patient's associative processes into predictable patterns without awareness of how it happened. The implied thought or response seems to come up autonomously within patients, as if it were their own inner response rather than a suggestion initiated by the therapist. Psychological implication is thus a way of structuring and directing patients' associative processes when they cannot do it for themselves. The therapeutic use of this approach is obvious. If patients have problems because of the limitations of their ability to utilize their own resources, then implications are a way of bypassing these limitations.

If you sit down, then you can go into trance.

Any implication stated in the logical "if . . . then" form can be a useful way of structuring a suggestion. The introductory "if" phrase states a condition that is acceptable or easily accomplished by the patient so that a *Yes Set* is created for the suggestion that follows in the concluding "then" phrase.

Obviously, you are not going into a trance, now!

"Now" lasts only for a short while; the implication is that you will go into a trance as soon as "Now" is over.

Certainly, your arm won't be numb before I count to five.

Implies it will be numb after a count of five. In every psychological implication, there is a direction initially structured by the therapist and a response created by the patient.

In the above, we are initially structuring the implications that will direct the patient's associations and behavior in predictable directions. Exactly when the patient will go into trance or how numbness will be created, however, are responses mediated on an unconscious level by the patient. Consider the following examples:

Before you go into trance, you ought to be comfortable.

The most obvious implication is that one will go into trance after one is comfortable. The very process of getting comfortable, however, also evokes many unconscious adjustments of relaxation and not doing that are also important for initiating trance experience.

The very complexity of mental functioning,

A truism.

You go into a trance to find out,

A phrase which implies that the patient does have an important purpose in going into a trance.

A whole lot of things you can do.

This implies that it is not what the therapist can do but what the patient can do that is important.

And there are so many more than you dreamed of. [Pause.]

The pause implies that the patient's unconscious may make a search to find some of these individual things she was previously unaware of.

It is important in formulating psychological implications to realize that the therapist only provides a stimulus; the hypnotic aspect of psychological implications is created on an unconscious level by the listener. The most effective aspect of any suggestion is that which stirs the listener's own associations and mental processes into automatic action. It is this autonomous activity of the listener's own associations and mental processes that creates hypnotic experience.

There are, to be sure, crude and mostly ineffective uses of implication in everyday life, where the speaker in a very obvious manner attempts to cast negative implications or aspersions on the listener. In such crude usage the implication is obviously created entirely by the speaker. In our use of psychological implication, however, we mean something quite different. In the psychological climate of the therapeutic encounter the patient is understood to be the center of focus. Every psychological truth is consciously or unconsciously received by the patient for its possible application to himself. Psychological implication thus becomes a valuable indirect approach for evoking and ***Utilizing*** a patient's own associations to deal with his own problem.

This was well illustrated when a colleague referred a rebellious teenager to Erickson. He listened quietly to the lad's story and then initiated an important therapeutic development with one simple statement.

I don't know how your behavior will change.

The rebellious teenager was in no mood to accept advice from a doctor, and, in truth, Erickson really did not know how his behavior was going to change. By openly admitting that he did not know, Erickson disarmed the lad's resistance so he could momentarily experience an acceptance set. Erickson then managed to insert one implication in that moment of acceptance: "Your behavior will change." The boy was now left with the idea of change; his own associations and life experience would have to create exactly how that change was going to take place.

Exercises in Psychological Implication

1. Exercises in implication and clinical inference were Erickson's first approach in training Rossi. He dragged out old protocols, some of them 25 years old or more, and gave Rossi the exercise of reading the first page or two and then, by implication and inference, predict what was to follow. Another set of exercises was to study the first sketch of a character by Dostoevski or Thomas Mann and by implication infer what the character's fate would be in the novel. For a period of his life, Erickson enjoyed whodunit fiction for the same purpose. Study recordings of your own therapy sessions, particularly initial interviews, and explore the possible implications of each of the patient's remarks. Then study the implications of your own. How many are actually therapeutic?

2. Study recordings of hypnotic inductions, particularly your own. Learn to recognize the implications that are present in your voice

dynamics (such as intonations and pauses) as well as the content of your words.

3. Carefully construct sentences that (a) state a general psychological truth that (b) by implication initiates an inner search that will (c) evoke and mobilize the listener's own memories, associations, ideomotor and ideosensory responses, and so on.

4. Carefully write out hypnotic inductions formulating a series of psychological implications that can facilitate trance and each of the classical hypnotic phenomena.

Chapter Five

Therapeutic Binds and *Double Binds*

The concept of the Double Bind has been used in many ways. We use the terms bind and Double Bind in a very special and limited sense to describe forms of suggestion that offer patients the possibility of structuring their behavior in a therapeutic direction. A bind offers a free choice of two or more comparable alternatives—that is, whichever choice is made leads behavior in a desired direction. Therapeutic binds are tactful presentations of the possible alternate forms of constructive behavior that are available to the patient in a given situation. The patient is given free, voluntary choice between them; the patient usually feels bound, however, to accept one alternative.

Double Binds, by contrast, offer possibilities of behavior that are outside the patient's usual range of conscious choice and control. Since the original formulation of the ***Double Bind*** (Bateson et al., 1956) as a hypothesis about the nature and etiology of communication in schizophrenia, a number of authors have sought to ***Utilize*** the concept of the ***Double Bind*** to understand and facilitate psychotherapy and hypnosis (Haley, 1963; Watzlawick et al., 1967, 1974; Erickson & Rossi, 1975). Since we use the term in a very special and limited sense, we will present only an outline of how we conceptualize the ***Double Bind*** for an understanding of therapeutic trance and hypnotic suggestion.

The ***Double Bind*** arises out of the possibility of communicating on more than one level. We can (1) say something and (2) simultaneously comment on what we are saying. We may describe our primary message (1) as being on an object level of communication while the comment (2) is on a higher level of abstraction, which is usually called a secondary or metalevel of communication (a metacommunication). A peculiar situation arises when what is stated in a primary communication is restructured or cast into another frame of reference in the metacommunication.

In requesting an ideomotor response such as ***Hand Levitation***, for example, we (1) ask patients to let their hand lift but (2) to experience it as lifting in an involuntary manner. In requesting an ideosensory response, we may (1) ask patients to experience a hallucinatory sensation of warmth, but (2) it is usually understood that such an experience is outside patients' normal range of self-control. Therefore, patients must allow the warmth to develop on another, more involuntary level. We have many ways of saying or implying to patients that (1) something will happen, but (2) you won't do it with conscious intent, your unconscious will do it. We call this the conscious-unconscious ***Double Bind***: since consciousness cannot do it, the unconscious must do it on an involuntary level. Conscious intentionality and one's usual mental sets are placed in a bind that tends to depotentiate their activity; unconscious potentials now have an opportunity to intrude. The conscious-unconscious ***Double Bind*** is the essential basis of many of the therapeutic ***Double Binds*** discussed in the following sections.

In actual practice, the metacommunication that comments on the primary message, may take place without words: one may comment with a doubting tone of voice, a gesture or body movement, subtle social cues and contexts. Hidden implications or unconscious assumptions may also function as a metacommunication binding or qualifying what is said on the ordinary conversational level. Because of this the patient is usually not aware that conflicting messages are being received. The conflict is frequently enough to disrupt the patient's usual modes of functioning, however, so that more unconscious and involuntary processes are activated.

Ideally, our therapeutic ***Double Binds*** are mild quandaries that provide the patient with an opportunity for growth. These quandries are indirect hypnotic forms insofar as they tend to block or disrupt the patient's habitual attitudes and frames of reference so that choice is not easily made on a conscious, voluntary level. In this sense, a ***Double Bind*** may be operative whenever one's usual frames of reference cannot cope and one is forced to another level of functioning. Bateson (1975) has commented that this other level can be "a higher level of abstraction which may be more wise, more psychotic, more humorous, more religious, etc." We simply add that this other level can also be more autonomous or involuntary in its functioning; that is, outside the person's usual range of self-direction and control. Thus, we find that the therapeutic ***Double Bind*** can lead one to experience those altered states we characterize as trance so that previously unrealized potentials may become manifest.

In actual practice, there is an infinite range of situations that may or may not function as binds or ***Double Binds***, What is or is not a bind or ***Double Bind*** will depend very much on how it is received by the listener. What is a bind or ***Double Bind*** for one person may not be one for another. In the following sections, therefore, we will describe a number of formulations that may or many not lead a particular patient to experience a bind or ***Double Bind.*** These formulations are approaches to hypnotic experience; they cannot be regarded as techniques that invariably produce the same response in everyone. Humans are too complex and individual differences are simply too great to expect that the same words or situation will produce the same effect in everyone. Well-trained hypnotherapists have available many possible approaches to hypnotic experience. They offer them one after another to the patient and carefully evaluate which actually lead to the desired result. In clinical practice, we can only determine what was or was not a therapeutic bind or ***Double Bind*** in retrospect by studying the patient's response. The following formulations, therefore, offer only the possibility of therapeutic binds or ***Double Binds*** that may structure desired behavior.

The Bind and *Double Bind* Question

Binds are easily formed by questions that give the subject a free choice among comparable alternatives. Any choice, however, facilitates an approach toward a desired response. To facilitate the acceptance of the trance situation, a great number of possibilities exist, such as the following:

Would you like to experience a light, medium, or deep trance?

Would you like to go into trance sitting up or lying down?

Would you like to have your hands on your thighs or on the arms of the chair when you go into trance?

We could designate these questions as binds because while they do structure a trance situation, they can easily be answered by most people with their usual conscious sets. For some people, however, the second example could function as a ***Double Bind*** if it is found that they do, in fact, go into a trance when they sit or lie down in response to the question.

The following questions, by contrast, are more typically ***Double Binds*** because they cannot be answered with one's usual conscious sets. One must usually relax and allow more autonomous or unconscious functions to fulfill them. Such ***Double Bind*** questions are of particular interest for facilitating Erickson's experiential approach to hypnotic phenomena. By turning attention to one's subjective experience, one is focused inward in a manner that can lead easily to an experience of trance and hypnotic phenomena. This question approach is also particularly suitable for those subjects who respond to the initial phase of trance induction with hyper-alertness, anxiety, or tension. The question allows them to ***Utilize*** their conscious focus to facilitate the recognition of the suggested phenomena. The question ***Double Bind*** is thus, very useful for resistant subjects, who need to use their consciousness to maintain some control in the hypnotic situation. Consider these examples:

Will your right hand or your left begin to feel light first? Or will they both feel that lightness at the same time?

Will your right hand move or lift or shift to the side or press down first? Or will it be your left hand?

Do you begin to experience a numbness in the fingers or the back of the hand first?

What part of your body begins to feel most comfortable (warm, cool, heavy, etc.)?

These questions may function as ***Double Binds*** because a hypnotic suggestion in the form of an ideomotor or ideosensory response is being facilitated no matter which alternative is experienced. When naive subjects experience such phenomena for the first time, they are usually surprised and a bit delighted. Such phenomena are experiential proof that they can learn to develop latent potentials and altered modes of functioning for further therapeutic work.

The Time Bind and *Double Bind*

Time is an excellent dimension for formulating binding questions and situations.

Do you want to enter trance now or in a few minutes?

Would you like to go into trance quickly or slowly?

Will you be ready to get over that habit this week or the next?

These questions can be answered with one's usual frames of reference and may therefore be classified as binds that simply focus attention in the direction of a desired response. Whatever the patient's answer, however, they are being bound to make the therapeutic response—either now or later. With some subjects the first two questions may actually evoke the initial experiences of trance; for them the context of the hypnotherapeutic situation and the therapist's attitude of expectation that they will go into trance may function as metacommunications that activate autonomous processes leading them into trance experience.

Double Binds Utilizing time to evoke responses on a more autonomous level may be structured as follows:

Please let me know when that feeling of warmth develops in your hand.

Is that anesthesia proceeding quickly or slowly?

Take all the time you need to really learn how to experience that (any ideomotor or ideosensory response) in that special trance time where every moment in trance is equivalent to hours, days, or even weeks of regular time.

All of these questions and situations *Utilizing* time contain a strong psychological implication that the desired response will take place. Most hypnotic responses take time. In trance, subjects usually experience psychomotor retardation -- a lag between the time when a suggestion is given and when the subject is finally able to carry it out. The time bind capitalizes on this time lag and makes it an integral part of the hypnotic response.

A charming example of the possibility of a therapeutic ***Double Bind Utilizing*** time was offered to a six year-old boy by Erickson.

I know your father and mother have been asking you, Jimmy, to quit biting your nails. They don't seem to know that you're just a six year-old boy. And they don't seem to know that you will naturally quit biting your nails just before you're seven years-old. And they really don't know that! So when they tell you to stop biting your nails, just ignore them!

Of course, Jimmy did not know that Erickson knew that he would be seven in a few months. Erickson's words, uttered with sincere conviction and in a confidential tone implying that he was taking Jimmy into secret confidence, were enough to ***Double Bind*** Jimmy into giving up nail biting within two months in a way that the boy could not consciously understand. He could not understand, for example, how his pleasure in being permitted to ignore his parent's irritating demands that he stop biting his nails actually reinforced the ***Double Bind*** that activated his own internal resources to create a way of giving up nail biting on his own. As it turned out, Jimmy was later able to brag that he quit a whole month before he was seven years-old.

The Conscious-Unconscious *Double Bind*

Erickson frequently gives a preinduction talk about the differences between the functioning of the conscious mind and the unconscious mind. This prepares the patient for ***Double Binds*** that rest upon the fact that we cannot consciously control our unconscious. The conscious-unconscious ***Double Bind*** blocks the patient's usual voluntary modes of behavior so that responses must be mediated on a more autonomous or unconscious level. Any response to the following situations, for example, requires that the subject experience trance.

> **If your unconscious wants you to enter trance, your right hand will lift. Otherwise your left hand will lift.**
>
> **You don't even have to listen to me because your unconscious is here and can hear what it needs to to respond in just the right way.**
>
> **And it really doesn't matter what your conscious mind does because your unconscious automatically will do just what it needs to in order to achieve that anesthesia [age regression, catalepsy, etc.].**
>
> **You've said that your conscious mind is uncertain and confused. And that's because the conscious mind does forget. And yet we know the unconscious does have access to so many memories and images and experiences that it can make available to the conscious mind so you can solve that problem. And when will the unconscious make all those valuable learnings available to your conscious mind? Will it be in a dream? During the day? Will it come quickly or slowly? Today? Tomorrow?**

In this series of ***Double Binds,*** the therapist is using an open-ended approach. The therapist gives a number of truisms about psychological functioning, any one of which will help to solve the patient's problem. The value of this open-ended approach is that it gives the patient's unconscious the freedom to work in whatever way is most suitable for its own unique patterns of functioning.

This open-ended approach, together with the conscious-unconscious ***Double Bind***, is also the essence of one of Erickson's approaches to resistant patients. When combined with ideomotor signaling (as will be described in a later section) to indicate when the unconscious has made a satisfactory response or answered a question, the conscious-unconscious ***Double Bind*** becomes a reliable way of evoking hypnotic or involuntary responses in a manner that is usually acceptable to even the most resistant, frightened, or misinformed subject. In general, all the ***Double Bind*** approaches are excellent means for helping the so-called resistant patient bypass or resolve the erroneous ideas and the limitations of his belief system that have been impeding hypnotic responsiveness and therapeutic change.

Erickson introduced a series of interrelated ***Double Binds*** in this session that were all directed toward depotentiating conscious sets by emphasizing the potency of the unconscious over consciousness.

Consider the following:

> **But your conscious mind will keep it only with the consent of your unconscious mind.**
>
> **You don't need to listen to me. Your unconscious mind can listen to me without your knowledge.**
>
> **A person seeking therapy comes in and tells you one story that is believed fully at the conscious level and in nonverbal [unconscious] language can give you a story that is entirely different.**
> **And the unconscious mind has had little opportunity to give recognition to its own ways of understanding. [Implying it would be well to give the unconscious that opportunity now.]**
> **And your willingness to rely upon your unconscious mind to do anything that can be of interest or value to you as most important.**
>
> **Now there are many different ways in which the mind can function in which the unconscious can join with the conscious.**

Many different ways in which the unconscious can avoid the conscious mind without the conscious mind knowing that it has just received a gift.

If the reader studies the context of these remarks, it will be found that they are usually directed toward freeing the patient's capacity for functioning on an unconscious level to explore the many response potentials that have been excluded by consciousness. Learning to experience trance and the response potentials that are available in trance is thus directly related to the patient's ability to let go of the directing and limiting functions of his usual frames of reference. Erickson demonstrates an important approach to separating conscious from unconscious processes at the end of this session. He typically distracts patients for at least two to five minutes after the formal termination of trance because, unless a patient has been trained otherwise, it usually takes that long to fully separate trance and waking states. The distraction period allows the conscious associative connections to trance events to be broken. Being so broken, trance events tend to remain amnesic. This also helps make a recognizable demarcation between trance and wakefulness. This recognizable demarcation thus automatically ratifies the fact that the trance was "real."

We view the typical experimental approach to hypnosis where the investigator administers a standard scale of direct suggestions, and then immediately questions subjects about their experience as being destructive of the unique aspects of the first stages of learning how to experience trance. Such immediate questioning blurs the still delicate distinction between trance and waking states in subjects who are just learning how to let themselves experience trance. The experimenter's immediate questions unwittingly build associative bridges between the contents of the trance and the awake state. ***These associative bridges actually destroy the experience of trance as an altered state that is discontinuous from the ordinary awake state.***

It is an odd, but sadly true fact that consciousness usually does not recognize when it is in an altered state; people must learn to recognize the delicate and nascent experience of developing trance just as they must learn to recognize any other altered state (due to alcohol, drugs, toxemias, psychosis, etc.) It is also well established that the process of observation frequently interferes with the observed process. This is particularly true for psychology in general and hypnosis in particular. Making injudicious direct observations usually interferes with the trance phenomenon being investigated.

The Double Dissociation *Double Bind*

Erickson introduces another more complex ***Double Bind*** in this session to facilitate dissociation. Note the subtle interlocking of the following suggestions for dissociation that seem to cover all possibilities of response, while at the same time introducing the possibility of certain posthypnotic responses.

> **You can, as a person, awaken, but you do not need to awaken as a body.**
>
> **[Pause]**
>
> **You can awaken when your body awakes, but without a recognition of your body.**

In the first half of this statement, awakening as a person is dissociated from awakening as a body. In the second half, awakening as a person and body are dissociated from a recognition of the body. Because of this we may call this type of statement a double dissociation ***Double Bind.*** So complex is the total effect of this suggestion that it is not immediately obvious just what response possibilities are being suggested. The actual response possibilities are as follows:

> **You can as a person awaken, but you do not need to awaken as a body.**
>
> **You can as a person awaken, but you do not need to awaken as a body and recognize your body.**
>
> **You can as a person awaken, and you can as a body awaken, but without a recognition of your body.**

Hypnotic forms such as the double dissociation ***Double Bind*** have an exciting potential for exploring an individual's response abilities, as well as mediating suggestions. As with open-ended suggestions, double-dissociation ***Double Binds*** permit a certain amount of free choice that enables a subject's individuality to express itself in ways that are surprising even to the subject. Double dissociation ***Double Binds*** tend to confuse subjects' conscious mind and thus, depotentiate their habitual sets, biases, and learned limitations. Under these circumstances, the field is cleared for the possibility of creative processes to express themselves in a more autonomous and unconscious manner. We know from studies in neuropsychology (Luria, 1973) that the secondary and tertiary association areas of the parieto-temporo-occipital cortext are capable of synthesizing and mediating the same psychological function in many different ways. Hypnotic forms such as the double dissociation ***Double Bind*** may enable the subject to exercise and utilize the incredible potentials of these association areas in ways that are entirely new and outside the range of the subject's previous experience. Understood in this manner, the double dissociation ***Double Bind*** can be explored as a means of enhancing creativity rather than simply programming suggestions.

Another example illustrating possibilities of the double dissociation ***Double Bind*** follows:

> **You can write that material without knowing what it is then you can go back and discover you know what it is without knowing you've done it.**

Formulations such as the above for automatic writing with or without either a recognition of its meaning or that one has written it are not as arbitrary as they may seem. Studies of the secondary zones of the occipital cortex and optico-gnostic functions (Luria, 1973) illustrate that each of the above possibilities can occur naturally in the form of agnosias when there are specific organic disturbances to brain tissues. Each of these agnosias is possible only because a discrete mental mechanism for normal functioning has been disturbed when it appears. The agnosias are thus tags for identifying discrete mental mechanisms. A so-called suggestion in the form of a double dissociation ***Double Bind*** may be utilizing these same natural mental mechanisms. We hypothesize that these mental mechanisms can be turned on or off in trance even though they are usually autonomous in their functioning when a person is normally awake. From this point of view, we can conceptualize suggestion as something more than verbal magic. Adequately formulated hypnotic forms actually may be ***Utilizing*** natural processes of cortical functioning that are characteristic of the secondary and tertiary zones of cerebral organization. These processes are synthetic and integrative in their functioning and are responsible for processes of perception, experience, recognition, and knowing. Constructing hypnotic forms that can either block or facilitate these discrete mechanisms of the secondary and tertiary zones thus has the potential for vastly extending our understanding of cerebral functioning. This may be the neuropsychological basis for using hypnotic forms for altering human behavior and greatly expanding all forms of human experience.

A Hypothesis About Evoking Hypnotic Phenomena

Hypnotic forms such as the double dissociation ***Double Bind*** also suggest a more general hypothesis about the means by which traditional hypnotic phenomena can be evoked by dissociation, providing another hint about how new hypnotic phenomena can be developed. We may hypothesize that in general, a hypnotic phenomenon takes place simply by dissociating any behavior from its usual associational context. In our previous example, Erickson demonstrated how awakening as a body can be dissociated and separated from its usual associational context of awakening as a person. When he demonstrates how not recognizing one's body can be effected by dissociating the ability to see (or recognize one's body) from its usual associational context with awakening as a person, he is actually demonstrating how a negative hallucination can be evoked by a process of dissociation.

In a similar manner, the traditional hypnotic phenomena of catalepsy can be evoked by dissociating the ability to move a part of the body from its usual associational context of awakening; anesthesia by dissociating the ability to feel; amnesia by dissociating the ability to remember; and so on. The classical hypnotic phenomena of age regression, automatic writing, hallucinations and ***Time Distortion*** can all be understood as "normal" aspects of behavior that take place in an autonomous or hypnotic manner simply by separating them from their usual associational contexts. It is now an exercise for the therapist's ingenuity to locate those associational contexts from which any of these traditional behaviors can be dissociated to evoke hypnotic phenomena in any particular patient. We can naturally expect that there will be individual differences in the strength with which these various behaviors are attached to different associational contexts in different subjects. The therapist's task is to determine which behaviors can be most easily dissociated from which contexts in which patients. Whenever a behavior is successfully dissociated from its usual context, we have evoked a hypnotic phenomenon. As the therapist develops a facility for this approach, there will be room for evoking entirely new effects that have not yet been reported in the literature. An infinite number of hypnotic phenomena can be evoked for the purposes of basic research and therapy.

The Reverse Set *Double Bind*

Erickson learned something about the reverse se*t* ***Double Bind*** as a boy on the farm. He recounts the events as follows: (Erickson and Rossi. 1975).

> My first well-remembered intentional use of the Double Bind occurred in early boyhood. One winter day with the weather below zero, my father led a calf out of the barn to the water trough. After the calf had satisfied his thirst, they turned back to the barn, but at the doorway the calf stubbornly braced its feet and, despite my father's desperate pulling on the halter, he could not budge the animal. I was outside playing in the snow and, observing the impasse, began laughing heartily. My father challenged me to pull the calf into the barn. Recognizing the situation as one of unreasoning stubborn resistance on the part of the calf, I decided to let the calf have full opportunity to resist since that was what it apparently wished to do. Accordingly I presented the calf with a Double Bind by seizing it by the tail and pulling it away from the barn while my father continued to pull it inward. The calf promptly chose to resist the weaker of the two forces and dragged me into the barn.

> Psychiatric patients are often resistant and withhold vital information indefinitely. When I observe this, I emphatically admonish them that they are not to reveal that information this week, in fact, I am insistent that they withhold it until the latter part of next week. In the intensity of their subjective desire to resist, they fail to evaluate adequately my admonition; they do not recognize it as a Double Bind requiring them both to resist and to yield. If the intensity of their subjective resistance is sufficiently great they may take advantage of the Double Bind to disclose the resistant material without further delay. They thereby achieve their purpose of both communication and resistance. Patients rarely recognize the Double Bind when used on them, but they often comment on the ease they find in communicating and handling their feelings of resistance.

The reverse set ***Double Bind*** permits the subject both to resist and to yield! People with problems are, in fact, usually caught between conflicting impulses. They are caught in ambivalence between resisting and yielding to various impulses and trends within themselves. An effective approach to resolving this dilemma is to allow both the resistance and the yielding to be expressed. It does not make sense from a rational point of view—but it does make sense from an emotional point of view—to free and express all the impulses that were previously locked in mutual contradiction.

Another clear example of Erickson's use of the reverse set to cope with contradictory, defiant, negativistic, and resistant behavior was reported as an illustration of his utilization of the subject's own behavior to initiate trance (Erickson, 1966). The first step is to carefully challenge the subject in such a way that a reverse set is established; the subject is provoked to do the exact opposite of what Erickson says. In this description of his work, Erickson tells how he gradually introduces a series of suggestions the reverse of which will lead the subject to experience trance. This excerpt was taken from a longer write up of dealing with a heckler (one of the students) during a teaching demonstration.

> My utterances were carefully worded to elicit either verbally or by action an emphatic contradiction from the heckler, who was told that he had to remain silent; that he could not speak again, that he did not dare to stand up; that he could not again charge

fraud; that he dared not walk over to the aisle or up to the front of the auditorium; that he had to do whatever I demanded; that he had to sit down; that he had to return to his original seat; that he was afraid ; that he dared not risk being hypnotized; that he was a noisy coward; that he was afraid to look at the volunteer subjects sitting on the platform; that he had to take a seat in the back of the auditorium; that he had to leave the auditorium; that he did not dare to come up on the platform; that he was afraid to shake hands in a friendly fashion with the presenter (Erickson) ; that he did not dare to remain silent; that he was afraid to walk over to one of the chairs on the platform for volunteer subjects; that he was afraid to face the audience and to smile at them; that he dared not look at or listen to the presenter; that he could not sit in one of the chairs; that he would have to put his hands behind him instead of resting them on his thighs; that he dared not experience Hand Levitation; that he was afraid to close his eyes; that he had to remain awake; that he was afraid to go into a trance; that he had to hurry off the platform; that he could not remain and go into a trance; that he could not even develop a light trance; that he dared not go into a deep trance, etc.

The student disputed by word or action every step of the procedure with considerable ease until he was forced into silence. With his dissents then limited to action alone, and caught in his own pattern of contradiction, it became relatively easy to induce a somnabulistic trance state. He was then employed as the demonstration subject for the lecture most effectively.

The next weekend, he sought out Erickson, gave an account of his extensive personal unhappiness and unpopularity and requested psychotherapy. In this he progressed with phenomenal rapidity and success.

This technique, in part or in toto, has been used repeatedly in various modifications, especially with defiant, resistive patients, particularly with incorrigible juvenile delinquents. Its significance lies in the utilization of the patient's ambivalences and the opportunity such an approach affords the patient to achieve successfully contradictory goals, with the feeling that these derived out of the unexpected but adequate use of his own behavior. This need to meet fully the demands of the patient, however manifested, ought never to be minimized.

The Non Sequitur *Double Bind*

Erickson uses non sequiturs or illogic as ***Double Binds***. Non sequiturs and illogic tend to bind, immobilize or disrupt a person's conscious sets so that choice and behavior tend to be mediated on a more involuntary level. To the child who does not want to go to bed, he might first employ a time bind:

Would you rather go to sleep at 8:00 or 8:15?

Of course the child chooses the lesser of the two evils and agrees to go to bed at 8:15. If there is any further difficulty, Erickson might employ an illogical, but convincing ***Double Bind*** such as: "Do you wish to take a ***bath*** before going to bed, or would you rather put your pajamas on in the ***bathroom***?" In such a non sequitur ***Double Bind***, there is a similarity in the content of the alternatives offered, even though there is no logical connection. One could get vertigo trying to figure out the sense of such a proposition. Even though it is impossible to figure out, one tends to go along with it when it is expressed in a confident and convincing manner.

Contrasting Therapeutic and Schizogenic *Double Bind*

The relation between Erickson's therapeutic use of the ***Double Bind*** and the studies of it by Bateson (1972) in the genesis of schizophrenia offers an interesting study of similarities and contrasts. We list them side by side for comparison.

Table 1 (10.5.T.1) Bateson Schizogenic vs Erickson Therapeutic *Double Bind*

The Bateson Schizogenic ***Double Bind***	The Erickson Therapeutic ***Double Bind***
Two or more persons: The child "victim" is usually ensnared by mother or a combination of parents and siblings.	Two or more persons: Usually patient and therapist are ensconsced in a positive relationship.
Repeated experience of the same ***Double Bind*** rather than one simple traumatic event.	One or more forms: of the ***Double Bind*** are offered until one is found that works.
A primary negative injunction: "Do not do so-and-so or I will punish you."	A primary positive injunction: "I agree that you should continue doing such and such."
A secondary injunction conflicting with the first at a more abstract [meta] level and like the first, enforced by punishments or signals that threaten survival.	A secondary positive suggestion at the more abstract level that facilitates a creative interaction between the primary (conscious) and metacommunication (unconscious).
A tertiary negative injunction prohibiting the victim from escaping the field.	A tertiary positive understanding (rapport, transference) that binds the patient to his therapeutic task, but leaves him free to leave if he chooses.
Finally, the complete set of ingredients is no longer necessary when the victim has learned to perceive his universe in ***Double Bind*** patterns.	The patient leaves therapy when his behavior change frees him from transference and the evoked ***Double Binds.***

It may be noted in summary that the schizogenic ***Double Bind*** uses negative injunctions that are enforced at the metalevel, or abstract level, which is outside the victim's control and from which there is no escape. Watzlawick et al. (1967) have illustrated the therapeutic application of the ***Double Binds*** closely modeled on Bateson's formulation wherein the patient is bound to a course of behavior change with no means of escape. Such ***Double Binds*** are admittedly difficult to formulate, however. Erickson's ***Double Binds,*** by contrast, appear to be looser in their formulation on the primary message level but more complex in utilizing many aspects of the patient's unconscious dynamics simultaneously on the metacommunicative level.

Erickson's therapeutic ***Double Binds*** always emphasize positive agreement on the level of metacommunication while offering possibilities that can be refused on the primary message level if they are not appropriate. Erickson has stated, "While I put the patient into a ***Double Bind*** they also sense, unconsciously, that I will never, never hold them to it. They know I will yield anytime. I will then put them in another ***Double Bind*** in some other situation to see if they can put it to constructive use because it meets their needs more adequately." For Erickson, then, the ***Double Bind*** is a useful device that offers a patient possibilities for constructive change. If one ***Double Bind*** does not fit, he will try another and another until he finds one that does.

The Unconscious and Metacommunication

Throughout this discussion of the varieties of ***Double Bind,*** the reader may have noted the ease with which we could use the terms "unconscious" and "metacommunication" in the same place. These terms may, in fact, be in the process of becoming interchangeable. This suggests we may be witnessing a fundamental change in our world view of depth psychology whereby we are developing a new and more efficient nomenclature. Philosophers have never liked the term "unconscious," it was the academic and philosophical rejection of this term that impeded the early acceptance of Freud's psychoanalysis. The use of the term "unconscious" still divides academic and experimentally oriented psychologists from clinicians as well as doctors in physical medicine from psychiatry. The term "metacommunication," however, was developed within a mathematico-logical framework, and as such, it fits in with the world view of the research scientist as well as the clinician. It may well be that we are on the threshold of a new zeitgeist wherein we will revise the terms of depth psychology to make for a better fit with current conceptions in mathematics, cybernetics, and systems theory.

EXERCISES WITH *DOUBLE BINDS*

1. Construct your own original list of a variety of ***Double Binds*** with a positive metacommunication to do the following:

    a. Structure a trance situation

    b. Structure each of the classical hypnotic phenomena

    c. Ratify trance

    d. Structure therapeutic alternatives for a variety of clinical problems (e.g., phobias, compulsions, depression, anxiety, habit problems).

    e. Structure corrective action in various emergency situations

    f. Structure learning, creative imagination, and problem solving

    g. Structure relations between the conscious and unconscious

    h. Devise experimental situations to test which of your original ***Double Binds*** are most effective

2. Explore the dynamics of ***Double Binds*** with negative metacommunications that engender the following:

    a. Competitive situations

    b. Exploitive situations (economic, social, etc.)

3. What experimental situations can you devise to explore the relation between ***Double Binds*** and such sociological catastrophes as wars and depressions and such psychological problems as neurosis, psychosis, and phobias?

Chapter Six

Open-Ended Suggestion

Erickson ends the commentary to this session with an important admission. He frequently uses a buckshot approach that offers the patient many possibilities of response in an open-ended manner; thus, the patient's own unconscious can select just what experience is most appropriate at that time. How different this is from the older authoritarian approaches that belabor the patient with highly specific direct commands and suggestions! By offering suggestions in such manner, he achieves three important goals:

1. There is no possibility of a patient failing on a suggestion since all responses are defined as admissible hypnotic phenomena

2. Patients' response abilities, and hierarchy of responses are explored to provide clues as to what behaviors are available for the achievement of therapeutic goals

3. Since anything the patients do is defined as a satisfactory hypnotic response, they cannot resist or withdraw from the situation. Whatever they do tends to propel them further into the hypnotic situation of following suggestions.

In his 1964 paper on his technique with resistant patients, for example, Erickson manages to effect a dissociation between the conscious and unconscious while defining practically any possible response on the conscious level as a valid hypnotic phenomenon. As Erickson explained it, he used the terms "conscious mind and unconscious mind" thus offering a second intimation is given of dissociation.) In part, he describes it as follows:

> Now when you came into this room you brought into it both of your minds, that is, the front of your mind and the back of your mind . . . Now, I really don't care if you listen to me with your conscious mind, because it doesn't understand your problem anyway or you wouldn't be here, so I just want to talk to your unconscious mind because it's here and close enough to hear me so you can let your conscious mind listen to the street noises or the planes overhead or the typing in the next room. Or you can think about any thoughts that come to your conscious mind, systematic thoughts, random thoughts because all I want to do is to talk to your unconscious mind and it will listen to me because it is within hearing distance even if your conscious mind does get bored .

In these few sentences, the reader can observe not only how these suggestions admit and define practically anything the conscious mind can do as a valid hypnotic response, but also Erickson's simultaneous use of truisms, dissociation, implication, ***Double Binds***, and finally even an approach to depotentiating consciousness with boredom. This open-ended approach of simultaneously using many possible means of effecting trance and suggestions is highly characteristic of Erickson's style. We will study many illustrations of this open-ended approach in each of the following sessions.

Exercises with Open-Ended Suggestions

1. Begin the practice of formulating suggestions in an open-ended manner that admits and defines any possible responses as acceptable. This is particularly important in the induction of trance, where both the therapist's and patient's fears of failure are most pronounced. Formulating induction suggestions in an open-ended manner allows both parties to relax. A premium is placed on exploration and on a convergence of expectations in the patient and therapist that greatly facilitates rapport and therapeutic progress.

(Sacerdote, 1970).

2. When in doubt about where a patient is in trance or what can be experienced, formulate suggestions in an open-ended manner that admits any kind of response as adequate

.

3. When in doubt about a patient's readiness to experience a particular phenomenon, formulate open-ended suggestions that admit any degree of that response as adequate. It will be useful for the beginning hypnotherapist to know and learn to recognize all possible degrees or increments of response for all the classical hypnotic phenomena.

4. Learn to formulate therapeutic suggestions in an open-ended manner that admits no possibility of failure.

Suggestions Covering All Possibilities of a Class of Responses

Closely related to open-ended suggestions, but opposite in direction, are suggestions that are carefully formulated to cover all possibilities of a class of responses. While open-ended suggestions accept any response as valid, suggestions covering all possibilities of a class of responses usually restrict the patient to a narrow range of acceptable possibilities. The open-ended suggestion admits an essay of any possible response that allows the patient's originality to become manifest. Suggestions covering all possibilities of a class of responses restrict the patient to a relatively narrow range of choices within which he can respond. Erickson (1952/2021) illustrates this approach in his ***Hand Levitation*** technique of induction as follows:

Shortly your right hand, or it may be your left hand, will begin to lift up, or it may press down, or it may not move at all, but we will wait to see just what happens.

Maybe the thumb will be first, or you may feel something happening in your little finger, but the really important thing is not whether your hand lifts up or presses down or just remains still; rather, it is your ability to sense fully whatever feelings may develop in your hand.

While open-ended suggestions are useful in exploring a patient's response potentials, the suggestions that cover all possibilities of a class of responses are more useful when we wish to funnel a patient's responses in one definite direction. To move a subject in the direction of experiencing anesthesia, for example, one could proceed with suggestions covering all possibilities of a class of responses somewhat as follows:

> **Now you can notice just where that arm is feeling something and where it is not. Just where it may tingle or be numb or not feel anything at all.**

When the patient indicates there are areas where the arm is numb or without sensation, the therapist can then proceed with exploratory questions that allow the anesthesia to spread to the desired area. To explore the possibility of alterations in visual perception and for positive or negative hallucinations one could proceed somewhat as follows:

> **And now or in a few moments when your unconscious is ready there maybe a blankness or a haziness in your visual field.**
>
> **And how will that haziness develop? Will there be a fog or shadows? And when will the shadows begin to arrange themselves into definite forms?**
>
> **Will your eyes be open or closed?**
>
> **It will be interesting to find out whether it will be hazy or foggy or blurred. Or will things be unusually bright, sharp, and clear when you open your eyes? Will there be an alteration of the color background?**
>
> **Will some things be unusually clear and other things not seen at all? You can wonder and wait comfortably as that develops.**

This series of suggestions admits just about any possibility of a response in altered visual perception as a successful and interesting experience. It helps patient and therapist explore what response potentials for altered perception are available to the patient at this particular time and place.

Exercises in Covering All Possibilities of a Class of Responses

1. Plan how you could formulate suggestions covering all possibilities of a class of responses to funnel the patient's responsivity toward the experience of each of the classical hypnotic phenomena. Erickson provides an unusually clear example of this with ***Time Distortion*** in the next chapter.

2. It can be interesting to practice suggestions covering all possibilities of a class of responses in common everyday situations such as dining, recreation, shopping and so on. Suggestions outlining the possibilities of the ***what, where*** and ***when*** of such activities can enhance freedom of choice for your partner.

Chapter Seven

Ideomotor Signaling

Ideomotor signaling may be the most useful hypnotic form discovered within the past half-century. Erickson (1961/2021) has reviewed the series of discoveries that led him from the use of automatic writing to his development of Hand Levitation and finally ideomotor signaling during the 1920s and 1930s. The reader should be able to recognize where conscious-unconscious Double Binds are being formulated. In formulating or applying these, use words appropriate to the subject's educational or intelligence level. Erickson (1964) has outlined a complete introduction to ideomotor signaling for facilitating trance induction, trance deepening, and communication in trance with the following words.

Something everybody knows is that people can communicate verbally or by sign language. The commonest sign language, of course, is when you nod your head "Yes" or "No." Anybody can do that.

One can signal "come" with the forefinger, or wave "bye-bye" with the hand. The finger signal in a way means "Yes, come here," and waving the hand means really "No, don't stay." In other words one can use the head, the finger or the hand to mean either yes or no. We all do it. So can you.

Sometimes when we listen to a person we may be nodding or shaking the head not knowing it in either agreement or disagreement. It would be just as easy to do it with the finger or the hand. Now, I would like to ask your unconscious mind a question that can be answered with a simple "Yes" or "No." It's a question that only your unconscious mind can answer.

Neither your conscious mind nor my conscious mind, nor, for that matter, even my unconscious mind knows the answer. Only your unconscious mind knows which answer can be communicated, and it will have to think either a yes or a no answer. It could be by a nod or a shake of the head, a lifting of the index finger, let us say, the right index finger for the "Yes" answer, the left index for a "No" since that is usually the case for the right-handed person and vice versa for the left-handed person. Or the right hand could lift or the left hand could lift. But only your unconscious mind knows what the answer will be when I ask for that "Yes" or "No" answer. And not even your unconscious mind will know, when, the question is asked, whether it will answer with a head movement, or a finger movement, and your unconscious mind will have to think through that question and to decide, after it has formulated its own answer, just how it will answer.

All of this explanation is essentially a series of suggestions so worded that responsive ideomotor behavior is made contingent upon an inevitable occurrence, namely, that the subject will have to think and to decide without there being an actual request for ideomotor responses. The implication only is there, and implications are difficult to resist.

We believe that for such ideomotor signaling to be truly autonomous and unconscious, patients should be in trance or distracted in one way or another so they will not have an opportunity to observe their own movements. Because of this, Erickson frequently prefers to look for automatic head nodding or shaking where patients are least likely to observe themselves. It is surprising how often patients will nod or shake their heads to contradict their own verbal statements even without any formal instruction about ideomotor signaling. Frequently, it is avery slow and slight but persistent head nodding or shaking that distinguishes the movements as coming from an unconscious level. These slow, abbreviated movements should be distinguished from larger and more rapid head movements that are more consciously used as a way of emphasizing what is being said verbally.

We prefer to ***Utilize*** a patient's own natural means of ideomotor signaling whenever possible. Whatever natural and automatic movements a patient makes in ordinary conversation can be studied for their metacommunicative value. Besides the more obvious head and hand movements, eye blinking (slow or rapid), body shifting, leg movements, arm position (e.g., crossed over one another as a defense), lip wetting, swallowing, facial cues such as frowning and tensions around the mouth and jaw can be studied for their commentary on what is being said verbally.

Since Erickson's introduction of ideomotor signaling other investigators (LeCron, 1954; Cheek & LeCron, 1968) have explored its usefulness in facilitating a variety of hypnotic phenomena. A most important aspect of sound hypnotic work is to know where the subject is at all times. Many subjects are reluctant to speak in trance, and when they do so their usual patterns of waking associations and behavior may be aroused, thus tending to suppress the autonomous aspects of trance experience. Ideomotor signaling appears to be a response system that can function more autonomously than speech. As such, ideomotor signaling is a more convenient form of communicating during trance. Subjects comment that it is easier to move a finger or hand or nod a head in trance than to talk. It tends to ratify the reality of their trance as an altered state when they realize their ideomotor signals are autonomous: they are experienced as taking place spontaneously without making any conscious effort to move.

In practice, there are many possible relations between awareness, volition and ideomotor signals. Initially, many subjects realize they "know" or can "feel" what movement will take place before it does. Because of this they are not certain whether the ideomotor movement was truly autonomous or whether they actually helped it. With deepening experience of trance, there is less awareness of the movements, and they are accepted as being more truly autonomous. With other subjects, perhaps those who are already experiencing trance without realizing it (the ***Common Everyday Trance*** wherein one's attention is fixed and focused so that the surrounding reality is ignored, such as when one is absorbed in listening to an interesting speaker, watching a movie, reading a book), the ideomotor movements come autonomously entirely as a surprise. These subjects are fascinated with them and wonder what responses will be given. The ideomotor movement obviously comes before they "know" what the answer will be. Other subjects tend to experience ideosensory responses before the actual ideomotor movement. They will "feel" an itch, prickliness, warmth, or some other sensation in the finger before it moves.

An uncritical view of ideomotor signaling takes such movements as the "true response of the unconscious." This is particularly the case when patients say one thing verbally but contradict themselves with ideomotor signals. Although there is much clinical experience to suggest that such contradictions are important clues about conflicts that the patient may not be aware of, there is to date no controlled experimental research that confirms this view. Because of this it is better at this stage of our understanding to view ideomotor signals simply as another response system that must be studied and checked—just as any other verbal or nonverbal form of communication must be. Ideomotor signals are particularly interesting in trance work because they are a system of communication that is compatible with the autonomous aspects of trance experience.

Exercises With Ideomotor Signaling

1. Study the historical aspects of ideomotor signaling in the form of the thought reading experiments of the 19th century (Drayton, 1899), mediumistic phenomena such as table turning and the Ouiji board (Bramwell, 1921), the Chevreul pendulum (Weitzenhoffer, 1957), etc. Much of the so-called occult and psychic phenomena may be understood as involuntary muscular movements and ideomotor and ideosensory responses that are unconsciously sent and received.

2. Study all varieties of apparently involuntary muscular movements as forms of ideomotor signaling in everyday life. Notice how people will unconsciously nod or shake their heads and move their lips, hands, and fingers when engaged in internal dialogue. Learn to read faces; learn to recognize the minute facial movements that indicate changes in mood and feeling. Study body posture and movements as nonverbal forms of communication (Birdwhistell, 1952, 1971; Scheflen, 1974).

3. Plan how you can introduce ideomotor signaling as a natural form of autonomous communication during trance in ways that can fit the individuality of each patient.

4. Learn to formulate suggestions so that the patient will give ideomotor signals when an internal response (experiencing warmth, anesthesia, hallucinations, etc.) has been experienced. Ideomotor signals can be combined with the implied directive to set up a communication system that can greatly facilitate trance training and the experience of all the classical hypnotic phenomena.

5. Plan and carry out carefully controlled clinical and experimental situations to evaluate the reliability and validity of ideomotor and ideosensory signaling.

Chapter Eight

The *Handshake* Induction

Erickson continues his indirect approaches in this session with the addition of his nonverbal handshake induction. A major problem in helping Dr. S learn to experience trance is to loosen the highly intellectualized and rigidly structured reality orientation she has constructed in her many years of formal education. The nonverbal techniques (Erickson, 1964/2022a) are particularly suitable for this task since they distract and promote the confusion that Erickson now acknowledges as a basic process in his approaches to induction.

Dr. S immediately experiences catalepsy, the fogging phenomenon, restricted awareness and comfort which are among the classical indicators of trance. By the end of this session, she is reviewing and possibly recovering forgotten memories; surprisingly, she is also beginning to experience a spontaneous anesthesia that was not suggested. Erickson likes to point out that it is in the spontaneous experience of such classical phenomena (along with other psycho-physiological indicators such as diminished pulse, and respiration) that can be taken as the most valid criteria for the reality of trance as an altered state.

This session brought to the fore two potent indirect approaches that were not identified earlier: conditional suggestions and compound suggestions. Erickson had been using them all along, of course, but this is the first time the Rossi had noticed them. Also noticed for the first time was the routine reliance on the ratification of trance phenomena as an indirect means of reinforcing suggestions.

Erickson's use of the term "ratification" is similar but not identical to the term "reinforcement" in psychological theory. Ratification refers specifically to the patient's belief system. To ratify something means to confirm (reinforce) that something has occurred. Specifically, in hypnotic work Erickson uses the word "ratify" with regard to hypnotic phenomenon he wants patients to experience and believe they are experiencing. To ratify the trance is to help patients realize and believe they did experience trance. To ratify the regression means that patients will later acknowledge that they did indeed experience a regression.

Session 3: Handshake Induction with Dr. S

This is the third trance session with Dr. S as a subject and Ernest Rossi (ER) as an active observer.

MHE: Now silently,
mentally,
count backwards
from 20 to 1.
You can begin the count,
now.

[Erickson shakes hands with Dr. S, but lingers before releasing her hand. Gradually, and with seeming hesitation, he alternately applies and releases pressure with his fingers on different parts of her hand. Dr. S is not even sure when he finally disengages his hand. Her hand is left in a cataleptic position in midair. During this handshake, Erickson looks toward her face but focuses on the wall behind her. She looks at his face and seemingly tries to capture his gaze or note whether or not he is actually looking at her. She seems a bit disconcerted by his faraway gaze.]

MHE: Her disconcerted feeling is a mixture of her imperfect touch with reality. It is her intellectual awareness that something has happened and her puzzlement about what did happen. She is not really comfortable about it; she is trying to resolve it and is experiencing difficulty in resolving it. That is a sophisticated subject's reaction.

ER: That is an intellectually sophisticated subject's reaction to trance induction?

MHE: Yes. That is a very common reaction.

MHE: Do you think you're awake?
[Said without altering his faraway gaze past her.]

ER: Now you ask this question that is so characteristic of you: "Do you think you are awake?" Why?

MHE: It means, "There is a good possibility that you are asleep and don't know it."

ER: That's the implication.

MHE: It arouses strong doubts in them, and it makes them very uncertain. If a stranger comes up to you and says, "Do you know me?" it makes you question and search through this memory and that.

ER: So, it puts the person in perplexity.

MHE: Yes, perplexity, and it emphasizes the conditional trance. It gives body to the trance.

ER: I see. It begins to reinforce the trance, which her disconcerted feeling indicated was already beginning. The ***Handshake*** induction wherein she is not sure when you remove your hand, then, begins a process of puzzlement about what is real and not real. The dynamics of this induction is essentially a kind of ***Confusion Technique.***

MHE: Yes, it is a ***Confusion Technique***. In all my techniques, almost all, there is a confusion. It is a confusion within them.

> **Dr. S: I never really know.**
> **[Laughs]**

ER: This immediate response reaffirms and ratifies the beginning trance.

MHE: When she says, "I never," she unwittingly attaches it to all other contexts with you. Only she doesn't know she is doing that. When you "don't know," you are admitting you want to know and you are willing to let the other person direct you.

ER: I believe this is a very important point you are making. When she says, "I never really know" [with you], it may seem like a simple casual statement, but you believe it is an exact statement of her relation to you even though she herself does not realize the significance of her statement. Actually, she is making a metacommunication; she is communicating about her communication to you. Most metacommunications are made unconsciously (Bateson, 1972).

Dr. S.: I am. I guess — I'm a little fogged up.
[Pause]

MHE: The fogging is a dimming of reality.

MHE: Do you really think you're awake?

MHE: My asking the question also implies: you're different, you are in a different state now. But, she doesn't know I'm implying that.

ER: The doubt you have in your voice when you ask this question, implying an altered state, it turns in into a ***Double Bind*** : if she answers "Yes" she is acknowledging only that she ***thought*** she was awake but must now reconsider in the light of your doubt; if she answers "No" she admits she was not awake. You are again catapulting her into trance without her knowing why. It is these ***unobserved*** maneuvers on your part that are so effective in inducing trance and facilitating the acceptance of suggestions. They are effective because they structure contexts (metacommunications) and initiate associations in a manner that circumvents patients' conscious sets and all their usual objections, biases, and limitations.

Dr. S: No. [Laughs] I'm really comfortable.
[Pause]

[Erickson continues to look toward her, but focuses beyond.]

Dr. S: You're staring. [Laughs]

MHE: Her statement about comfort is a way of reassuring herself. You have to be altered in some way to have a reason for talking about your comfort. It also implies she is going to stay in that state and intensify it.

That is what you are avoiding saying to the subject but get the subject to say themselves.

ER: "I'm comfortable and I'm going to stay here and get more and more comfortable," which means going more and more into trance. She is structuring her own self suggestion. It is characteristic of your approach that you structure circumstances so the patient makes the appropriate self-suggestions rather than you making a direct suggestion and risking the attendant possibility that the patient might reject it. It is much more effective if you can structure their associative processes without their awareness that you are doing it.

MHE: That's right. There is no need to say, "You are going in deeper and deeper."

ER: Now, just as catalepsy or stopped vision is a characteristic of trance, would you say that comfort is a characteristic of trance?

MHE: Yes, because you said you're comfortable, you are going to make even the uncomfortable chair comfortable. That requires cooperative activity on your part.

ER: So, we can say that ***comfort and wanting to make yourself comfortable are characteristic of trance?***

MHE: Yes. Since it is awfully uncomfortable to lose reality, you have to replace that reality with another.

ER: That other reality is ***comfort***.

MHE: That is correct.

ER: She also laughs at that point.

MHE: The laugh is a defensive reaction, and you don't have to defend yourself unless there is a threat.

ER: Which is the loss of outer reality.

> **Dr. S: I feel kind of funny since my left eye muscle kind of winks closed.**

MHE: Here, she is only able to muster up enough awareness about one eye.

ER: She is not cognizant of the fact that her awareness is actually limited to her left eye at this point. It is from just such apparently innocuous remarks that you make important inferences about the patient's consciousness.

> **MHE: [To ER, but without altering the faraway gaze past Dr. S.]**
> **Notice the silent waiting,**
> **the expectancy in her.**
> **So far,**
> **as the patient knows you are not**
> **pressuring,**
> **you're waiting.**
> **You are letting the patient**
> **discover how she can**
> **enter the trance.**

MHE: You can't ***wait*** for something without knowing it is going to happen.

ER: Your waiting has the hidden implication that trance will happen. It is only an implication but it actually structures behavior without the patient being aware of it. You have structured an expectancy in her that may initiate her into a response attentiveness to any minimal changes in herself. The structured expectancy facilitates her trance awareness to the minimal changed that can be the first signs of a new hypnotic experience.

> **[Dr. S plays absent-mindedly with her dress and touches the back of one hand with the other.]**

> **MHE: You notice how**
> **occasionally**
> **she feels herself**
> **or she drags herself**
> **out of the developing trance**
> **by looking over at you?**

MHE: She plays with her dress, but even that is not real enough now, so she goes to touching her hand.

ER: The casual behavior of touching of her own hand is a stereotyped effort to reestablish the reality that is now being rapidly dissociated. Actually, it is an indication of self-absorption and a restricted awareness of anything outside herself. That, of course, is a way of defining trance experience.

> **MHE: Now, the next thing**
> **for her to do**
> **is actually to develop**
> **a hallucination of,**
> **let us say,**
> **a specific landscape.**

One that
she has not seen previously.
But a landscape
she would like.
[Pause]
Now,
who knows what
she would put
in a landscape?
Birds,
trees,
bushes,
rocks.

ER: Why the remark about a landscape she has not seen previously?

MHE: I could see she was searching through her memory, but to have her make something I would like to turn her in on herself still more. By naming the specifics of birds and trees, I focus her attention more closely and more narrowly. I can direct her attention without saying exactly how.

ER: I've had difficulty in my beginning work with hypnosis in knowing just where the patient is. That's because I've not learned to put her in some definite place as you do. This is what you meant when you mentioned that you hold a patient firmly to her task.

MHE: It is very important
for her to develop
a specific hallucination
and to retain it
and be able
to describe it.
[Pause]

MHE: It is very important that she do something specific here. It is important that she does something, something "specific." And for heavens sake, what is it?

ER: Oh, I see, you are readying her for work now, of learning to visually hallucinate. She thinks: "I've got some important work to do. Okay, but what is it?"

MHE: That's right. Making her increasingly more interested in the work she will now do.

ER: Is there a paradox here? In the induction, the purpose was to dissociate her conscious mind so it would not interfere, yet here you are instructing it. Are you focusing the conscious on the unconscious?

MHE: No, the conscious mind is to give full cooperation to the unconscious. You're feeding it to the unconscious.

ER: You have gathered up all her conscious awareness and are giving its energy to the unconscious?

MHE: Yes.

> [Erickson now describes one of his current cases, where the patient's conscious mind is not yet ready to handle certain insights that are being formulated in the unconscious. The patient is producing symbolic drawings and writings that his conscious mind cannot yet understand.]

[Next, Erickson gives a detailed 20-minute case history of a former patient who painted a landscape he saw in hypnotic trance and the relevance of this landscape for his personal dynamics. He appears to be talking to ER. Dr. S sits quietly, apparently going deeper into trance.]

MHE: What happens
in creating
a hallucination
related to the past?
A scene of Dr. S
as a little girl
enjoying something
she long ago forgot.
[Pause]
And I would like that scene
to come into being,
be real.
And I want Dr. S
to begin that scene,
feeling,
sensing,
thinking
as that situation was
years ago.
And there will be
no memory
of the intervening years
since then.
So Dr. S can be
a little girl
happily playing,
something long forgotten.
And now you can regress
and enter into that.
[Pause]

[At this time, Dr. S's children were actually playing outside the office in Erickson's backyard, so we inside could hear their laughter and the faint hubbub of their voices]

ER: You give these case histories while the patient is in a trance so they can learn by association; they learn to identify vicariously with that case history, and they tend to do similar things.

MHE: Yes. She had some age regression there in which she had some fantasies of her childhood and some of the wishes of her adult life and some of its realities.

[**Editors' note:** ***Therapist's voice in patient's inner experience.***]

MHE: In my voice,
you can hear
the whispering wind,
the rustle of leaves.
[Pause]
And then my voice
becomes that of some neighbor,
adult friend,
relative,
someone known.

ER: She was learning by association in listening to her children, and here you merge your voice with her inner experience.

MHE: That's right. How do you merge your voice with a patient's inner experience? You use words that ordinary life has taught you: "The whispering wind." We have all had whispering experiences.

ER: So that puts you into associative contact with something whispering and close.

MHE: And close: I'm not asking her to do anything she doesn't want to. It could be a friend, relative, anyone known.

> **MHE: You will in due course**
> **say something**
> **long forgotten**
> **now remembered.**
> **[Pause]**
> **A very happy memory.**
> **And then the next year**
> **you will remember,**
> **and the year after that,**
> **and the year after that,**
> **and time is passing rapidly**

MHE: When is "in due course"?

ER: It could be any time.

MHE: That's right.

ER: You are trying to lift a specific amnesia here? You're making an effort to have her recover forgotten memories?

MHE: Yes.

ER: With that last phrase, you are adding the possibility of time distortion?

MHE: Yes.

> **MHE: and you are growing**
> **[Pause]**
> **becoming a big girl.**

MHE: This ratifies the regression because she can only be big now if she was little earlier.

ER: Even if it was only for a fraction of a second, a mere flash of an early memory, she is now ratifying it, no matter how much or how little there was.

> **MHE: And someday**
> **you will meet some stranger**
> **and you will be able**
> **to tell him about it.**
> **And when you meet**
> **that stranger,**
> **you will tell him**
> **about the beautiful landscape.**

MHE: Every women has a past in which she wanted to meet a stranger.

ER: You are picking up a specific motivation there.

MHE: But you have not defined it, you are still letting her make her own definition of it.

ER: By focusing in and accompanying her, using words with both general and specific meaning, you are tapping into a very intimate channel of her mind, not just a banal or general reality. It is a general reality you know every woman has had, and yet, each woman has a specific experience with a stranger. You're safe in suggesting a general category, a stranger, but it will elicit a individual and specific memory in her, as it will in every woman.

MHE: There is a general problem for the beginning therapist here. You start patients in a train of association, but they drift along their own currents of thought, and frequently leave the therapist stranded far back. Then the patient gets furious because the therapist tries to barge in—in the wrong way. He hasn't used words that allow him to accompany the patient. To do this, ***we use words that have both a general and a very specific personal significance.*** Every woman wants to meet a stranger in her girlhood, teenage years, her early adult life. That stranger who would eventually become someone very specific, her lover, her husband.

ER: These words with both a general meaning and specific personal significance allow you to focus and accompany patients into very personal associations even though you may not know exactly what they are experiencing.

MHE: And now in progression
come through the years
until you reach
October 1972.

MHE: You're asking the patient to progress from time A to B and C. That ratifies that the years of A through C were real. So, in a way you are ratifying the age regression.

MHE: And when you get there
when you get to
the right date

[Pause]
you will arouse
with full memory.

ER: When you make arousing from the trance contingent upon reaching the current date, you are again ratifying that she must have been in the past to progress to the present to wake up. In general, you try to associate your suggestions with any inevitable behavior that is about to occur. One of your favorite examples is, "Don't ***enter trance*** (suggested behavior) until you sit all the way down in that chair," (inevitable as the patient approaches the chair). Every mother has said, "Shut the door (suggested behavior) on your way out" (inevitable as the child approaches the door).

MHE: You will realize
hypnosis was employed,
you will not remember
going into a trance.
It isn't necessary
to remember
going into a trance.
[Pause]

ER: This appears to be a simple dissociation ***Double Bind*** to facilitate an amnesia. You dissociate the memory of going into trance from its normal context of "You will realize hypnosis was employed." You then reinforce the dissociation by remarking, "It is not necessary to remember going into a trance."

Dr. S: Um. [She reorients to her body by stretching a bit, touching her face, etc.]

MHE: Do you think you can go in a trance this morning?

Dr. S: Humm?

MHE: Do you think you can go into a trance this morning?

Dr. S: Uh, yeah, I guess I did. Do I think I can again?

MHE: Humm?

Dr. S: Yeah, I guess I could.

ER: When she asks, "Do I think I can again?" it means that she realizes she was just in a trance. Therefore, your posthypnotic suggestion that she forget that hypnosis was just employed failed.

MHE: Except, it did not really fail. She is just "realizing" the trance. You can realize there was a yesterday, but not exactly what you did yesterday.

ER: Amnesia may be present for many things you did yesterday even though you realize there was a yesterday. So, the general category of trance experience is recalled, but not necessarily the specific contents. She is following your suggestion very literally when you said in the last section, that she could, "***realize*** hypnosis was employed . . . you will ***not remember*** going into a trance." There is a subtle, but very real difference between "realizing" and "remembering." You do not bother testing the amnesia at this point because she is still so close to the trance that she could build associative bridges to it, and thus, destroy the possibility of fulfilling your suggestion for amnesia.

MHE: That's right.

MHE: What memories come to mind?

Dr. S: Being in Maine, by the ocean, looking at the starfish and things.

MHE: In Maine?

Dr. S: Yeah, and my uncle, a lobster fisherman, told me to get up at five the next morning to go out on the beach with him.

MHE: All right, now what has happened to you this morning?

Dr. S: I guess I went back to that scene when I was 12 years old.

MHE: How do you mean, you went back?

Dr. S: I guess I remembered it.

MHE: How tall were you?

Dr. S: Five-one or five-two.

MHE: Why did you say your uncle?

Dr. S: Oh, he didn't talk much. I did wake up the next morning and went with him.

MHE: Are you awake yet?

ER: Why are you asking all these specific questions here?

MHE: You ask specific questions in therapy when you don't know where the patient's problem is. I'm exploring I'm opening up many different aspects.

ER: I see. Perhaps there was an emotional problem associated with this memory.

MHE: Yes. If there is a problem here, some of these questions may give her an opportunity to talk about it. But here, she just treats them as straightforward questions.

> **Dr. S: [Laughs] I, I think so, yes.**
>
> **MHE: How did you go into a trance this morning?**
>
> **Dr. S: Well you took my hand or something.**
>
> **MHE: What's the "or something"?**
>
> **Dr. S: Well, I never know what you are doing. Yes, you took my hand and looked at me.**
>
> **MHE: Is that the best description you can give?**

MHE: By asking her these questions, I'm also facilitating amnesia.

ER: How? You mean asking her how she went into trance is a distraction or an unimportant detail that is going to help her forget what actually happened in trance?

MHE: Yes. It's a distraction. When she is so vague as to say, "Or something," it indicates her memory is being contracted.

ER: When she says, "I never know what you are doing," she is admitting the success of your confusion approach, and the way it limits her conscious awareness.

Dr. S: Yes, I think so. I'm not familiar with that. I was looking at you but got embarrassed looking so I looked at the top of your hair. Then it started fogging up.

MHE: Explain that fogging.

Dr. S: Well, it kind of gets foggy. It's cloudy or foggy, not quite in focus. Like it's distant, like by the ocean it gets foggy. You can't concentrate on a point any longer . . . That might have brought back that scene because that looks like the fog of the ocean . . . It was distorted for a minute. Like you could see in that glass.
[Dr. S again points out the irregularly cut glass piece of art on Erickson's desk, which he frequently uses a fixation point for inducing hypnosis.]
Things are distorted and elongated.

MHE: What time is it?

Dr. S: Unfortunately, I just looked. It is ten of 11, but it did seem longer.

ER: This report of fogging was a classical sign of hypnosis in the older literature and I've recently learned that gypsies characteristically see fog or clouds in their crystal balls just before the visions. You have described it as a characteristic of the white background subjects apparently experience when they have "stopped vision" in deep trance (Erickson, 1967/2021). What is the meaning of such fogging?

MHE: Fog comes in when you get away from external reality. It is a way of occluding reality. It makes you feel all alone just as you feel alone when you walk out on a foggy day.

MHE: Do you think you're awake yet?

Dr. S: Well, I feel slightly distant but I feel basically awake I think, I don't know. Yes, I am.

ER: She has been awake and now you begin to cast doubt upon her awake state with this ***Double Bind*** question. Is this an indirect trance induction?

MHE: That's right.

ER: The distant feeling she immediately describes is, of course, the first indication that another trance is beginning.

MHE: Going into trance is like going away because you are going distant from external reality.

MHE: Now direct your attention
to your right hand.
[Pause]
Your right hand
may have a tendency
to move upward.
[Pause]
It begins to quiver
and move up
toward your face.

[Dr. S's arm does begin to levitate to her face.]

[Pause]
When your hand
touches your face,
you can take
a deep breath,
and go deeply asleep,

and be unable
to lower your hand.

MHE: You see. she is looking ***at a hand.*** Where is the rest of her?

ER: The implication is that she has lost the rest of her body. So this is effecting a dissociation, and a dissociation is a characteristic of trance. So, as soon as this begins to take place, you've got a trance. You used a ***Hand Levitation.***

MHE: But you are not laboriously saying, "Cease to see the rest of your body."

ER: Which would only arouse the typical response, "I can't." You give suggestions for dissociation by implication.

MHE: Your arm will feel
entirely comfortable,
at ease,
or it may lose
all feeling,
or it may develop
a wooden feeling,
a feeling of not
being your arm.
I'd like to have
you interested
in discovering
your way of handling
that arm.
[Pause as Dr. S's hand levitates to her face.]

ER: Here you give her many possible options about what her subjective experience may be as she holds her hand by her face. This allows her to *Utilize* whatever subjective means she has to implement your suggestion. You facilitate a direct suggestion, as "be unable to lower your hand," by covering (or appearing to cover) all possibilities of subjective experience to support it. You substitute an interesting piece of self-exploration for what might otherwise be a boring or tedious task.

MHE: Of course
something has happened
to your left hand,
and that will remain,
and when you awaken
you will have lost
all control
of your right arm.
[Pause]
And I want you
to be curious
about that dissociation
of your right arm—
the nature
and character of it—
because everybody handles
the situation slightly differently.
[Pause]
Your arm will remain
immobile.

ER: Did you notice something happening to her left hand, or was that an indirect suggestion?

MHE: I'm really telling her, "Let something happen to your left hand." The implication is that it will imitate the right hand. The implication is also present that she doesn't know what's happened to her left hand.

ER: This indirect way of giving suggestions deepens trance.

MHE: It always deepens trance. Dr. S offers me the handicap of intellectual desire to keep her knowledge available for use with her own patients.

ER: That's a handicap because you'd rather not have her consciousness so active. You would rather see how her individual differences are manifest in a spontaneous manner.

MHE: She's got to find out her differences and she can't dispute them.

ER: This is fascinating! You use implication as an indirect form of suggestion to set behavior in motion that will help her explore her own individual differences in dealing with the situation. You are really not manipulating and controlling her. Rather, you are ***offering*** suggestions in such a way that her own unique response potentials become manifest in a manner that can be surprising and informative to both of you. Even while immobilizing her arm in what might appear to be a conventional catalepsy, you are actually leaving room for the exploration of human potentials. It is actually the subjective process by which she immobilizes her arm that will reveal whether she has a latent talent for anesthesia ("it may lose all feeling"), comfort, rigidity, ideosensory responses ("wooden feeling"), or whatever.

> **MHE: And I can count**
> **backward from 20 to 1**
> **in any way I wish.**
> **At the count of one**
> **you will awaken,**
> **but your arm won't.**
> **[Pause]**
> **20, 15, 10, 5, 4, 3, 2, 1.**

ER: You frequently associate awakening with a posthypnotic suggestion. This is another form of contingent suggestion in which the inevitable behavior of awakening is made contingent on the posthypnotic suggestion that, "your arm won't [awaken]."

Dr. S: Humm.

[Laughs as she notices her right hand immobile by her face. She reaches up with her left hand and rubs the back of her right hand.]

MHE: Why did you rub it?

Dr. S: Because it feels numb.

ER: It is easy to miss this "numbness" or analgesia that is unobtrusively indicated by the casual way she rubs the back of her hand. Your question about it brings the admission that it is actually numb. She is thus following a very casual suggestion for a possible analgesia you administered earlier in your "suggestions covering all possibilities of a class of responses." This posthypnotic analgesia is also a consequence of the dissociation implied in the awakening suggestions you just gave, "At the count of one you will awaken but your arm won't." This is an excellent example of how you can administer two or more mutually reinforcing suggestions to reinforce one process.

MHE: Now, what's happening to your left arm?

Dr. S: Right arm is still stiff.

MHE: Something is happening to your left hand.

Dr. S: [Laughs as she notices her left hand getting a bit stiff and immobile.]

ER: She is apparently awake at this point, but when you ask this question, is it indirectly inducing another trance?

MHE: Yes.

ER: The suggestion proper. Naturally, she quickly acknowledges that her arm is tired, thus ratifying that the trance condition was different from the awake state. This also contains the implication that one can do different things in trance.

ER: This seems to be an excellent way of inducing a trance in an indirect manner so that Dr. S does not even recognize a trance is being induced. You simply ask an innocent question about what's happening to her left arm. In response, she cannot help, but focus her attention on that arm. Your question is actually an implied suggestion that something will happen, and when something does happen (whether its a movement, an awareness of a sensation, or whatever), that something announces the beginning of a dissociation (because it appears to happen by itself without the subject's conscious volition), and dissociation, of course, is a major feature of trance experience.

MHE: And the subject takes credit for it. You're not telling the subject to "do this, do that." So many therapists tell their patients how to think and how to feel. That is awfully wrong.

ER: It is more effective to induce the trance in a way the patient can take credit for.

MHE: It takes you by surprise?

Dr. S: It does feel a bit tingly.

MHE: This question is also a statement.

ER: You reinforce ***Surprise*** and by implication a state of confusion, so you—

MHE: Reinforce the trance!

> **MHE: It's going to happen, and you'll have no control over what happens.**
>
> **Dr. S: I don't remember your telling me anything about it, so I don't know what's going to happen.**
>
> **[Notices how left hand is getting stiffer in a midair pose]**
>
> **MHE: You may have an idea of what's happening.**
>
> **[It was gradually becoming evident that her left hand was becoming immobile.]**

ER: This is a compound suggestion that is very typical of your style. The truism in the first part, "It's going to happen," opens a ***Yes Set*** that tends to facilitate acceptance of your strongly directive suggestion in the second part, "You'll have no control over what happens." The casual way you said this was so disarming that at the time I did not even recognize that you were making a strong suggestion for dissociation.

> **Dr. S: Well, it feels a little strange, like my hand feels it is falling asleep or something. I'm not sure myself, but my left hand is getting a little numb too.**
>
> **MHE: Now, try to discover what is happening so you can define what is happening to that hand.**

Dr. S: Well, it feels a little numb.

MHE: Something else is happening.

Dr. S: Well, its moving a little too.

MHE: [Turning to ER] Actually, of course, its moving around is a form of resistance at this time.
[Pause]

ER: Your suggestion that she will have "no control over what happens," initiates a process of confusion and finally a catalepsy and an associated anesthesia.

MHE: The aside at the end is actually an indirect suggestion that something is happening.

ER: I see. Your remarks to me are actually indirect suggestions to her.

MHE: You can discover
what's happening
to your arm
through your elbow
and then through your wrist.
[Pause]
You see
what has happened.
First there was
extreme mobility
in the entire left arm,
and then less at the elbow,
and then finally growing immobility
down to the wrist,
and then finally the fingers.

So your arm
got fixed
bit by bit.
[Pause]
Now what do you suppose
is the next thing
you will do?

MHE: Patients all have their own patterns of experiencing hypnotic phenomenon in a segmental manner. It is not important that she knows how she does it, but this sort of description allows me to stay with her. Staying with your patient is so important.

ER: So, this was an indirect trance induction by simply suggesting that something was happening to her left arm. What you found happening was a gradually spreading immobility (catalepsy) and numbness (anesthesia.) These responses are a highly individual matter, and much of the skill of the therapist is in discovering their spontaneous manifestation. Having established those hypnotic phenomena, you end by asking another question, "What do you suppose is the next thing you will do?" That question sets the stage for another open-ended exploration of whatever other hypnotic phenomena she may be ready to experience.

MHE: Can you figure it out?

Dr. S: I feel a little odd at this point

MHE: [Turning to ER] You are probably aware of what's going to happen.

[Turning to Dr. S] Of course,
you are aware
that you
are not
fully awake.

MHE: If she's got to "figure it out," that affirms that something is happening.

ER: She responds to your question with further dissociation indicated by the "odd" feeling. These two statements catapult her into trance by fostering doubt about her mental state.

MHE: Yes.

Dr. S: Would it be all right if I put my arm down?

MHE: Then your eyes will shut.
[Pause]

ER: This is another contingent suggestion: you associate your suggested behavior ("your eyes will shut") with an inevitable behavior that is about to occur (putting her arm down). Your suggestion rides piggyback on the patient's own motivation. You *Utilize* her wish to do one thing to have her accept another suggestion that will maintain trance.

MHE: I want your arms to be very comfortable,
and then you can awaken comfortably,
and you can awaken only after you open your eyes.
[Looking at ER] And no matter what the trance state is, when they have had their eyes open, you have them close their eyes first and then open them to awaken.
That comes from a lifetime of experience.

[Dr. S awakens and reorients to her body by stretching a bit, touching her face, patting her hair, adjusting her skirt.]

MHE: And how do you feel now?

Dr. S: Fine.

MHE: Tired?

Dr. S: No, fine.

MHE: Now while awake, hold your arm up in that same awkward position and see how tired it gets.

[Dr. S holds her arm up and soon acknowledges that it is getting tired.]

In this session, for example, when Dr. S was beginning to feel her arm getting stiff, immobile, and what she described as "tingly," Erickson reinforced the tendency toward dissociation with a compound suggestion.

MHE: It is going to happen

ER: This is the first statement of an obvious truism since it is in fact happening as Dr. S herself demonstrates and describes.

MHE: and

ER: The conjunctive "and" connects the two statements.

MHE: You'll have no control over what happens.

ER: The second statement contains the suggestion proper that will reinforce her current experience of dissociation.

[A much more complex compound suggestion with many implications is in the last statement Erickson makes in this session.]

MHE: Now while awake

ER: This strongly indicates that trance has terminated and reinforces her state of awakeness. Since she really knows trance has terminated, this is also a truism that opens her for what follows.

MHE: hold your arm in that same awkward position

ER: The word "hold" implies she must make an effort, and "awkward" implies it will be difficult. This strongly sets up the likelihood that the suggestion proper, which follows, will actually happen.

MHE: and

ER: The conjunctive "and" associates the following suggestion with the previous truisms (that she is awake and can hold her arm in that awkward position.)

MHE: see how tired it gets.

ER: The suggestion proper. Naturally, she quickly acknowledges that her arm is tired, thus ratifying that the trance condition was different from the awake state. This also contains the implication that one can do different things in trance.

MHE: You have them close their eyes because there is a whole lifetime of experience of having their eyes closed before they awaken.

ER: Again you ***Utilize*** a habitual built-in mechanism for your own purpose. What experiences have you had here? Has anyone ever left your office in trance? How long have you kept people in trance?

MHE: People have gone out of the office and then walked back in and said, "You'd better awaken me."

> [Dr. Erickson now recounts a few instances where he allowed especially competent hypnotic subjects to remain in trance for as long as they required to solve a particular problem—in one case for two weeks. They would go about their normal everyday activity without anyone detecting their trance state. The purpose of the trance was to enable them to continuously work out some inner problem.]

ER: You ratify the trance by having her "while awake, hold your arm up in that same awkward position and see how tired it gets." This, of course, is an instruction that contains a strong suggestion that her hand will get tired. Since the hand gets tired more rapidly when awake, that ratifies she must have been in a trance earlier.

[**Editors' note:** ***Dr. S awakens slowly as ER and MHE further discuss the dynamics of trance before concluding for the day.***]

ER: You said earlier that in almost all your induction techniques, ***Confusion*** is something that breaks up their reality orientation. It breaks their tie to normal awakeness?

MHE: Yes. You know, ordinarily, what is what about yourself and the other person. When confused, you suddenly become concerned about who you are and the other person seems to be fading.

ER: *Confusion* is an opening wedge to trance?

MHE: Yes. If you are uncertain about yourself, you can't be certain about anything else.

ER: Actually, they are getting a lot of their reality sense from you and if you throw doubt into them?

MHE: It spills over into their doubt about all reality. If you are uncertain about something, you tend to avoid it.

ER: I see! They start withdrawing from reality if they are uncertain about it.

MHE: That's right! They don't know what it (reality) is.

ER: If you then add to that the suggestion of a pleasant inner reality, they'd rather go to it.

MHE: Anything is better than that state of doubt.

ER: Especially, if you are up in front of an audience with everyone looking at you.

MHE: You want to get out of that situation, but there is no place except trance.

ER: That is why hypnosis works so well in front of an audience. That is where the stage hypnotist gets a lot of his leverage.

MHE: Yes. He merely capitalizes on that, and he makes it deliberately unpleasant by his aggressive manner and the various tricks he employs. They will do anything to escape from that.

> [Erickson gives examples of how he created unpleasant situations to catapult patients into trance. Some of these are outlined in Rossi's 1973a paper, "Psychological Shocks and Creative Moments in Psychotherapy."]

ER: So, this ***Confusion*** is the basis of many of your nonverbal pantomime techniques, would you say?

MHE: That's right.

ER: It is the basis of staring or looking through the subject. These are all ways of disconcerting the subject, ways of making them have doubts about themselves.

MHE: They begin to wonder but they don't know what they are wondering about. That is very confusing!

ER: Even in something as simple as eye fixation: you focus on that spot, but if you keep focusing on that spot, sooner or later your eyes are going to get tired, you are going to get blurred vision. All these things induce***Confusion***.

MHE: That's right.

ER: So, *Confusion* really is at the basis of all induction techniques?

MHE: It is the basis of all good techniques. Just as in something as simple as closing the eyes. Most workers in hypnosis do not know that as the subject closes the eyes, the subject is cutting off the visual field and is really losing something, but he doesn't know what he is losing. He thinks he is just closing his eyes.

ER: There are many things happening when we close our eyes, many realities we must give up.

MHE: In focusing on a spot, you automatically cut down on peripheral vision. Then the spot gets larger as it occupies all the field of vision. You know a spot can't get larger, yet, it does!

ER: So, that is again distorting reality and throwing them into *Confusion*.

MHE: They don't know what to do. So then, the therapist can tell them what to do. He lays out the ground for the subject to traverse, review, organize.

ER: So, can we make a summary statement that the basis of good hypnotic induction is *Confusion*?

MHE: *Confusion* about the surrounding reality which in ordinary life is always clear. If the surrounding reality becomes unclear, they want it cleared up by being told something (e.g., I don't know where I am in this city: where am I? I don't recognize this place: what is it?)

ER: That automatically tends to promote a regression, incidentally. It associates them to the time when they were children and asked such questions.

MHE: That's right! And you are not demanding it, but you are eliciting a receptive attitude, and your most innocent question can be interpreted by them. If you know how to ask questions, you ask them in such a fashion that they will pick out the thing you want.

ER: So, ***Confusion*** is the most basic phenomenon of induction?

MHE: We'll call it: The dimming of outer reality. When outer reality becomes dimmed, you get confused.

ER: So, we can summarize the dynamics of induction with a flow diagram:

Figure 1 (10.8.F.1) Trance Induction Diagram

DIMMING OF OUTER REALITY

↓

CONFUSION

↓

RECEPTIVITY TO CLARIFYING SUGGESTIONS

↓

TRANCE WORK PROPER

Chapter Nine

Dynamics of the *Handshake* Induction

The Handshake induction is one of the most fascinating and effective procedures developed by Erickson for initiating trance. It is essentially a surprise that interrupts a subject's habitual framework to initiate a momentary confusion. A receptivity for clarifying suggestions is thus initiated with an expectancy for further stimuli and direction. In a letter to Weitzenhoffer in 1975, Erickson described his approach to the Handshake Induction as a means of initiating catalepsy. When he released the subject's hand, it would remain fixed in a cataleptic position or would keep moving in any direction he initiated. He used this approach as a test to assess hypnotic susceptibility and as an induction procedure. The prerequisites for a successful Handshake induction are a willingness on the part of the subject to be approached, an appropriate situation and the suitability of the situation for a continuation of the experience. An edited version of Erickson's outline of the whole process and some variations is as follows.

> ***Initiation***: When I begin by shaking hands, I do so normally. The "hypnotic touch" then begins when I let loose. The letting loose becomes transformed from a firm grip into a gentle touch by the thumb, a lingering drawing away of the little finger, a faint brushing of the subject's hand with the middle finger — just enough vague sensation to attract the attention. As the subject gives attention to the touch of your thumb, you shift to a touch with your little finger. As your

subject's attention follows that, you shift to a touch with your middle finger and then again to the thumb.

This arousal of attention is merely an arousal without constituting a stimulus for a response.

The subject's withdrawal from the handshake is arrested by this attention arousal, which establishes a waiting set, an expectancy.

Then almost, but not quite simultaneously (to ensure separate neural recognition), you touch the undersurface of the hand (wrist) so gently that it barely suggests an upward push. This is followed by a similar utterly slight downward touch and then, I sever contact so gently that the subject does not know exactly when—and the subject's hand is left going neither up nor down, but cataleptic. Sometimes, I give a lateral and medial touch, so that the hand is even more rigidly cataleptic.

Termination: If you don't want your subjects to know what you are doing, you simply distract their attention, usually by some appropriate remark, and casually terminate. Sometimes they remark, "What did you say? I got absentminded there for a moment and wasn't paying attention to anything." This is slightly distressing to the subjects and indicative of the fact that their attention was so focused and fixated on the peculiar hand stimuli that they were momentarily entranced so they did not hear what was said.

Utilization: Any ***Utilization*** leads to increasing trance depth. All ***Utilization*** should proceed as a continuation or extension of the initial procedure. Much can be done nonverbally. For example, if any subjects are just looking blankly at me, I may slowly shift my gaze downward, causing them to look at their hand, which I touch as if to say, "Look at this spot." This intensifies the trance state. Then, whether the subjects are looking at you or at their hand or just staring blankly, you can use your left hand to touch their elevated right hand from above or the side—so long as you merely give the suggestion of downward movement. Occasionally, a downward nudge or push is required. If a strong push or nudge is required, check for anesthesia.

There are several colleagues who won't shake hands with me, unless

I reassure them first, because they developed a profound glove anesthesia when I used this procedure on them. I shook hands with them, looked them in the eyes, slowly, yet rapidly immobilized my facial expression, and then focused my eyes on a spot far behind them. I then slowly and imperceptibly, removed my hand from theirs and slowly moved to one side out of their direct line of vision.

I have had it described variously, but the following is one of the most graphic:

"I had heard about you and I wanted to meet you and you looked so interested and you shook hands so warmly. All of a sudden my arm was gone and your face changed and got so far away. Then the left side of your head began to disappear, and I could see only the right side of your face until that slowly vanished also."

At that moment, the subject's eyes were fixed straight ahead, so that when I moved to the left out of his line of vision, the left side of my face "disappeared" first and then the right side also.

"Your face slowly came back, you came close and smiled and said you would like to use me Saturday afternoon. Then, I noticed my hand and asked you about it because I couldn't feel my whole arm. You just said to keep it that way just a little while for the experiencc."

You give that elevated right hand, (now cataleptic in the handshake position,) the suggestion of a downward movement with a light touch. At the same time, with your other hand, you give a gentle touch indicating an upward movement for the subject's left hand. Then, you have his left hand lifting, right hand lowering. When right hand reaches the lap, it will stop. The upward course of the left hand may stop or it may continue. I am likely to give it another touch and direct it toward the face so that some part will touch one eye. That effects eye closure and is very effective in inducing a deep trance without a single word having been spoken.

There are other nonverbal suggestions. For example, what if my subject makes no response to my efforts with his right hand and the situation looks hopeless? If he is not looking at my face, my slow, gentle out-of-keeping-with-the-situation movements (remember: out-of-keeping) compel him to look at my face. I freeze my expression, refocus my gaze, and by slow head movements direct his gaze to his left hand toward which my right hand is slowly, apparently purposelessly moving. As my right hand touches his left with a slight, gentle, upward movement, my left hand with very gentle firmness, just barely enough, presses down on his right hand for a moment until it moves. Thus, I confirm and reaffirm the downward movement of his right hand, a suggestion he accepts along with the tactile suggestion of left Hand Levitation. This upward movement is augmented by the facts that he has been breathing in time with me and that my right hand gives his left hand that upward touch at the moment when he is beginning an inspiration. This is further reinforced by whatever peripheral vision he has that notes the upward movement of my body as I inhale and as I slowly lift my body and head up and backward, when I give his left hand that upward touch.

Erickson's description of his ***Handshake*** induction is a bit breathtaking to the beginner. How does one keep all of that in mind? How does one develop such a gentle touch and such skill? Above all, how does one learn to ***Utilize*** whatever happens in the situation as a means of further focusing the subject's attention and inner involvement, so that trance develops? Obviously, a certain amount of dedication and patience are required to develop such skill. It is much more than a matter of simply shaking hands in a certain way. Shaking hands is simply a context in which Erickson makes contact with a person. He then ***Utilizes*** this context to fix attention inward and so set the situation for the possible development of trance.

As he shakes hands, Erickson is himself fully focused on where the subject's attention is. Initially, the subject's attention is on a conventional social encounter. Then, with the unexpected touches as their hand is released, there is a momentary confusion and their attention is rapidly focused on his hand. At this point, "resistant" subjects might rapidly withdraw their hand and end the situation. Subjects who are ready to experience trance will be curious about what is happening. Their attention is fixed and they remain open and ready for further directing stimuli. The directing touches are so gentle and unusual that subjects' cognition has no way of evaluating them; the subjects have been given a rapid series of nonverbal cues to keep their hand fixed in one position, but they are not aware of it. Their hand responds to the directing touches for immobility, but they do not know why. It is simply a case of an automatic response on a kinesthetic level that initially defies conscious analysis because the subjects have had no previous experience with it. The directing touches for movement are responded to on the same level with a similar gap in awareness and understanding.

The subjects find themselves responding in an unusual way without knowing why. Their attention is now directed inward in an intense search for an answer or for some orientation. This inner direction and search is the basic nature of trance. Subjects may become so preoccupied in their inner search that the usual sensory-perceptual processes of our normal reality orientation are momentarily suspended. The subjects may then experience an anesthesia, a lacuna in vision or audition, a time distortion, a deja vu, a sense of disorientation or vertigo, and so on. At this moment, the subjects are open for further verbal or nonverbal suggestions that can intensify the inner search (trance) in one direction or another.

Exercises in the Nonverbal Approaches

1. The keys to learning nonverbal approaches to trance induction are observation, patience, and learning one step at a time. One can begin learning the Handshake Induction by developing a habit of carefully observing a person's eyes and face as you are shaking hands with them in a normal way. The next stage might be to practice releasing the hand a bit slower then usual. Then learn how

to definitely hesitate in releasing the hand, carefully watching the subject's face to "read" the nonverbal responses (e.g., confusion, expectancy) to your hesitation. As your experience develops, even at this level you will begin to recognize who may be a good subject by the degree receptivity to your hesitation. The subject who stays with you and allows you to set the pace of the handshake is evidently more sensitive and responsive than the person who rushes off.

The next step might be only to release the hand halfway, so the subject is momentarily confused. You can then practice letting go of the rest of the hand so gently that the subject does not recognize when the release took place, the hand remaining momentarily suspended in midair. You can sometimes heighten this effect by speaking very softly so the subject's attention is further divided in trying to attend to you. The final stage is learning to add the directing touches as nonverbal stimuli for immobility (catalepsy) or movement (Handshake Induction). Sacerdote (1970) had described and analyzed a similar procedure for inducing catalepsy in a nonverbal manner.

2. What other nonverbal touch situations of everyday life can you learn to Utilize to fix and focus attention inward to initiate trance?

Chapter Ten

Compound Suggestions: The Paradigms of Acceptance Set, Reinforcement, or Symbolic Logic

A surprisingly simple aspect of Erickson's approach is his use of compound suggestions. The compound suggestion in its simplest form is made up of two statements connected with an "and" or a slight pause. One statement is typically an obvious truism that initiates an accepting or Yes Set, the other statement is the suggestion proper.

MHE: Just look at one spot
and I'm going
to talk to you.

ER: In this example, the therapist has control over his own behavior ("I'm going to talk to you"), and by simply talking he can actually reinforce the suggestion, "Look at one spot."

MHE: There's nothing
that is really important
except the activity
of the unconscious mind
and that can be
whatever your

unconscious mind
desires.

ER: The importance of unconscious activity is suggested and then reinforced by an obvious truism of its independent activity.

MHE: We know the unconscious
can dream
and you can easily forget
that dream.

ER: This indirect suggestion to dream is itself a scientific truism. It is further reinforced by the truism that one can forget a dream. Merely mentioning, "You can easily forget," is also an indirect suggestion for amnesia.

MHE: You have altered
your rate of breathing,
your pulse,
and your blood pressure.
Without knowing it
you are demonstrating
the immobility
that a good hypnotic subject
can show.

ER: After an initial period of trance induction, when a subject is in fact very quiet, this statement about altered body functioning is a truism opening a *Yes* or *Acceptance Set* that permits the therapist to indirectly suggest "you are . . . a good hypnotic subject."

MHE: You can continue
enjoying
relaxing comfortably

for a few moments
and after you awaken
you can relate
one or two things
you are willing to share
and you can let the rest
remain within
the unconscious
where it can continue
its constructive work.

ER: At the end of a satisfactory hypnotherapeutic session the reward of relaxing comfort tends to reinforce all that happened previously. An *Acceptance Set* for the posthypnotic suggestion to both recall and forget is "You can let the rest remain in the unconscious". This is also an indirect suggestion for amnesia, permitting the unconscious to continue therapy on its own, free from the limiting and biasing influence of both the therapist's and patient's conscious sets.

It is clear from these examples that compound statements consist of two parts:

1. A truism consisting of an acceptable fact that can establish an Acceptance Set for the suggestion or reinforce it. If the truism has motivating properties for the patient, it is even more effective.

2. A suggestion proper that can appear before or after the truism. When the truism comes before the suggestion in a compound statement, it initiates a Yes Set or Acceptance Set for the suggestion that follows. When the truism follows the suggestion in a compound statement, the truism is in a position to function as a reinforcer of the suggestion.

As can be seen from the above examples, Erickson uses both forms. It will be a matter of future research to determine if both forms are equally effective. If they are, it would indicate that the commutative law (wherein the positions of the truism and suggestion may be reversed), so common in symbolic logic, may also apply to our usage of compound statements. This would imply that these hypnotic forms follow the types of laws found in symbolic logic (Henle, 1962). If it is found that the reinforcement form (wherein the truism follows the suggestion) is more effective, then it would appear that the classical laws of learning theory are more appropriate for our understanding of compound statements in hypnosis. If it is found that the *Acceptance Set* form (wherein the truism precedes the suggestion) is more effective, then it would be evidence that positive expectancy, deemed so important by Erickson, is in fact the more significant factor in hypnotic suggestion.

Compound Statements: The Paradigm of Shock and Creative Moments

Another provocative and interesting form of compound suggestion *Utilizes* a model of shock and its resultant creative moment (Rossi, 1973a), during which an unconscious search is initiated within the patient's associative processes. (Erickson and Rossi, 1975). A few examples are as follows:

MHE: Now the first step,
of course,
is to untangle your legs
[Pause]
and
untangle your hands.

ER: Erickson initiated hypnosis with an attractive, but rigid woman with this casually offered statement that is subtly shocking because of the sexual implications of "untangle your legs." The pause allows the shock to set in and initiate a creative moment with its rapid array of indistinct, confusing, and half-formulated questions which evoke a high level of added unconscious activity searching for the proper implication. The second half, "untangle your hands," makes the above sex shock retroactively acceptable. The sexual allusion is now rationalized as something that was not really intended. The shock effect, however, remains in force on an unconscious level. Mentioning "untangle" a second time now shunts the high level of mental activity initiated by the sex shock into other associative networks and pathways to "untangle" and open more exploratory sets on many levels.

MHE: I can listen to the whispering
[Pause]
of the wind in the woods.

ER: There can be a shock reaction to the word "whispering," which, of course, has many implications on many levels (secrets, sex, etc.). The pause allows the shock and a creative moment to initiate a high level of unconscious search. The "wind in the woods" then makes the above innocuous while developing a poetic mood for allegorical work evocative of daydream, fantasy, and other trance-oriented activity.

MHE: Secrets,
feelings,
behavior.
You would rather not talk about
[Pause]
can be examined privately
and objectively
in your own mind
in your own trance
[Pause]
for help with the problem at hand.

ER: "Secrets" is another shock word, initiating a creative moment within the safety of trance. The pause allows the shock and inner search for highly emotional memories to be activated. The potentially disturbing memories are then made relatively safe by now defining the situation as a "private" and "objective" evaluation. Another pause allows this safe investigation to proceed. Further positive reinforcement is then added with the final phrase assuring that this activity will "help with the problem at hand."

In these examples, a pause is the critical element, allowing a creative moment to develop in response to the first shock portion of the compound statement. This first shock portion of the hypnotic suggestion is obviously most useful for initiating a high level of mental activity and search that can then be discharged into the associative networks opened by the second portion. In effect, then, this form of suggestion allows one to initiate a high level of mental activity and then focus it in a predetermined manner on a problem area.

Exercises in Compound Suggestions

1. In this section, we have introduced an approach for analyzing compound suggestions. It can be seen that much fundamental research needs to be done to determine whether compound statements function according to the paradigms of Acceptance Set, learning theory, or symbolic logic (or all three!) The researcher can explore these questions by designing and executing controlled studies to study the relative effectiveness of these paradigms. The clinically oriented reader can explore this question by constructing both types of compound suggestions for use in workshop practice to facilitate the acceptance of suggestions. It may be found that some clinicians are more effective with one form or another as a function of their personal style of verbalization, voice dynamics, and other characteristics.

2. Review tape recordings of therapy sessions to study the natural compounds in the patient's and therapist's speech. As a patient describes a personal problem, study his compounds to gain insights into the association patterns that give rise to complexes, symptoms, and so on. As the therapist talks to a patient, what patterns of ideation and behavior are being consciously or unconsciously reinforced by the natural compounds in his speech?

3. Construct hypnotic inductions designed to associate suggestions with truisms that are particularly acceptable to individual patients. Plan how the various hypnotic phenomena can also be associated with such truisms in compound statements that are easy to accept.

Contingent Suggestions and Associational Networks

Another form of compound suggestion is used when Erickson arranges conditions such that a patient's normal flow of voluntary responses is made contingent on the execution of a hypnotic suggestion. A hypnotic response that may be low in a patient's behavioral hierarchy is associated with a pattern of responses high on the patient's behavioral repertory and usually already in the process of taking place. Patients find that the momentum of ongoing behavior is too difficult to stop so they simply add the hypnotic suggestion as an acceptable conditional for the completion of the pattern of behavior that is already begun and pressing for completion. The contingent suggestion simply hitchhikes onto patients' ongoing flow of behavior. Responses that are inevitable and most likely to occur are made contingent on the execution of the hypnotic response. Erickson, thus, interlaces his suggestions into the patient's natural flow of responses in a way that causes hardly a ripple of demur.

The simplest form of contingent suggestion may be mother's injunction, "***Shut the door*** on your way out!" as a child is running out the door. The already occurring flow of behavior, "on your way out" is made contingent upon "shut the door," since the mother is actually implying, "You can't go out ***unless*** you shut the door." Other examples used to systematically deepen trance are as follows:

> **Your eyes will get tired and close all by themselves as you continue looking at that spot.**
>
> **You will find yourself becoming more relaxed and comfortable as you continue sitting there with your eyes closed.**
>
> **As you feel that deepening comfort you recognize you don't have to move, talk, or let anything bother you.**
>
> **As the rest of your body maintains that immobility, so characteristic of a good hypnotic subject, your right hand will move the pencil across the page, writing automatically something you would like to experience in trance.**

Associating suggestions in such interlocking chains creates a network of mutually reinforcing directives that gradually form a new self-consistent inner reality called trance. It is the construction of such interlocking networks of associations that gives body or substance to trance as an altered state of consciousness with its own guideposts, rules, and reality.

A more complex form of contingent suggestion is in the example Erickson has used on numerous occasions in front of large groups with a subject he was inducing trance in for the first time as well as in private practice with patients who were well trained in trance. As the person approached his chair, Erickson would say, "Don't enter trance until you sit all the way down in that chair, there."

Don't enter trance

MHE: Use of the negative "Don't" to disarm possible resistance against the suggestion to "enter trance."

until

MHE: A form of the contingent that now reintroduces the possibility of trance in what may be a form acceptable to the patient.

you sit all the way down

ER: As part of the ongoing flow of inevitable behavior, this establishes a ***Yes Set*** or accepting set for the preceding.

in that chair

ER: An acceptable directive that puts another immediate positive valence on all the preceding.

there.

MHE: "There" implies that if they do sit in that chair, they are accepting the choice of going into trance. It is understood that there are other chairs they can sit in and not go into trance.

This complex contingent suggestion thus follows this general paradigm:

A negative -> a suggestion -> a contingent -> ongoing flow of behavior.

A classical example of an associational network built up of interlocking chains of contingent suggestions that led to a dramatic experience of visual hallucinations, amnesia, and posthypnotic suggestion was Erickson's approach to inducing trance in a resistant member of an audience.

Example of a Contingent Suggestion in Trance

On one occasion a dentist urged his wife to volunteer as a demonstration subject, so she could learn to experience trance. She adamantly refused and even tried to hide in her seat behind a pillar in the auditorium. Erickson spied her and proceeded as follows:

MHE: I like volunteers and I also like to pick my volunteers.

ER: This compound statement introduces the agreeable word "volunteer" and makes everyone a potential volunteer.

MHE: The one I'd like to pick is the pretty girl wearing the white hat who keeps hiding behind the pillar.

Subject: All the way from Colorado Springs, my husband urged me to act as a subject. I told him I didn't want to.

MHE: Now, notice that you thought you didn't want to.

MHE: The implication of this remark is to place her not wanting to volunteer into the past with "thought you didn't want to." This phrase is also a ***Double Bind*** because it contains another implication: "thought you don't want to," on a conscious level can imply that you really wanted to on an unconscious level.

> **MHE: And now that you've come out entirely from behind that pillar, you might as well come all the way to the platform.**

ER: This is a contingent suggestion where "come all the way up" is hitch-hiked onto her ongoing behavior of coming out from behind the pillar.

> **Subject: [As she steps forward] But I don't want to.**
>
> **MHE: While you continue to come forward please, don't go into a trance until you sit all the way down in this chair.**

MHE: Another contingent suggestion ***Utilizing*** the negative "don't" to permit a recognition and expression of her negative attitude, while yet defusing it.

> **MHE: As you are on the platform, you know you are not in a deep trance,**

MHE: A truism and a reassurance that she is not in deep trance. This implies she may be in light or moderate trance.

> **MHE: but you are getting closer to that chair**

MHE: In conjunction with the previous sentence, this implies she is going into trance the closer she gets to the chair.

MHE: and you are beginning to recognize you don't care

ER: "Beginning" initiates a process of inner search that now ***Utilizes*** her negative "don't care" attitude . . .

MHE: whether or not you are going into trance.

ER: . . . to shift her into the possibility of "you are going into trance."

MHE: The closer you get, the more you can recognize the comfort of going into a trance.

ER: Another contingent suggestion to which is added the positive motivation of "comfort."

MHE: But don't go all the way in until you sit all the way down in the chair.

ER: The classic contingent suggestion described earlier.

MHE: All the way down. [Said as she is in the process of sitting down.]

ER: This is a two-level communication; it is a statement with double meaning: (1) Sit "all the way down" and (2) go "all the way down" into trance. Her behavior of sitting down means she is accepting the statement on level 1, but as she sits she is also without realizing it accepting the suggestion to go into trance on level 2.

MHE: I associated every one of her forward movements with the development of another fraction of trance by interlocking every piece of ongoing behavior with another easily acceptable suggestion.

MHE: You are all the way down
in the chair
all the way from Colorado Springs.

ER: In a curious way, this implies that every movement from Colorado Springs was an inexorable movement toward her current trance experience. This deepens the significance of her trance by giving it a long history.

MHE: You knew you did not want to go into a trance.
You knew you would prefer something else.
As you think it over

ER: A series of three truisms leading up to the following suggestion.

MHE: there is something else.

ER: A suggestion proper that again puts her on an inner search.

MHE: So why don't you look at it?

ER: An open-ended question focusing her attention. This is also an indirect suggestion ("Look at") for the possible experience of a visual hallucination.

Subject: [Looking at a blank wall] I get so much pleasure watching those skiers through my kitchen window.

ER: She responds literally to the above and "watches those skiers" with the "pleasure" Erickson has suggested a while back.

MHE: What else enhances it?

ER: Another open-ended question that allows her to bring in more personally enhancing associations.

Subject: I always keep the hi-fi on while I watch the skiers. That is the easiest way to wash the dishes.

ER: She adds the music from the hi-fi player that also belongs to her experience. The easiest way to enable hallucinatory behavior is to evoke the patient's own associations rather than an arbitrary item.

[At this point the husband stands up in the audience and says the following.]

Husband: Yes, she washes the dishes while watching the skiers come down the mountainside by our kitchen window.

[The husband then sends a message up to Erickson expressing the wish that he would initiate her into hypnotic training for childbirth.]

MHE: I think you might like to include hypnosis in your future.

ER: This is an open-ended suggestion that gives her new options for future behavior.

MHE: Suppose you ask me about it after you are awake.

ER: This is a posthypnotic suggestion that allows her the possibility of bringing up her own wishes and needs regarding future hypnotic work. It would be both unethical and highly destructive of the possibility of future trance work to introduce specific suggestions about hypnotic training for childbirth without first getting her request for it when she is awake.

Subject: [She awakens and looks around the platform.] I told my husband I would not volunteer as a hypnotic subject!

I was hiding behind that pillar and now I'm here?! I must have been in a trance.

MHE: Isn't it remarkable how comfortable you feel?

ER: A question that is a truism (comfort is characteristic of trance) evokes positive feelings to depotentiate her reactive anger.

Subject: What did I do in trance?

ER: Implying an amnesia.

MHE: You would really like to know, wouldn't you?

ER: This brings forth the memory-traces of her trance experience, so they are ready to enter consciousness.

Subject: I certainly would!

MHE: Just look there!

[As Erickson looks and points meaningfully at the blank wall she was looking at when she first hallucinated.]

Subject: Oh, they are skiing!

[She continues actively hallucinating the skiers, describing their movements.]

ER: Her strong motivation is here *Utilized* by providing a channel for experiencing those memory traces consciously in the form of a visual hallucination with her eyes open, staring at that same wall. Trance was reinduced by a *Surprise Approach* that allowed the memory traces to discharge in hallucinatory form.

[Subject is then reawakened with an amnesia for this second trance.]

MHE: What do you suppose, when you first came up to the platform, you did in that trance?

Subject: [Subject mentions that she probably saw skiers and again repeated all the details about the skiers as if she had not discussed them before. She then goes on to wonder aloud if she might not have a use for hypnosis in the future.]

ER: She is now following the posthypnotic suggestion about the possibility of including hypnosis in her future.

MHE: Well, you are married.

Subject: Well, I intend to have children. [Subject then discusses the possibility of Utilizing hypnosis in childbirth. Years later, she very successfully did so.]

ER: The association about marriage naturally evokes a connection between marriage—childbirth—hypnosis.

Exercises with Contingent Suggestions

1. The value of observing regularities in patients' behavior which was emphasized in chapter 1, will now be apparent. The effectiveness of contingent suggestions depends in great part on their being appropriately timed and associated with regular patterns of ongoing behavior. The more a patient is locked into a certain pattern of behavior, the more powerful a vehicle will it be for the appropriately hitchhiked suggestion.

Formulate both simple and complex contingent suggestions that you could associate with any fairly automatic ongoing patterns of everyday behavior you've observed in individual patients. This can be as simple as encouraging a patient to continue any ongoing pattern of associations or behavior. Gradually learn how to add modifying suggestions and finally suggestions to structure further therapeutic responses.

2. Plan how you could utilize simple and complex contingent suggestions for facilitating psychotherapeutic responses.

3. Construct associational networks that will facilitate hypnotic induction as well as any particular hypnotic phenomenon. Erickson's work on the construction of artificial complexes and experimental neurosis (Erickson, 1944) is of particular value for studying his method of formulating associational networks. The formulation of such associational networks may be the clearest illustration of the construction of hypnotic realities.

Multiple Tasks and Serial Suggestions

As we have seen, it is frequently more effective to offer two or more hypnotic suggestions rather than one. Often the momentum of doing one easy task will help a more difficult one along—as is the case with contingent suggestions.

A series or chain of interlocking suggestions is another effective method for structuring a pattern of behavior. The performance of one item serves as a cue and stimulus for the next. Erickson frequently used such series during the early years of his learning and experimentation with hypnotic realities. He would have experimental subjects in a laboratory imagine and "mentally go through the process step by step and in correct order" of reaching for an imaginary piece of fruit on an imaginary table (Erickson, 1964/2022a). If one were actually to reach out and pick up a piece of real fruit, a series of stimulus-response interactions with the real objects outside of one's skin would be required. If one performs this task mentally, however, one is interacting entirely within one's own mind with memories of sensory stimuli, perceptual patterns, kinesthetic cues, etc. This inner focus and ***Utilization*** of one's own mental programs is the essence of trance experience. To put subjects on any sort of mental task requiring a series of steps ***Utilizing*** their own internal programs, therefore, is another valuable hypnotic form.

Because of this Erickson frequently gives serial, multiple, or compound tasks just as he makes compound statements. His favorite word appears to be "and." "And" allows him to connect suggestions into series so that they mutually reinforce each other, while at the same time maintaining the subject within a concentrated inner focus.

The fixing and focusing of attention inward on an imaginary task is thus an indirect means of inducing trance. This inner trance-inducing focus is easily accomplished by having subjects review a series of early memories, visualizing a series of scenes or a movie (for visual types), listening to inner music (especially for those with music training), and so on. This is the basis for the fantasy and visualization approaches to inducing trance (the "house-tree-person" or "blackboard" visualizations, etc.)

A chain of casual, ***Naturalistic*** suggestions forming an associational network is particularly effective for facilitating posthypnotic behavior. The following example from one of Erickson's early seminars (Erickson, 1939/2010) is particularly effective because this series of suggestions about cigarettes is a ***Naturalistic*** one in the sense that it ***Utilizes*** typical patterns of behavior and motivation common to all cigarette smokers. The subject simply floats along on a natural chain of behavioral events that are already more or less built in.

After awakening the subject would (A) notice Dr. D searching vainly through his pockets for a package of cigarettes, and (B) the subject would then proffer his own pack, and (C) Dr. D absentmindedly would forget to return the cigarettes, whereupon the subject would feel very eager to recover them because he had no others.

The ***Naturalistic*** or "built-in" aspect of this series of suggestions capitalizes on the automatic and partially unconscious manner with which habitual behavioral patterns are carried out. The early stages of trance training are greatly facilitated by ***Utilizing*** behavioral patterns that the subject is very familiar with. These require little or no conscious effort and thus are not likely to interfere with the still fragile nature of early trance experience.

Exercises with Multiple Tasks and Serial Suggestions

1. Formulate hypnotic inductions wherein the subject is kept busy with two or more tasks. While (A) looking at that spot the subject is enjoined to (B) notice whatever sensations develop in the eyelids. While (A) watching the hand levitating (B) the unconscious can bring forth all the associations and memories needed to solve a problem.

2. Formulate multiple tasks that are to be carried out on two levels, the conscious and unconscious, so that Double Binds become operative.

3. Formulate serial suggestions that lead step by step to the experience of dissociation and each of the classical hypnotic phenomena.

4. Formulate serial suggestions and associational networks that can facilitate posthypnotic behavior by Utilizing the subject's own natural behavioral patterns.

Chapter Eleven

Mutual Trance Induction

The first one begins with a surprise for Dr. S, and develops into a more complex demonstration. The second example involves a different more experienced subject. One of Erickson's favorite methods of training a hypnotic subject is to give the novice an opportunity to observe a more experienced subject in trance. But on this occasion, Erickson does something more: he orchestrates a mutual trance induction where two subjects interact in such a way that they facilitate each others' experience of trance. This section contains two examples of mutual trance induction.

In this session, Erickson begins by pointing out many of the psycho-physiological indications of beginning trance. He then has an opportunity to discuss a number of other outstanding characteristics of trance: patient's subjective feelings of distance; patient's inner reality and rapport, patient's change in voice quality and learning to speak in trance. The need for careful and continual observation of the patient is further emphasized when Erickson outlines the significance of pulsations that can be observed in different parts of the patient's body. He is particularly careful to note indications of distress in the patient's behavior. There are various subtle approaches to making inquiries about this distress that will safeguard the integrity of the patient's inner balance between conscious and unconscious knowing.

Of particular significance in this session is the clarification of Erickson's view of trance as an active state of unconscious learning. He points out that it took one of his subjects (a hospitalized mental patient) 200 hours to get to the point that he was able to do something more than just sit there. Yet, the patient is not expected to direct himself consciously, as is usually the case when one is awake. The learning is not of the intellectual sort that is practiced in school. The momentum for this mental activity is to come from the unconscious. It proceeds autonomously and is experiential rather than intellectual learning. Erickson points out that most of Dr. S's learning has been of the intellectual sort, but in hypnotic work she can learn best by letting go and experiencing. Learning spontaneously through one's own inner experience is then described as another way of deepening trance.

Session 4: Surprise and Mutual Trance Induction with Dr. S and Dr. H

As a surprise, Dr. H, a highly experienced hypnotic subject currently in therapy with Dr. Erickson, was invited to join ER and Dr. S for this session.

ER: What is the function of S*urprise* in your work?

MHE: The function of S*urprise* is this. The patient comes to you with a certain mental set, and they expect you to get into that set. If you surprise them, they let loose of their mental set and you can frame another mental set for them.

ER: You're dislodging the erroneous conscious sets that are giving them problems.

MHE: Yes. That's also what you do with ***Confusion Technique.***

> **MHE: Now I'm just going to look at her. I want both of you**
> **[ER and Dr. H] to observe her blink reflex.**
> **[Pause of 30 seconds as all three watch Dr. S.]**

MHE: In talking about Dr. S here, I am actually giving her indirect suggestions. I here note many of the criteria of beginning trance as soon as she manifests them in a seemingly spontaneous manner.

ER: This is one of your favorite approaches to indirect suggestion: you say things to an audience or talk about another person's experience as a way of initiating trains of associations in the patient that may eventually culminate in hypnotic responsiveness. It is an indirect form of ideomotor or ideosensory suggestion.

> **MHE: There was a slight quiver of her eyelids.**
> **Along with that quiver**
> **is an ironing out of facial muscles.**
> **There's an alteration in the breathing.**
> **There's also a lowering of blood pressure.**
> **Also a slowing of the heart rate.**
> **There's a loss of reflexes.**
> **She's aware that I am speaking about her to you.**
> **Now there is a slight change in rhythm.**
> **And she's beginning to drift**
> **right into a deep trance state.**

MHE: Everything I say about Dr. S is also a suggestion to Dr. H, but he did not know it. Every suggestion I made to Dr. S elicits some understanding in Dr. H, and that understanding requires that he act it out for himself to some degree.

ER: That is the basic principle of ideomotor activity in hypnosis. You ***Utilize*** it here to initiate an hypnotic induction in Dr. H without his being aware of it.

[Erickson here describes his typical procedure of demonstrating hypnosis with several naive subjects in front of an audience. He would surround a resistant subject with cooperative subjects, demonstrating the various phenomenon until the resistant subject was influenced by the hypnotic "atmosphere" all around him. The resistant subject would soon exhibit a "look of surprise" as he began to feel influenced and Erickson would reinforce this by remarking how "interesting" and "charming" the feelings were. Very often those who were initially afraid would go all the more deeply into trance once they got around their fear with this approach.]

MHE: And she's removing herself from this reality
to go into a different reality
where ER's reality and Dr. H's reality is changed
and mine is becoming less and less important.
And my voice?
I don't know exactly how
she hears it.
Maybe as a distant sound
which she does not feel a need to hear.
I am close enough to her
for her to hear me.
From that loss or change in body motility,
you can follow it,
it can tell you something about the character and ideation
that's going
through her mind.

[Mrs. Erickson was called. She comes in and is told to try to hush up Dr. S's children, who are playing loudly outside the office.]

MHE: To separate her from our reality [The tri-part reality shared by MHE, ER, and Dr. H] helps deepen the trance by focusing her in on her own reality.

ER: I see! If the hypnotherapist is interrupted in the middle of a session and has to speak to a mailman or plumber who knocked on the door, it can deepen the patient's trance reality because they are excluded and left alone with their own internal reality.

MHE: I discovered the hard way. Part of my early experience was in subjects always awakening, and I had a lot of difficulty. I'd have one subject in one room and another in another room, and they would awaken when I left the room. I discovered I had to leave them in a certain way, so they would maintain their trance state. I had to assure them they were not being deserted. They could rely upon me to return to them; I was only temporarily absent. At first I told them that verbally, and later I learned how to use nonverbal cues.

ER: Like what?

MHE: "I'm here, you are here" [Erickson demonstrates how by repeating this formula in different positions throughout the room the subject would get the idea that he was always in rapport with them, no matter where he was actually located.] When I moved away I'd say, "No matter where I am I will always be here." People don't know how much they know about the locus of a voice (Erickson, 1973).

ER: It's all unconscious learning.

MHE: Yes.

[Erickson here refers to a manuscript he was writing (Erickson, 1973) about how he actually produced seasickness in hypnotic subjects simply by changing the locus of his voice by bobbing and weaving up and down and back and forth, mimicking the changing locus a voice would have on a ship in rough waters.]

ER: How are you feeling right now, Dr. S?

Dr. S: Hummm, fine [Very softly as if very far away].

ER: Can you describe anything of your state of awareness to us?

MHE:People have a lifetime of learning that talking in your sleep is socially unacceptable. It's surprising how many people fear they will betray themselves by speaking in their sleep or trance.

ER: So you have to give patients special instruction and reassurance about their ability to speak in trance. And you do that simply by asking how they are feeling.

MHE: I've already used words like "comfort" and "fine," so when she uses the word "fine," I also know she is following my suggestions to feel comfort.

Dr. S: I can hear you. [Remote automaton like voice.]

[Pause]

ER: To what do you attribute the automaton like or faraway quality of her voice?

MHE: It's due to a different muscle tone. Her face is ironed out, there is greater plasticity and relaxation of all the muscles, including those controlling voice.

Dr. S: [Laughs] You're tickling me. [Personal voice as if she is nearly awake.]

[Actually the microphone cord inadvertently was bobbing against her knee as ER was adjusting it.]
ER: That was quite by accident, it was the microphone cord. How did you experience that tickling?

Dr. S: I thought maybe you were doing it to see if I would get out of this state. [Much laughter.] I know Mrs. Erickson came in and she stepped on my toe, but it did not hurt. [Even more laughter all around.]

ER: What's your state of awareness right now?

Dr. S: Oh, I'm coming awake.

ER: Fully awake?

MHE: She has this awakening reaction because I had not given her any specific instructions to disregard all extraneous stimuli while in trance. You need to know that any alien stimulus can enter into the trance situation, and you need to learn to deal with it. Mrs. Erickson may be in a deep trance when the phone rings, and she may answer it while remaining in trance. If it's an unfamiliar voice on the phone, she will wake right up, but if she knows who it is, she may remain in trance altering her voice so the person will not notice she is in trance. But if the other person is one of my hypnotic subjects, they will recognize the trance.

Dr. S: Oh, I'm back but slightly distant.

[Pause]

MHE: That feeling of "distance" is a sign of trance. Nobody has really explained that sense of being distant.

ER: How would you explain it? Every speaker in front of an audience has a sense that the audience is with me or not with me; they are distant from me. The feeling of distance then is due to feeling the lack of a shared-world-in-common (Rossi, 1972/2000).

MHE: Yes.

> **MHE: Dr. S has had the opportunity of discovering she can do that work. Now I have the right to be as stupid as possible.**
> **It isn't requisite for me**
> **to understand all.**
> **There can be progressive**
> **understanding on your part,**
> **on Dr. H's part,**
> **on the others' part.**
> **[Pause]**
> **And Dr. H need not be frightened**
> **about hate**
> **or frightened of the word: love.**
> **You're terrified**
> **of new understandings**
> **of those words.**
> **[Pause]**

ER: By saying that you "have the right to be as stupid as possible" you are making an exaggerated and humorous suggestion about how little you need to understand consciously. This implies that Dr. S and Dr. H need not use consciousness at this point either. Later, they can develop their conscious understanding, but for now let the unconscious handle things. You then address a few therapeutically relevant words to Dr. H about being "frightened" and so on.

> **MHE: And ER and Dr. S have come to join us this time.**
> **They called to find out if they could come,**

and I knew it would be to their advantage
and to your advantage (Dr. H)
to have them here.

ER: You apparently felt from nonverbal clues that Dr. H needed some reassurance at this point so you simply talk about the pragmatic aspect of this joint session. You then emphasize that it would be to everyone's mutual advantage to be together.

MHE: Yes. Notice I use a different tone of voice for "your" when referring to Dr. H and a different direction of voice.

ER: These voice cues are automatically and correctly interpreted by Dr. S and Dr. H, so they always know when you are referring to each even though you use the impersonal pronoun.

MHE: Because
I could effect an interplay
that would be extremely valuable
for you,
for Herbie (Dr. H),
for ER
and for Dr. S.

ER: When you do extensive work with some patients, as you have with Dr. H, you sometimes give them another name in trance. Why?

[Erickson gives many examples from everyday life where one person—lover, mate, parent, or child—may give another person a pet name to evoke a particular mood or aspect of their relationship. A child will say "Father" or "Dad" or "Daddy" on different occasions to constellate different aspects of the relationship with father. In trance, the patient may experience a particular ego state that the therapist wants to label with a special name so he can help the patient return to it later.]

Rapport in Mutual Hypnosis

[Dr. H had been watching Dr. S very carefully, presumably to study her state of awareness. At the moment Herbie is mentioned, however, his watching becomes more of a fixed stare. Dr. S seems to notice this, and they silently and deeply look into each other's eyes in a fixed, unblinking manner.]

MHE: ER can watch Dr. S and you (Dr. H) can discover certain things.
[Pause]

[Dr. S and Dr. H alternately blink. Dr. S's eyelids finally flutter and close, and then Dr. H's eyes close also.]

And Dr. S has made a new discovery,
but then you (Dr. H) too
have made a new discovery.
[Pause]

ER: You arrange a hypnotic atmosphere where both are sitting quietly in rapt attention and thus gradually developing a light trance. Now as they look at each other they automatically mimic each other's hypnotic behavior (e.g., the staring and eye blinking) and thereby go deeper into trance.

MHE: Yes. At this point Dr. H's distance was much greater than Dr. S's.

ER: You mean he was further into trance?

MHE: He was further away. Dr. H tended to go into a reality that included himself and me but excluding Dr. S and you.

ER: So, here you were trying to bring Dr. S and me into his inner reality more. But how could you tell he was tending to exclude Dr. S and me? Was he turning away from us and orienting bodily toward you?

MHE: A person could be looking right at you, yet you know they are not paying attention to you without their even knowing they are not paying attention.

ER: Yes, they will have that faraway look in their eyes.

MHE: But can you define that "faraway look" in precise terms?

ER: That would be difficult. Then you are saying that this comes with experience. By now it is almost an unconscious intuitive knowledge on your part.

MHE: Yes.

> **MHE: Now both of you want**
> **profound trances**
> **with hallucinations of the real**
> **and of the unreal**
> **and the organization of amorphous things.**
> **Amorphous things, amorphous emotions, relationships,**
> **and identities.**

[Pause]

MHE: By saying "***both*** of you want profound trances," I'm here beginning to effect a separation between them.

ER: You're saying that to each of them as separate people?

MHE: Yes. ***Each of them can have their own trance with its own individual meaning for each.*** For Dr. H as a patient, it is important to experience his diffuse emotions as part of his therapy. For Dr. S as a therapist in training, it is important to learn to recognize amorphous emotions and relationships she will later be called upon to cope with professionally.

ER: The same words will have different meanings for different people. This corresponds to your frequent use of certain words that will have different meanings at different levels within the same personality.

MHE: And when you spend time,
time can be of varying intensity.
It can be condensed,
it can be expanded,
so you can review a lifetime history in a few seconds time.
[Pause]
Those few seconds can be expanded
into
years.
Also a few days can be condensed
into a moment.
For both of you
it's a matter of your education
[Pause]
in dealing with patients
that you can take a patient's pain

and teach a patient to experience all of the pain
as a momentary passing twinge.
It can be very sharp only momentarily
even though it lasts all day.
Both of you want to learn how to expand time,
expand awareness,
and both of you need to know
that there is such a thing as
a contraction of time, feeling, pain, emotion.
A pleasing lecture of an hour's duration may seem like
it has barely begun when the hour is over.
Or in a boring lecture the chair begins to hurt,
and you get tired, and you wonder
when the hour will be up.
Both of you have had that experience in the past.
You know when you've had those experiences.
Now you're going to apply them to yourselves
in a way that helps your understanding of yourself
and your understanding of others.
[Pause]

MHE: *Time Distortion* will be useful to both of them here in their different contexts.

ER: You suggest all possible types of *Time Distortion* (condensation and expansion) that may operate to whatever degree the patient finds himself using. You are thus following your basic technique of suggesting all possible responses, so that it is almost impossible for the suggestion to fail. Whatever the patient experiences has been covered by your inclusive suggestion and can thus be counted as a success.

MHE: Again here the matter of education will be taken in a different way by each of them. And so on for much of this material.

ER: You use common everyday truisms that both
of these well educated subjects are certain to have experienced to induce a *Yes Set* to enhance the plausibility and acceptability of your suggestions.

MHE: And you both realize
thoroughly
that the hypnotic state
is not really induced by me
but by yourselves.
[Pause]
And Dr. H saw Dr. S do something with her eyelids,
and then he repeated it.
And Dr. S, in watching Dr. H,
in turn repeated what Dr. H did,
and she went into a trance.
Then Dr. H went into a trance also.
As far as ER is concerned
he has learned that
the proximity of one hypnotic subject to another
does the same thing as is expressed
in folk language:
Monkey see, monkey do
which is a way of understanding
children;
they see, they do.
[Pause]
There is no importance in my talking to you;
time will just pass
and I can do as I wish.
[Pause]

ER: Here you are putting the responsibility for trance learning on the subjects, so they will not be passively dependent on the hypnotherapist.

MHE: Yes. When they know they are doing it, they know they can alter their own behavior.

ER: So that's an important way of reducing the magic and motivating them further in the direction of therapeutic self change. The therapist provides the patient with a setting and opportunity to do creative work. Trance is actually an active process wherein the unconscious is active, but not directed by the conscious mind. Is that right?

MHE: That's right.

ER: This is one of your important contributions to modern hypnosis: getting away from the automaton concept of the hypnotic state to conceptualize hypnosis as a state of very active inner learning that takes place autonomously. Is that right?

MHE: Yes.

ER: In a trance state, you have released the unconscious to do its own work without interference from consciousness.

MHE: And to do it in accord with the experimental learning of the subject.

ER: Previously hypnosis was thought of as a state where the subject passively received therapeutic suggestions.

MHE: By being told what to do and when to do it.

ER: But your approach is frequently the opposite of that. You just let the subject get into a trance state where he can do his own inner work.

> **MHE: Now each of you is learning something**
> **pertaining to yourselves.**
> **You are developing your own psychological techniques of psychotherapy**
> **without knowing that you are developing them.**
> **Dr. H now realizes**
> **his tremendous response to the visual stimuli Dr. S gave him.**
> **And Dr. S realizes that also.**
> **[Pause]**

ER: Here, for example, you are instructing them to do their own inner learning, their own inner work for themselves. They are not just to sit there passively. Could this be some of the difficulty Dr. S is experiencing? She doesn't have the idea yet of doing her own inner work, she is being too passive.

MHE: She tells us she's been skipping around, just looking.

ER: That's characteristic of many subjects I'm learning to work with. They are just hopping around. But that is not the state you are looking for.

MHE: It took one of my subjects 200 hours to learn. He would just sit there. Dr. S has been a student, a scholar. She learns intellectually, but she doesn't know how to learn something experientially. I've got to explain to her that she is to learn by experience.

> **MHE: [to ER] Notice that pulsation [in Dr. S's face].**
> **Now I'm going to talk to ER, so you need not pay any attention.**

ER: Do you want to comment on the pulsations?

MHE: In watching the face in the trance state, there are various places you can note the pulsation. It isn't necessary for you to use your fingers on the wrist. Use your eyes on the patient's ankle, neck, temple. Watch the changing pulsations. Often fluctuations can tell you things. You learn to correlate pulsations with muscle tonus. You can suddenly realize that increased pulsations means there exists a greater tonicity in muscles. You can't really see the muscle tonicity develop until it develops to a certain degree but from more rapid pulses you know the muscle is tighter. Now a slower pulse brings about a lessening of tonicity. Body behavior in all parts of the body should be under your observation.

MHE: You also look for signs of perspiration, pallor, changes in facial expression, any signs of distress. You're careful at such times.

ER: When you note those distress signals you become very careful about what you are saying. It could be traumatic.

MHE: That's right.

ER: So even while a person is in trance, you are careful about what might filter into their conscious mind.

MHE: You don't push at such times.

ER: How about when trance has terminated? Do you question them about their trance distress then?

MHE: Only in the most general terms.

[Erickson now gives a demonstration of how he will gently imitate the head movements a patient made in trance while saying, "How about here, there, up, down, from this to that," etc.]

ER: If it's safe for the conscious mind to deal with the material, consciousness will pick up your most general hints. If it is not safe, it will not understand what you're getting at.

[MHE completely ignores Dr. H and Dr. S for about 10 minutes. He talks to ER about certain manuscripts on his desk, which they are working on together.]

MHE: I think I will let Dr. H awaken first.
Now Dr. H, take your time,
count backwards from 20 to 1,
awakening 1/20th at each count.
Begin to count now.
[Pause]

[Dr. H awakens and reorients his body.]

Now Dr. S, I want you to begin counting silently,
mentally from 20 to 1 and begin to count now.
[Pause]

[She awakens and reorients her body.]

ER: It's rather remarkable they both took the same amount of time to awaken.

MHE: You see, when you're working with subjects, you let them have an opportunity to experience their trance state without necessarily giving them anything to do. You leave them to their own devices. It deepens the trance. They become more aware of what they can do. They become more facile in their capacities.

ER: It becomes a period of free learning for the subjects when you leave them to their own devices.

MHE: Yes:

ER: But Dr. S has been getting irritated with you because she may not know how to deepen the trance by herself.

MHE: It's not something you learn to do consciously, it happens spontaneously; you only know later that it happened.

> [Erickson here gives other examples of spontaneous unconscious behavior such as putting more salt on your food on a hot day without realizing it. When people, even young children, move to a warmer climate, they learn this spontaneously on an unconscious level.]

ER: This again emphasizes that therapeutic trance is a state of active learning that takes place autonomously without conscious intervention.

Chapter Twelve

The *Surprise Technique*

Erickson frequently utilizes Surprise to shake people out of their habitual patterns of association in an effort to facilitate their natural patterns of unconscious creativity. The problem with offering direct suggestions is that unless they are carefully integrated with the patient's inner experience, they may interfere with the autonomous and creative aspect of trance experience. If trance is a focus of a few inner realities that move by themselves, then the therapist's direct suggestion may come as an intrusion on that autonomous inner flow. The direct suggestion might inadvertently activate the patient's conscious intention to try to do something on a voluntary level. By asking patients simply to "wait for a surprise," on the other hand, we are allowing them to remain in quiesence while unconscious processes gradually mobilize a truly autonomous response.

Surprise is an agreeable word to most people. It conjures up many associations of pleasant childhood experiences and surprise parties and gifts. The ego is usually receptive to a surprise. A surprise always implies that the subject will have no control—and that, of course, facilitates autonomous functioning. The word "surprise" is thus a conditioned cue for most people to give up control and to be curious about the pleasant thing that is going to happen to them.

MHE: Or would you like to have it as a surprise?

Now or later?

ER: That question actually implies a pleasant experience will happen. To that agreed upon surprise is added another surprise.

MHE: Shortly
I'm going to lift your hand
in the air.
What happens
after that
is going to surprise you.

MHE: When the subject goes through all the possible surprises, what can surprise them?

ER: An unusual thing.

MHE: And what unusual thing is there? The hand could stay there and the subject cannot put it down.

MHE: You are pretty well aware of all the things you can do,
but the most surprising experience you can have is to discover
that you can't stand up... now.

ER: The first part of this statement is a truism: the subject knows what she can do. The surprise about not being able to stand up comes as a shock that tends to depotentiate her usual conscious sets and facilitate the immobility of the lower body. This surprise is thus another classical example of not doing. The drawn-out emphasis on the word "n o w" evokes a curiosity response from the subject, who says to herself: "What does that mean? Is anything happening? What has happened?" These questions allow an opening and time for the autonomous process of immobility to develop. The typical subject then begins to move the top part of her body to test the suggestion but leaves the bottom part from the waist down immobile. Frequently, the therapist can give the subject a surprise slap on the thigh, so she can experience the further surprise of a caudal analgesia.

Another example of the ***Surprise*** was related by Erickson as he discussed his permissive approach in allowing patients to express their own variations to a ***Hand Levitation*** approach:

> The therapist's attitude should be completely permissive so a patient can respond in any way to Hand Levitation—even by pushing down harder and harder. I'm thinking of a certain college student who did that. After he did that long enough I said, "It's rather interesting—at least it is to me. I think it will be up to you when you discover that you can't stop pushing down."
>
> He thought he was resisting. The idea that he couldn't stop took him completely by surprise and it was a full-grown idea when it hit him. That would be something he would be interested in. He would be surprised! He couldn't be surprised unless he couldn't stop pushing down. Not being able to stop pushing down was made contingent upon the idea of interest and a surprise. He found to his surprise that he couldn't stop pushing down and he asked, "What happened?"
>
> I said, "At least your arms have gone into a trance. Can you stand up?"
>
> Can he? That simple question elaborated "At least your arms have gone into a trance," and extended it to his feet. Of course, he couldn't stand up.
>
> There was only one conclusion to reach: his body was in a trance because he no longer had control over it. That apparently was what he wanted—to regard hypnosis as a condition in which you have no control over yourself.

The shock and ***Surprise*** this student experienced must have been all the more upsetting since he obviously had a high investment in not following suggestions, as is indicated by his pushing his hand down when it was suggested that it levitate. In this case Erickson states, "Not being able to stop pushing down was made contingent upon the idea of interest and surprise." Erickson did, in fact, succeed in evoking interest, shock, and surprise with his provocative statement, "It's rather interesting—at least it is to me. I think it will be to you when you discover that you can't stop pushing down." He evoked a shock and surprise that momentarily suspended the student's belief system. In that precise moment, he added his own self suggestion suggestion, "You discover that you can't stop pushing down."

CONFUSION
due to shock, stress, uncertainty, etc.

↓

UNSTRUCTURING
of usual frames of reference

↓

RESTRUCTURING
needed

↓

RECEPTIVITY
to therapeutic suggestions

Exercises with *Surprise*

1. Surprise has a number of possible functions in hypnotic work.
a. Shock and Surprise can momentarily depotentiate an individual's habitual mental sets, so that perception and understanding may be spontaneously reorganized in a new way.
b. An anticipation of a pleasant surprise has motivating properties and leaves the individual open, aware, expectant of something. That something can be either a new insight from within or an important suggestion from the therapist.
c. The anticipation of a pleasant surprise allows the ego to relax so that more autonomous processes can function in a way compatible with trance.

Plan how you could utilize the above characteristics of Surprise to enhance an experience of each of the classical hypnotic phenomena.

2. To learn something about a person's fundamental world view and habitual frames of reference, ask about their most "surprising life experience." And what would be the most surprising thing that could happen to them?

3. Once you understand something about a person's world view, plan how you could say or do a simple and innocent thing that is a bit outside that world view so the person is shocked and surprised. Of course, tact and good taste are required for such adventures. With experience, you can learn to elicit a double-take and a laugh from people as they spontaneously reorganize their perceptions and/or accept a suggestion you offer them at that critical moment of surprise when there is a momentary suspension of their habitual sets and patterns of understanding. This kind of approach is used by professional comedians and some skillful orators.

THE CONFUSION-RESTRUCTURING APPROACH

A major theme reiterated again and again in the most surprising contexts by Erickson is that the patient "does not know" what is happening. Of course, consciousness is at all times limited. Consciousness focuses on this or that, ever shifting from moment to moment. At any given moment, it can only be focused on a limited range of information. Erickson ***Utilizes*** this limitation by continually introducing changes in areas outside that momentary focus of consciousness. If he can be sure that the patient's consciousness is focused in area A, then he will introduce a change in area B. When the patient's consciousness returns to refocus on B, the patient is in for a ***Surprise***: an unexpected change has been introduced. This ***Surprise*** throws off patients' usual reality sense, they become confused, and they reach for and accept any suggestions that the therapist can introduce to restructure the lost reality.

In Chapter 1, we discussed how Erickson did not find hyper-suggestibility characteristic of trance (Erickson, 1932/2010). We can now more clearly understand what he meant. Under the shock and ***Surprise*** of many of the older authoritarian approaches to hypnotic induction, it is obvious how the confusion-need-for-restructuring mechanism operated so automatically that it appeared as if the patient was hyper-suggestible in trance. This so-called hyper-suggestibility, however, is actually the automatic acceptance of any acceptable restructuring that will end the intolerable confusion that has been effected by the hypnotic induction or any means of unstructuring the ego's usual frames of reference.

The basic process required for the acceptance of suggestions by the confusion-restructuring approach, then, is as follows:

The reader can understand the above as intervening steps between stages two and three of the flow diagram presented in the previous chapter on Confusion in the Dynamics of Trance Induction. Acceptance of the therapist's suggestions will be in direct proportion to both the optimal degree of unstructuring and the appropriateness of the therapist's suggestions for restructuring a particular patient in a therapeutic manner. What people can accept as restructuring is very much a function of their therapeutic needs and goals.

Erickson uses this basic method of confusion-restructuring in therapy as well as in inducing hypnosis and facilitating the acceptance of suggestions. He has described many instances where he uses shock, (Rossi, 1973b) for example, to unsettle a patient's problem so the patient will grasp therapeutic suggestions to restructure a now shaken sense of reality.

A rather dramatic example of Erickson's use of confusion-restructuring in induction is in the situation where a nurse reluctantly came to the front of an audience to serve as a demonstration subject. As she approached Erickson he confused her as to which chair she should sit in by unexpectedly directing her alternately from one chair to another. (He directed her nonverbally to one chair while verbally indicating another.) When she was thoroughly perplexed, he finally said, "Go into a trance as you sit all the way down," and simultaneously indicated clearly which chair she should sit in.

Such approaches are obviously only suitable for therapists with quick wits and some practical experience. There are, however, many types of confusion-need-for-restructuring situations in everyday life and psychotherapy that can be creatively ***Utilized*** by any therapist. The momentary confusion of a loud noise or unexpected event, for example, produces a momentary gap in understanding that requires an explanatory suggestion. Erickson is continually playful in the way he introduces puzzles and oddities in the therapy situation that confound the mind so it will be receptive to suggestion. He will ask someone a beguilingly simple mathematical question, or drag out some fascinating esoterica from a Believe It or Not article (A popular trivia publication that reports unusual phenomena). By such simple means, he confounds the usual limiting sets of consciousness and awakens a need for explanation and restructuring. A ***Yes Set*** or accepting set is established, and the patient is grateful for anything new the therapist can then introduce.

Readers will have to determine for themselves the degree to which these various levels of confusion-restructuring can be used comfortably in their own therapeutic practice. A simple awareness of the confusion-restructuring process can be of immense value regardless of how the therapist feels about purposely provoking confusion. Most patients bring in enough confusion of their own which they want therapy to resolve! Rather than viewing such confusions negatively as indicators of pathology or problems, however, the therapist can look upon them as opportunities to help patients restructure their world.

Exercises in Confusion and Restructuring

1. Surprise, confusion, and restructuring are all intimately related processes. To learn to Utilize them creatively in therapy requires a certain flexibility in the therapist's world view. Creatively-oriented therapists will therefore seek out life experiences that will enable them to continually break out of the limitations of his own habitual framework (Rossi, 1972).

2. Uncertainty, ambivalence, and confusion are typical complaints of people who come to therapy. These are frequently treated as symptoms the therapist is supposed to remove. We can now understand how they are actually a preliminary stage for the possible creative change and growth of the personality (Rossi, 1972/2000; Rossi, 1973a). Learn to recognize in these complaints the outlines of what is changing in a patient's world view and how that change can be facilitated in a growth-enhancing manner.

Therapeutic Trance as a State of Active Unconscious Learning

Erickson makes it clear that therapeutic trance is a state of active learning on an unconscious level; that is, learning without the intervention of conscious purpose and design. Trance experience may be likened to that of the dream wherein mental events usually proceed autonomously.

There may be a question here as to whether this is true learning (in the sense of an acquisition of new responses,) or merely automatic behavior on an unconscious level. The proof of new learning must always lie in the results: Does the patient actually evidence new response capacities as a result of his hypnotic experience?

Erickson continually emphasizes learning without awareness. In this induction section, for example, he says to Dr. H and Dr. S, "You are developing your own psychological techniques of psychotherapy without knowing that you are developing them." He clearly believes that such learning can take place more effectively and creatively in an altered state, when many of the usual biases and preconceptions of the patient's conscious frame of reference are not active. Therapeutic trance is thus a condition wherein the usual biases and distractions of consciousness are minimized, so that new learning can take place most efficiently.

This view is entirely consistent with what is known about the creative process in general (Rossi, 1968, 1972/2000; Ghiselin, 1952), wherein it is recognized that consciousness is only a receiving station for the new combinations of the creative process that actually take place on an unconscious level. It is also consistent with the early hypnotherapeutic approaches of Liebeault, Bernheim, and Braid (Tinterow, 1970), who would sometimes place patients in a healing trance for a short time and then "wake" them up without any further direct suggestions about exactly how the therapy was to take place. The "healing atmosphere" provided by such early workers together with the belief system of their times functioned as indirect and nonverbal suggestions to set in motion creative, autonomous processes within their patients that could effect a "cure." Modern 20th-century man is handicapped, however, by a materialistic, and overly rationalistic belief system that tends to downgrade the functioning of these autonomous ther-apeutic processes. Modern man has an unfortunate hubris of consciousness (Jung, 1960) wherein he believes everything mental can be accomplished on a conscious and voluntary level. Such voluntary efforts frequently get in the way of natural healing processes. To cope with these misguided con-scious efforts, Erickson developed indirect approaches such as confusion and restructuring as a means of confounding patients' conscious limita-tions, so their unconscious has an opportunity to create new solutions.

Chapter Thirteen

Trance Learning By Association

In this session, Erickson again uses a more accomplished subject, Mrs. L, to demonstrate hypnotic responsiveness so that Dr. S can learn by association. Erickson begins with a Surprise: he asks Dr. S to perform her first hypnotic induction on another person. She does this surprisingly well, in a way that is original while still Utilizing a number of basic principles of hypnotic induction. The significance of this surprise request is that it prevented Dr. S from rehearsing ahead of time. It forced Dr. S to rely on her intuition and the unconscious learning she has acquired thus far in her personal experiencing of trance. Erickson encouraged her to learn to use experiential rather than intellectual knowledge.

In this session, Erickson returns to the theme of unconscious learning as a basic issue in doing genuine trance work. He comments that Dr. S still "doesn't quite trust her unconscious mind to do all the learning necessary." He clearly means that during trance the patient is learning without the usual mode of ego consciousness. Consciousness is not necessary for learning. Indeed, Erickson prefers learning to take place without the biasing intervention of consciousness.

In experimental psychology, it has been demonstrated that learning can indeed take place without awareness (e.g., latent learning). Such learning without awareness is Erickson's preferred way of working with patients in trance. Erickson has commented on the fact that much of what passes for hypnosis in the experimental literature, where a short induction of a few minutes' duration is followed by standardized suggestions (that do not take into account or meaningfully ***Utilize*** patients' individual differences), is actually a mixture wherein the patient uses conscious volition mixed with unconscious learning. This reliance on conscious volition and direction is the mark of an inadequately trained hypnotic subject. Such subjects will quickly reach a limit in the degree to which they can experience genuine hypnotic phenomena because their conscious sets and learned limitations interfere with the efficient functioning of unconscious mechanisms.

Two indirect approaches to ***Utilizing*** such unconscious mechanisms are clarified in this session: the implied directive and questions. These approaches have been developed by Erickson and others in clinical hypnosis. It will be fascinating and important to study the parameters of these approaches with more controlled laboratory studies as well as further field and clinical investigations. We are just now beginning to appreciate the complexity and vastly unrealized potential for using language to effect therapeutic goals.

In this session, Erickson requested Mrs. L, an excellent hypnotherapeutic subject with whom he has worked before, to be present. In a ***Surprise*** move, he asks Dr. S to hypnotize Mrs. L. This is the first occasion on which Erickson is able to observe work with hypnosis as an operator. Dr. S begins by addressing her suggestions to the subject.

Session 5: A Practice Mutual Trance Induction with Dr. S and Mrs. L

Dr. S: Close your eyes, relax, and imagine yourself in a fantasy spot which you liked very much.
[Pause]
Either by a lake or river, just some place you like.
[Pause]
You manage to get more and more relaxed. Take a deep breath and relax.

[Mrs. L does take a deep breath at this point.]

You start feeling more and more comfortable.
[Pause]

MHE: "Imagine yourself in a fantasy spot," makes it very personal. "Either by a lake or a river," now introduces reality. It becomes the patient's reality when she adds "just some place you like." "Take a deep breath," is a very safe suggestion because any patient has to breathe.

ER: Yes, so Dr. S is safe in going along with what Mrs. L is naturally doing.

MHE: And you can add any adjective you want, in this case a "deep breath." The adjective "deep" is a suggestion that is facilitated by being associated with an inevitable response: The patient will have to breathe.

ER: So, this was an excellent progression of suggestions that Dr. S used here:

MHE: Yes. But those suggestions take Mrs. L far away from this room. They take her to some specific memory, but Dr. S doesn't know which.

ER: That's the problem. A really experienced operator would know exactly where the patient was being placed unless a general exploration was wanted.

Dr. S: You'll find this world your very own world that you'll like very much.
[Pause]

Okay. Let's try a few signals, Okay?
[Pause]
Let this be the "Yes" finger right here.

[Dr. S taps Mrs. L's right forefinger.]

MHE: Given what goes just before, why shouldn't she like this world very much? You're not telling her to like it, you're just stating an obvious fact. The subject is not obeying like an automation. She will here simply agree that she does indeed like this place and feel Dr. S respects her.

ER: So again, Dr. S is doing very well here. She initiates an experience of relaxation and comfort in a place Mrs. L likes. She then announces that Mrs. L "will find this world . . . you'll like very much." This is actually a hypnotic repetition: Dr. S sets up a pleasant experience and then says it is a pleasant experience. Mrs. L, immersed as she is in the experience, however, does not recognize the repetition; she simply feels comfortable and respected as well since Dr. S is seemingly so correct in describing her inner experience.

Dr. S: And when you are feeling very peaceful
and comfortable, you can concentrate on "Yes"
and you may notice that finger float up.
OK, you can do that now. You can concentrate on "Yes."

[Pause as one of Mrs. L's fingers levitates.]

That's right.

MHE: "You can concentrate," is a statement of fact. It is not a command. If I say, "You can," it implies, "you can do that or something else." It is not a direct order. It is an inoffensive way of directing.

ER: So whether Dr. S realizes it or not, she has been learning something in her personal hypnotic work with you: She's learned how to use implication and indirect suggestions.

> **Dr. S: You are going to find that each time that you may want to spend a few minutes by yourself, relaxing, feeling very comfortable and serene, that you can go back to this feeling, you can put yourself into this world anytime that you like. There are times when you really need this serene feeling.**
> **[Pause]**
> **OK, now, anytime that you would like to come back and join us, you can**
> **just take a deep breath, stretch.**
>
> **[Mrs. L awakens, stretches, reorients to her body. A general conversation takes place for about five minutes. Erickson then undertakes to hypnotize Mrs. L.]**

MHE: Yes. "Times when you really need." What times? You're naturally going to have some memories of some times. So this is her own exploration. She will explore, but Dr. S has not told her to explore.

ER: So again, in a very indirect and innocuous way Dr. S has sent Mrs. L on an exploratory trip.

MHE: Self-exploratory and yet, not for the purpose of seeking names, etc., but for seeking serenity.

ER: It seems that Dr. S has been learning something about the indirect approach to suggestion in her work with you.

Erickson Induction by Recapitulation

MHE: I would like to have you do today what you did yesterday.

[Pause. Mrs. L's six week-old baby begins crying very loudly in the background, but Mrs. L pays no heed.]

You can make your own count from 1 to 20.

Now you know that today's a change

and go very deeply into a trance,

ER: In this simple introductory statement, you are recapitulating previous successful hypnotic work, and you're thereby reactivating associations that will facilitate your present hypnotic work.

ER: Why did you talk of "change" here?

MHE: The baby crying out there was not present when I worked with Mrs. L previously. Therefore, she had better change herself, so that she could accommodate this new stimuli without being disturbed.

ER: Without telling her directly that she supposed to ignore her baby today.

MHE: I gave her enough credit to know what I meant by "change."

ER: If you had said directly, "Ignore your baby's crying," she would certainly have resisted.

MHE: What woman wouldn't?

> **MHE: and you learned the other day**
> **how you could lose the ability**
> **to stand up.**
> **Now you can lose the ability**
> **to keep**
> **your right hand**
> **on your thigh**

ER: You don't command her, "You will not be able to stand up!" You just emphasize a natural behavior since we all can lose the ability to stand at one time or other. It's relatively easy to lose an ability. In trance, it is much easier ***not to do something*** rather than making all the effort to do something.

MHE: That's one thing people don't know about themselves. They don't know they can lose the ability to stand up. They don't know they can lose the ability to speak. Yet, it happens all the time, as when they remark, "I stood there like an idiot unable to say anything in that situation. I didn't know enough to say anything!"

> **MHE: because no matter what you do**
> **it will move up toward your face.**
>
> **[Mrs. L's hand does begin to levitate smoothly toward her face.]**
>
> **You can have the experience of being all alone**
> **with only a voice.**
> **My voice.**

And soon you won't even know whether your eyes are open or closed.
You don't need to know.
And now your hand is stuck to your face.
[Pause]
You can go back to Columbia.

[Columbia is a peaceful location that Mrs. L had referred to in previous work with Erickson. This also carries an implication of change.]

MHE: The patient's common reaction here is, "It will not move up to my face!" But, they will be doing something and "no matter what" they do, they wind up touching their face. There is an ever-continuing threat. For example, "Try harder!" No matter how hard they try to keep their eyes open, you know they will close sooner or later.

ER: *This is the logic of many induction suggestions: What the operator says is always a foregone conclusion.* Subjects do not realize that the resistance they are attempting is impossible, and they then attribute their failure to resist as giving in to the operator's power of suggestions.

MHE: Another example would be, "You don't know when you're going to change your rate of breathing."

ER: Sooner or later everyone will change their breathing rate. You thereby also develop a set for "change" which is so important for therapy, and at the same time you depotentiate consciousness by saying, "You don't know."

MHE: I would like you to learn
that no matter what any person believes,

your belief,
your unconscious belief,
your unconscious knowledge,
is all that counts.
[Pause]
In the course of living from infancy on,
you acquired knowledge,
but you could not keep all that knowledge in the foreground of your mind.
[Pause]
In the development of the human being,
learning in the unconscious
became available in any time of need.
When you need to feel comfort, you can feel comfort.
When you have a need for relaxation,
you can have it.

ER: Here again, you are emphasizing the importance of the unconscious at the expense of the conscious.

MHE: Yes,

ER: In referring to the acquisition of knowledge from infancy and the potential availability of such knowledge, you are making an effort to activate association pathways to unconscious learning and knowledge that can be *Utilized* in dealing with current problems. You closely associate this suggestion with the ordinary ones for comfort and relaxation that have been successful with Dr. S. This association of a new suggestion with one that has been previously successful tends to facilitate the new suggestion.

MHE: And many times in the past
you have been able to hear something
and to forget it immediately.
[Pause]

It is a common experience.
When being introduced,
you shake hands and go on to the next person.
And wonder what Mrs. Jones' name is
[Pause]
while you are shaking hands with Mrs. Smith.
Your mind has that
knowledge,
and you don't even need
to know that you have it.
[Pause]
Months later, you can meet Mrs. Jones on the street and spontaneously call
her by her name.
You don't even need to know when or where you met,
for when the occasion arises,
your unconscious will supply that knowledge.

ER: Here you begin to elicit forgetting mechanisms by leading her into association pathways where forgetting is likely to occur. This is very typical of you; you rarely give direct suggestions. In one of your early papers, you even say of your experience with thousands of trances that "hyper-suggestibility was not noticed" (Erickson, 1932/2010). Is it possible you don't believe that hyper-suggestibility is characteristic of trance? You substitute the gradual elicitation of natural mental and behavioral mechanisms by verbal and non-verbal associations for the so-called phenomenon of hyper-suggestibility of trance. Hyper-suggestibility is actually an artifact?

MHE: Yes. It's just called hyper-suggestibility.

ER: But it's really natural mental and behavioral mechanisms the operator has succeeded in leading a patient into. The art of hypnosis is the skill with which the therapist succeeds in evoking these natural mechanisms for a specific therapeutic purpose.

MHE: As soon as you know
only you and I,
or you and my voice are here,
your right hand will descend to your thigh
[Pause as her hand begins to descend]
here is only here,
nothing more.
[Pause]
You don't even need to know your name.
As you learned a long time ago
you are me,
and me was everything.
[Pause]
I would like to have you count backward from 20 to 1,
and begin the count right now.

ER: This is a subtle form of directive where you don't actually tell her to do something, but you assume something will be done. You then only give her the option of signaling when it is done. The giving of the signal when it is done actually seems to have both motivating and reinforcing properties on the implied directive.

MHE: A parallel with ordinary behavior is when you eat or drink until you are satisfied. ***You will know*** when the eating and drinking are done.

ER: Do you agree that "the implied directive" is a good name for this?

MHE: Yes. I'm not telling her to ignore the presence of others in the room. No one can do that. But you can limit your awareness. We all have had extensive training in limiting our awareness.

ER: We can limit our awareness to a book, a movie, etc. Actually that is another way of describing concentration: the mind focuses on one limited area and omits everything else.

[Mrs. L opens her eyes, but does not reorient to her body. Therefore, she is still in trance.]

MHE: Tell us what you think we've experienced.
[Pause. Mrs. L's baby continues crying very loudly.]

Mrs. L: We were talking and we were very comfortable.

MHE: Do you hear your daughter?

Mrs. L: Yes.

MHE: How do you feel about that?

Mrs. L: Comfortable.

MHE: Does it distress you?

Mrs. L: Somewhat, but I don't want to help her right now.

MHE: That's an odd feeling, isn't it?

Mrs. L: Yes.

MHE: It's a nice thing to learn
because it will teach you objectivity,
which will enable you to do right things at the right time
in the right way.
A little exercise by your daughter
is good for her.

ER: Because she did not reorient to her body we know she was still in trance even though she opened her eyes.

MHE: The fact that she still is "comfortable" and does not want to bother helping her crying daughter also verifies the trance state. There is something lacking there in the total awareness of the self and the situation.

ER: Showing that she is in an altered state.

MHE: An altered state, and she knows it! A person in trance doesn't feel certain things that are appropriate.

ER: So, this helps us to understand trance as an altered state.

MHE: Yes. Her verbal statement means: I know the baby should be attended to, but I don't feel like it; the momentum does not exist to lead me to the effort to attend to her.

ER: In trance, the motivating properties of stimuli are lost?

MHE: There is a limitation of what would normally be spontaneous behavior.

ER: There is a limitation of the ego's executive function of relating appropriately to the outside world. They do not relate to the outside world except through the therapist.

MHE: You really think you are awake, don't you?

Mrs. L: No.

MHE: That's right, you don't.
[Pause]

ER: You are affirming the trance with this ***Double Bind*** question?

MHE: Yes. I'm proving the trance exists.

MHE: Who is here?

Mrs. L: You are.

MHE: Who else?

Mrs. L: I don't know.

MHE: Is your daughter's voice here?

Mrs. L: Yes.

MHE: That's a nice sound, isn't it?

Mrs. L: Yes.

MHE: How do you feel about being in a trance with your eyes wide open?

Mrs. L: I like this better. Because then I know what is going on.

MHE: And what is going on? Are you enjoying yourself?

Mrs. L: Yes.

ER: Her response of not knowing who else is here is actually a negative hallucination; she is apparently unaware that Dr. S and I are seated right next to her, well within her range of vision. So here she has lost the ability to be aware of our presence, which you earlier suggested to her in the form of the implied directive.

MHE: What am I doing?

Mrs. L: Talking.

MHE: Anything else?
Mrs. L: Looking at me.

MHE: Anything else?

Mrs. L: No.

MHE: And how are you seeing me?

Mrs. L: With my eyes.

MHE: What else do you see?

Mrs. L: That book.

ER: The literalism of these responses ("talking," "looking at me," "with my eyes") is a classical indication of deep trance. You might appear to be having a casual conversation, but you are actually making a careful evaluation of her mental state.

MHE: Can you look and not see?

Mrs. L: Yes.

MHE: And we can be all alone here.
[Pause]
Or someone named Dr. S can join us.

ER: Posing a suggestion indirectly in the form of a question carries less risk of failure. If they cannot accomplish the suggestion they simply say "No" and nothing is lost. We don't know if she actually did experience a negative hallucination of not seeing here since you did not test it.

MHE: Look at Dr. S. Tell Dr. S to count to 20.

Mrs. L: Count to 20, Dr. S.
MHE: And to take a deep breath at the count of 20.

Mrs. L: Take a deep breath at the count of 20.
[Pause]

MHE: What change do you notice in her?

Mrs. L: She breathes slower,
her head lowers,
her eyes are closed.
[Pause]

MHE: What else do you notice?

Mrs. L: She is relaxed,
her hands are on her legs.

MHE: Do you think she knows her hands are there?

Mrs. L: I don't know.

ER: Now, with Mrs. L in trance, why are you suggesting that she hypnotize Dr. S?

MHE: I've had subjects determined not to go into a trance even though they volunteered. I let them express their resistance, and then I tell them to hypnotize someone else. When they hypnotize someone else, they start wanting their own hypnotic trance to develop.

ER: So, you've changed their set from resisting trance to wanting trance by making them an operator.

MHE: They now want a trance, but it's not been defined necessarily as trance in another.

ER: This is an interesting example of how you indirectly enhance motivation for trance experience. At some unconscious or preverbal level, an individual does not distinguish between "wanting a trance" for oneself or another. Wanting a trance for someone else will, by association, evoke partial aspects of trance in oneself and therefore enhance the possibility that one will more easily experience a trance if given an opportunity at that time. You were treating Dr. S as a resistant subject here?

MHE: Oh, yes. Her resistance isn't toward me or toward learning. ***She just doesn't quite trust her unconscious mind to do all the learning necessary.***

ER: Her conscious mind keeps coming in during her trance efforts.

MHE: To make sure.

ER: This is a typical problem many intellectually trained professional people will have in experiencing trance and learning on an unconscious level.

> **MHE: You don't need to know where your hands are.**
>
> **Dr. S doesn't need to know where hers are.**
> **[Pause]**

ER: Here again, you use not knowing: "You don't need to know where your hands are." You don't try to directly suggest, "Have no awareness of your hands." You simply point out that she need not know where they are.

This *Utilizes* that everyday mental mechanism where we don't actually have to know where our hands are such as when we watch TV or a movie, for example.

MHE: When driving a car you don't always have to have your foot on the brake. You don't need your best dress today. There are a lot of don'ts in life.

ER: You keep emphasizing all those "don'ts" and things you don't need; it's a means of relaxing the directing and controlling functions of the patient's ego.

MHE: By using established learning patterns.

ER: So instead of giving direct suggestions, you use established learning patterns that are already present in the subject.

MHE: And in some way
I want you to see someone
who is someone between you and me
whom you haven't seen in many years.

[ER was actually seated between MHE and Dr. S. Mrs. L opens her eyes and studies ER very carefully, and then with a slightly incredulous look she begins to talk with ER, who gradually assumes the role of John which Dr. L gives to ER.]

Mrs. L: John!

MHE: Who is John?

Mrs. L: He is a friend from college.

MHE: Now, speak to him.

Mrs. L: Hi.

ER: Hi.

Mrs. L: How have you been doing?
ER: Pretty good.

Mrs. L: Are you still in the Air Force?

ER: I left.

Mrs. L: Where are you living now?

ER: Where would you expect?

Mrs. L: Puerto Rico?

ER: Yes.

[A general set of questions and answers now takes place between Mrs. L and ER playing the role of John.]

ER: You never did positive visual hallucinatory work with Mrs. L before. Did you know she was going to respond so well to it?

MHE: She is a very good subject. She is a very gentle, soft personality, simple and uncomplicated. Such a personality does not feel insecure when you offer them something.

ER: You don't command or apparently even suggest: ***you offer*** and thus, ***Utilize*** her own inner needs and motivation. You've also built up your successful suggestion with her by first evoking a series of easier phenomena. You had her remain undisturbed by her crying child, lose the ability to stand, engage in ***Hand Levitation***, forgetting and negative visual hallucination before you felt sure enough to attempt a positive visual hallucination. This positive hallucination may be actually more in the nature of an illusion since she is actually seeing me and distorting my image to fit the image of her friend John. Presumably the next step would be a genuine visual hallucination of seeing something out there in space without any reality props.

MHE: Now listen to what I say carefully
and really understand what I say.

MHE: "Do you ***really*** understand?" means "distrust your conscious understanding."

ER: You're throwing doubt on the conscious mind again even though you seem to be saying the opposite.

MHE: That's right! "Do you ***really*** understand!" implies a strong doubt. To say, "And you will ***really*** understand" means the same as "you don't really understand." It has the same meaning either way you state it, positively or negatively.

MHE: Why did John just leave!
He did, you know.

Mrs. L: He went back home!

MHE: Where was he sitting!

Mrs. L: On a chair.

MHE: Can you look over in the direction of the place where he was sitting!

[Mrs. L now looks at the seat of the chair still occupied by ER. Her looking at the seat is in marked contrast to the way she looked at his face when she was talking to him earlier when she

projected John on him. Looking at the seat as she is suggests that she is now not seeing ER sitting there.]

MHE: What kind of chair was he sitting on?

Mrs. L: A green chair.

MHE: Tell me when you think he left.

Mrs. L: A few minutes ago.

MHE: Was he willing to go?

Mrs. L: Yes.

MHE: Why was he willing to go?

Mrs. L: He wasn't needed anymore.

MHE: Did you enjoy seeing him?

Mrs. L: Yes.

MHE: I'm emphasizing John was here. He had to be here in order to leave.

ER: So, you're ratifying the fact that she has just had an hallucinatory experience.

MHE: Yes. He can't leave unless he has been here.

ER: At the same time, you're telling her to make him disappear.

MHE: Yes. But you're making her affirm he was here.

ER: You ask, "Why did John just leave?" rather than simply tell her to erase the whole experience and run the risk of her denying that it ever happened in the first place. Actually, I've notices that all questions have a hypnotic effect insofar as they fixate and focus attention. Is this why you ask so many questions?

MHE: The patient needs help, and he does not know where to look, so I'd better focus his looking with a question.

> **MHE: Is there anyone else you would like to see that you haven't seen for a long time?**
>
> **Mrs. L: Yes.**
>
> **MHE: Who?**
>
> **Mrs. L: Bill. Bonjour.**
> **[Mrs. L begins to speak French to an hallucinated friend, Bill, who is now projected on ER. She now looks at ER's face as she speaks to him.]**
>
> **ER: [Playing the role of Bill] Let's speak English today.**
>
> **Mrs. L: No.**

ER: By asking this question about who *she* would like to see, you're *Utilizing* her internal memory banks and motivation to facilitate a hallucinatory experience.

> **ER: How come? Is it not possible for me to have learned English?**

Mrs. L: No.

MHE: Your French is rusty, Mrs. L. How come this person says some English words?

Mrs. L: He understands, he knows one or two words of English.
[Mrs. L frowns doubtfully and appears uneasy.]

MHE: Everything is fine, Mrs. L.
Very, very fine.
[Pause]
I want you to feel very pleased within yourself, would you?

ER: Since it did not fit her internal understanding of Bill, my suggestion that Bill could have learned English had no effect. Even though she is experiencing deep trance, an obviously impossible suggestion does not work. It arouses discomfort and resistance. Suggestions must match the patient's internal needs and patterns of learning and motivation to be effective.

MHE: Yes, this difficulty is a good example of that.

ER: You were quick to reassure her when she showed uneasiness about the inconsistency of her friend Bill knowing English.

MHE: Now listen to my words
very carefully.
Listen to them very carefully and understand them.
Do you think Mr. A will propose? [Mr. A is Mrs. L's husband of many years.]

Mrs. L: Yes.

MHE: What makes you think so?

Mrs. L: He loves me.

[Pause]

[Conversation wherein an age-regressed Mrs. L describes some of her husband's feelings for her as she experienced them before they were married.]

ER: You solicit her careful attention to prepare her for the subtle indirect suggestion that is to follow. By using the future tense here, you imply that Mrs. L's husband has not yet proposed. This reorients her to the past before she was married. So you've effected an age regression without any direct suggestion for it.

MHE: Yes. And here again when I say, "What makes you think so?"

MHE: Close your eyes,
and shortly I am going to awaken you,
and when I awaken you,
it will seem to you as if you had just sat down
and were waiting for me to begin.
Is that all right?

Mrs. L: Yes.

ER: By reorienting her to the time before we began trance work, you are effecting a possible amnesia for the trance work that just took place.

MHE: Now I am going to start the count
now: 20, 19, 18, 17, 16, 15, 14, 13, 12, 11, 10, 9, 8, 9, 10 11,
12, 13, 14, 15,
16, 15, 14, 13, 12, 11, 10, 9, 8, 7, 6, 5, 4, 3,
[Pause]
2,
[Pause]
1

How do you feel?

Mrs. L: Fine.

ER: Why do you do this counting reversal as you're waking her up?

MHE: You take them by surprise. They think you've made a mistake. And then they find as you count up toward 20, they are following the instruction to go deeper and deeper into trance. You reverse it downward again, and now they know from personal experience that they were deeper. They were lighter in trance and then deeper.

ER: You're proving the efficiency of counting to vary trance depth.

MHE: Yes. I've had patients tell me "that was an awful jerk when you reversed the count."

ER: That jerk proves and ratifies the trance.

MHE: That's their subjective proof of trance—not mine.

MHE: Are you ready to begin work?

Mrs. L: Okay.

MHE: What do you think we will do?

Mrs. L: I'm not sure what we are going to do. I suppose you want me to work with ER, so I will have a different experience. I don't know why the tape recorder.

MHE: You don't?

Mrs. L: No.

MHE: What is Dr. S doing?

Mrs. L: She looks like she's asleep.
MHE: Have you or I bored her that much?

Mrs. L: I doubt it.

MHE: Is she asleep?

Mrs. L: Yes.

ER: The fact that Mrs. L is successful in following this posthypnotic suggestion which Dr. S in part failed last session indicates that Mrs. L is more accomplished in trance learning. Allowing Dr. S to witness this while she is in the trance state makes it more likely that she will do it in the future.

[Dr. S makes motions as if to awaken]

MHE: Is her sleep stopping?

MHE: [To Dr. S] Go far away?

Dr. S: Yes.

MHE: Very far away.

[Dr. S now goes deeper into a trance while Erickson engages Mrs. L and ER in a casual conversation wherein it is learned that Mrs. L does not recall that she has been in a trance state. MHE now proceeds with Mrs. L as follows.]

ER: Dr. S was seemingly about to wake up here.

MHE: You use a direct authoritative suggestion in this situation where you see a patient in an uncertain state. When she is uncertain, you help her by taking over firmly. Just as when a child is uncertain about something, you say, "I'll tell you when to go... *Now*!" That's the same sort of thing. That is acceptable as help since patients have a long history of having accepted help in such circumstances.

ER: Direct authoritative suggestion works and helps when patients are uncertain, sitting on the fence. They are not really following a suggestion, they are just accepting a helpful push.

MHE: Have we done anything to you of which you are unaware?

Mrs. L: No.

MHE: Are you sure now?

Mrs. L: Positively.

MHE: Have you ever seen a dispute between the conscious and unconscious mind?
Now watch your right hand.
If I have done
a great deal with you
this morning,
your right hand will lift.

[Her hand begins to lift.]

Now, have I done
a great deal
with you this morning?

Mrs. L: A little.

MHE: How much?

[Her hand begins to lift more rapidly.]

Mrs. L: I don't know how to measure.

MHE: Do I know anything about you that I didn't know before?

Mrs. L: Yes.

MHE: What?

Mrs. L: You know that I went to Tunisia.

You know about some of my friends.

MHE: Could you tell me more?

Mrs. L: We were just talking about it.

MHE: When?

Mrs. L: Just a while ago.

Before I went to check the baby.

MHE: Can you tell me more than before?

Mrs. L: I think maybe.

MHE: What is your hand doing?

Mrs. L: Staying there.

MHE:: What?

Mrs. L: I think it is going up.

MHE: Why?

Mrs. L: I think you did more with me than I thought.
[Pause]
MHE: Do you believe yourself or your hand?

Mrs. L: My hand.

MHE: Have you forgotten what I did with you?
Consciously forgotten?

Mrs. L: Yes.

MHE: Did you see anybody here in the office today?

Mrs. L: Dr. Rossi.

MHE: Anybody else?

Mrs. L: Dr. S.

MHE: Here, you're teaching people by this conflict that their unconscious can do something that they did not know about. She herself is furnishing that evidence.

ER: So, you're proving the existence of the unconscious to her.

MHE: In the presence of her conscious mind, you demonstrate that the conscious can think one way and the unconscious another. You're going to have a chance to see and prove within yourself that they think differently.

ER: This is a highly important experience for patients to have: a demonstration of the existence of the unconscious. They would thereby tend to become more amenable to respecting and learning to relate to their unconscious. The therapist can then use ideomotor signaling to detect and monitor any sort of psychodynamic conflict in this way, as you have just done. There is a great need for clinically oriented research to develop new ways of using ideomotor signaling and to evaluate its validity in different situations.

MHE: Just as when you demonstrate to patients their motivation about stopping smoking. You ask them to put a few coins in a large bottle every time they would have lit up. A quarter or two when they would have bought a carton. Pretty soon the people who really want to quit see all that money piling up. That further motivates them to quit and save all that money. It also proves to them that they do want to quit. That is their proof. And when they fail to pile up the coins, that also is their proof that they don't want to quit.

ER: I see in this the possibility of a new therapeutic technique: Externalizing internal processes and motivations, so patients can relate to their inner dynamics in a concrete and easily comprehensible way. What patients do externally with the coins can be a reflection of what they do within themselves. The coins (or whatever other external gauge you attach to internal process requiring change) function as a cognitive feedback device altering the internal dynamics.

Ideomotor signaling appears to be an especially fine way of getting an assessment of internal processes and motivations because the autonomous aspect of the ideomotor movement is so convincing to the person who is experiencing it. In this example, Mrs. L actually believes the ideomotor movement of her hand more than her own conscious ideation.

MHE: Anybody else?

Mrs. L: John.

MHE: You saw him?

Mrs. L: Ummm.

MHE: Do you know you are in a trance right now?

Mrs. L: No.

MHE: You really can go into a trance
effectively.
You can enjoy
using your abilities

ER: She was awake; why was she going back into trance about here?

MHE: That's a thing you have to watch for. I noticed here that her face began to iron out and that there was more of a fixed, unblinking stare and a lessening of body mobility as she talked. ***Trance tends to be revivified when you review any hypnotic phenomenon that has occurred in the subjects.*** They begin to relive what they are talking about and begin to reexperience the trance, sometimes with and sometimes without their knowledge. So then you say, "You don't know you are in a trance?" And they don't know. So, you've just taught them it's possible to go into a trance without knowing it.

ER: That's a fantastic way of circumventing consciousness and remembering trance by association.

MHE: Yes.

ER: You revivify the trance by talking of trance events. Then you slip in the ***Double Bind*** question, "Do you know you are in a trance right now?" An answer of "Yes," means she knows, an answer of "No," means she does not ***know*** she was in trance. Both answers imply an acknowledgment of being in trance, only the knowledge of it was in question. The ***Double Bind*** reinforces trance further, so she recognizes that trance happened without her consciousness knowing exactly why. This demonstrates how little the conscious mind really knows. That is a very important learning because it enables her to recognize the value of exploring her unconscious and its capacities, which are greater than her conscious mind believes.

MHE: That's right.

> **MHE: A process that you don't know you have,**
> **but abilities that are in your unconscious mind.**
> **[Pause]**
> **Your eyes are wide open**
> **and adjusting so it won't get dark.**
> **[Pause]**

ER: Here again, you reinforce the idea that she has more ability than she believes. You're always building up the unconscious and the greater potentialities that people actually have while depotentiating their conscious mind with its limited beliefs about what can be accomplished. You allow a brief pause for that message to sink in, but then, before she can debate the matter, you immediately follow up with a self-evident truism about her eyes being open. The obvious truth of this must evoke a "Yes" within her that may now in part reinforce the previous suggestion about her unconscious abilities. You like to use statements of obvious truth to reinforce a previous suggestion. In your ***Interspersal Technique***, (Erickson, 1966b) you use a series of obvious truths to surround and thus reinforce every suggestion.

> **MHE: I am now going to awaken you**
> **and I want you to be very surprised**
> **you won't be able to bend your legs**

MHE: I'll take credit for awakening her, but she takes credit for going into trance.

ER: You're using the conditional suggestion format for this posthypnotic suggestion. The suggestion ("You won't be able to bend your legs") is paired with an inevitable occurrence ("I am now going to awaken you")

MHE: and you won't, will you?
[Pause]
You will see them but you won't be able to feel them
after I awaken you.
Agreed?
20, 19, 18, 15, 12, 10, 9, 8, 5, 3,
2,
1,
Are you ready to check on your daughter now?

Mrs. L: No

MHE: How do you really feel?
[Pause]

MHE: These shifts from the negative (won't) to the positive (will) and sometimes the shifts from positive to negative are keeping the patient in a constant state of movement. You change the mind this way and back.

ER: What's the value of keeping that constant movement?

MHE: You don't let the patients get a set. A mental set they can stay with.

ER: Why not?

MHE: You don't want them with ***their*** mental set.

ER: You keep them in movement, so they will have to grasp onto your mental set?

MHE: Yes, the mental set you want to work with. You keep them in flux so you can constantly orient them. But you aren't telling them, "I want you to pay attention to this one thing."

> **Mrs. L: My legs aren't awake.**
> **They don't work.**
>
> **MHE: How does that make you feel?**
>
> **Mrs. L: Awkward.**
>
> **MHE: How does that make you feel when your legs don't work?**
>
> **Mrs. L: Very limited.**
>
> **MHE: It doesn't distress you, does it?**
> **[Pause]**
>
> **MHE: And you can do that with any part of your body any time it is necessary.**
> **You can also use them any time it is necessary.**
> **Any time you need to you will be in full possession of your abilities. Do you understand that?**

MHE: She has a master's degree and yet, she uses this juvenile language here. Hypnotic subjects do regress to simpler forms of thinking, feeling, and behavior. Simpler, more youthful, less complicated forms.

ER: There is even more to this posthypnotic suggestion of not being able to stand: You are emphasizing ***not doing*** as a basic mode of hypnotic experience. You are giving her an experience in the basic notion that in trance: It is not the ego or the patient's usual waking patterns that accomplish the hypnotic suggestion.

In your paper on deep hypnosis, you said:

> "Deep hypnosis is that level of hypnosis that permits the subject to function adequately and directly at an unconscious level of awareness without interference by the conscious mind." (Erickson, 1952)

In a simple and subtle way, you then generalize this successful posthypnotic suggestion on her legs to include any other part of her body. You can greatly expand the area of any successful suggestion by this simple phenomenon of ***generalization***. It's a basic principle of learning theory as well as hypnosis.

MHE: Do you think you are wide awake?

Mrs. L: No.

MHE: That's right.
Close your eyes, and now this time you can awaken when I say, "one."
Now, one.

ER: She is still in a trance because she is now carrying out your earlier posthypnotic suggestion, "You won't be able to bend your legs." You have described (Erickson & Erickson, 1941) how carrying out a posthypnotic suggestion reinduces a momentary trance that can be ***Utilized*** to reestablish another trance. This illustrates the care one must occasionally take to awaken a subject when posthypnotic suggestions are used. You noticed at this point that even though you went through a formal "awakening" procedure by counting backward to one, she did not go through the typical awakening movements of stretching and so on, to reorient to her body. Therefore, she may not be really awake. This is confirmed when she acknowledges the posthypnotic suggestion with her statement about her legs not being awake. You therefore ask the ***Double Bind*** question about whether she "thinks" she is awake. Any answer (Yes or No), can imply she is still in trance. She readily admits she is still in trance, so you simply go about reawakening her again.

> **[Mrs. L now reorients to her body by moving her hands a bit, readjusting her legs, etc.]**
>
> **MHE: What is the different feeling you have now?**
> **[Pause]**
>
> **Mrs. L: I can do what I want, what my conscious mind is thinking about. Before, I could think about things but I didn't really feel like doing anything about it.**
>
> **MHE: That's right.**
> **Anything else you would like to add?**
>
> **Mrs. L: Well, when I am in a trance, I am much more relaxed, feeling, sort of good, except when I'm in a really deep trance, like I tend to lose the sense of balance a lot and I feel slightly awkward.**

ER: Are you confirming she is now awake as well as ratifying the trance by asking her what different feelings she has on awakening?

MHE: Yes. When you think about things, your body makes many ideo-motor movements. When children watch a movie, it's particularly obvious how they move about, thrusting this way and that, acting out the scene they are watching. Here, Mrs. L is saying, "I can do what I want, what my conscious mind is thinking about. In trance, I could think about things but I really didn't feel like doing anything about." In ordinary waking state, you start thinking about scratching your head and you immediately get subliminal movements in your fingers to do it. But in trance, you can think about it without subliminal movements.

ER: In the ordinary waking state, ideomotor movements are acted out, in trance they are not?

MHE: Yes.

ER: But how about finger signaling and ***Hand Levitation*** where you are using ideomotor movements to initiate or deepen trance?

MHE: That is where the operator is using ideomotor movements in a special fashion. You see a child watching a movie go through all the actions of what he is watching. But if you put him in a trance to hallucinate the same movie, he will watch it without body movements. He just sees.

ER: So there is a dissociation between ideation and that motor behavior in trance. That's why people are so quiet in trance. And that body stillness can be taken as a reliable indicator of trance.

MHE: Yes.

> **MHE: It's all right to feel that way, but you don't have to be off balance.**
> **You can feel any way you want to, but you don't have to be any way that you**
> **don't want to be.**
> **It is nice to feel warm when you are cold.**
> **It is nice to be cold when you are warm.**
> **How is it when you feel wet all over?**

Mrs. L: It makes me feel dry.

MHE: Describe that feeling for me.

MHE: If she can't think about walking and do it in the ordinary way (in the awake state), she loses her balance.

> [Erickson demonstrates how he cannot really think about moving his weak right arm without moving his left arm, which is not stronger. The differences in muscle is a long term consequence of the polio.]

MHE: I can't get any minimal movements in the right hand, so I can't even feel how I would move it if I could. Body feelings complement the thought of lifting the hand.

Now, Mrs. L has lost her sense of balance because she lost her body feeling in trance.

ER: She lost the sensory feedback the muscles give the mind, so she loses her sense of balance.

MHE: That's right! But if you instruct the person to have those movements, he can. When training a rifle team, I saw to it that they had certain types of subliminal body movements that were conductive to accurate shooting. When a shot putter got stuck on the shot put at 58 feet, I pointed out that his muscles did not know the difference between 58 feet and 58 feet and one-sixteenth of an inch. Roger Bannister broke the four-minute mile by reducing four minutes to 240 seconds because here 1/1000 of a second counts.

ER: This is all due to altering body feedback, altering the ideomotor connections. So, you can actually enhance physical abilities by breaking through conscious bias about limitations.

MHE: Yes, unrecognized conscious bias.

ER: Perhaps this is the secret of enhancing abilities in hypnosis: Breaking through the conscious bias of what our limitations are.

MHE: Yes. People say, "But I always eat cereal for breakfast! But we always have chicken on Sunday." These are all conscious biases. You can broaden your activity, however, if you recognize the bias. Experimentalists in hypnosis ought to know about the unlimited number of biases that everybody builds up.

ER: These biases are bedeviling their experiments, they are part of the source of individual differences, etc.

MHE: People who accomplish a great many things are people who have freed themselves from biases. These are the creative people.

ER: You can define creativity as freedom from the biases of the past. If you can break out of the sets of your forefathers, you can experience originality.

MHE: It's simply a conscious bias when people say they don't like cold. Sometimes it's good to feel cold—especially when you're too warm.

ER: So you're breaking through her conscious biases here and making her a more flexible person with these instructions. Then she picks up your idea of flexibility when she answers, "It makes me feel dry," to your query about wet.

MHE: Yes.

Mrs. L: It's kind of cold—no, I'm comfortable, but cold.

MHE: All right.
You can be dry now.
Now I am going to do something.
[Pause]
I want you to have a certain feeling
and a contrary knowledge.
I want you to feel naked from the waist up
even though you know
You are dressed from the waist up.
I want you to feel naked.
[Pause]

ER: She has been awake up to this point, but now she's going back into trance in a seemingly spontaneous manner here since she says "I'm comfortable." Why?

MHE: Because I have removed biases.

ER: Really? You protected her by reminding her that she is clothed, but then you surprised her by asking she feel naked. You have removed biases and conscious sets so she automatically slips into trance?

MHE: Biases are a part of our conscious living.

ER: They keep us conscious? Would you go as far as that?

MHE: They are not just biases, they are part of the way we experience the world.

ER: They are so much a part of the ground of our everyday experience that if we are deprived of them, we suddenly lose our conscious orientation. And that results in trance. So, by simply removing people's biases and preconceptions, they tend to go into trance. I find that so hard to believe!

MHE: You have given them a new kind of freedom in the trance state. With a few simple words you restore a sense of freedom, and that belongs to the trance state. They then begin to feel that freedom.

ER: Freedom from conscious bias is characteristic of the trance state. Can we then call this an indirect reinduction of trance by removing biases?

MHE: When you use the word "bias" it is so easily misunderstood. It is actually a common set.

ER: Removing a common set is what reinduces trance?

MHE: Yes. Another example is that when you have a subject talk about trance events and feelings, he slips back into trance. That's what Jay Haley means when he says I take a person in and out of trance without awareness of it.

> **MHE: Do you want ER to look at you?**
>
> **Mrs. L: No.**
> **[Mrs. L now covers her breasts with her arms crossed over them.]**

Do you want me to look at you?

Mrs. L: No.

MHE: To answer that question, she has got to feel naked.

ER: So, you are ratifying the hypnotic phenomenon of feeling naked. That's another example of the ***implied*** directive by asking a question that requires a hypnotic experience to have occurred!

MHE: That's right!

ER: You know these things are so subtle that I actually feel a bit dizzy, a bit not quite all here, in my effort to understand these things. I feel as if I'm in hypnosis right now. It's so hard to understand these things. I guess my old mental sets are breaking and my effort to grasp this new understanding makes me feel a little woozy!

MHE: She covers her breasts with her arms here. So, I dodge all the difficulties of directing her to being nude by simply asking that question.

ER: You dodge all the doubts she might have had about whether or not she really felt naked, etc.

MHE: I made it a ***fait accompli*** by asking that question.

ER: You use that ***fait accompli*** a lot by the careful use of questions.

MHE: That's right.

MHE: There is a contradiction, isn't there?

Mrs. L: I guess so.

MHE: It makes you uncomfortable, doesn't it?

Mrs. L: Yes.

MHE: It is a delightful thing to be able to use your mind consciously
[Pause]
and unconsciously.

[A few personal and identifying sentences are omitted here.]

MHE: What is the contradiction? She is getting nude for me (obeying the hypnotic suggestion), but she doesn't want me to look at her. She doesn't really get what I mean when she answers, "I guess so."

ER: Since she doesn't understand, you're again keeping her off balance.

MHE: I also discharge any great, discomfort by letting her know it's "delightful" to be contradictory insofar as you're able "to use your mind consciously and unconsciously" while it allows her to continue to be nude.

ER: You let her be comfortable with the contradiction and at the same time reinforce her being nude. You have her all tied up, she cannot move any which way but what you suggest.

MHE: The pause between "consciously and unconsciously" effects a separation between conscious and unconscious. It's delightful to use the conscious mind: to know you are naked. You used your unconscious mind to become naked.

ER: So, you let consciousness do something and unconsciousness do something, and they both cooperate in the task you're assigning.

MHE: That's right. She wants to be clothed. That's a conscious thing. She puts her arms over her breasts: that's a conscious thing. But she is nude and that nude feeling is from her unconscious, she got nude unconsciously.

ER: She got nude unconsciously through a feeling process rather than figuring it out with conscious logic. Feelings come from our unconscious.

MHE: Yes.

> **MHE: Dr. Rossi would like to do something**
> **which involves some rather complicated mental phenomena.**
> **Are you willing to do that?**
>
> **Mrs. L: Okay, except I don't have a good memory of my childhood.**
>
> **MHE: I'm glad you said that.**

ER: You're careful to get her permission here and give her a preparatory set for new work. I notice you always do this when you introduce something new. Mrs. L, in a manner that is all too typical, gives expression to one of the ways her conscious bias limits her ability to remember. You seize upon that self-limitation and seek to break through it.

> **MHE: If your unconscious**
> **thinks you have**
> **a far better memory**

of your childhood than you think,

[Mrs. L's hand does lift.]

MHE: You have a better memory
of your childhood
than you know about.
Do you mind looking back
at your childhood?
Mrs. L, close your eyes.
[Pause]
I would like to have you be puzzled by
something
that you can see.
I need some information first.
Did your father have a garden when you were very young?

Mrs. L: Yes.

MHE: All right.
I would like to have you
be puzzled by something
that you can see on the
other side of a garden.
[Pause]
It's a little girl.
She is a nice little girl.
Maybe she is doing something
she shouldn't be doing,
maybe she has dirty hands
or a dirty face.
I would like to have you clutch that child,
hold her
and
hold her.

ER: Her hand lifting demonstrates the difference between her conscious and limited view of herself and her unconscious's vaster degree of potentiality. In an indirect way, you are also depotentiating her conscious sets and assumptions by making a contradiction evident: A contradiction between her consciously expressed opinion and her arm levitation that implies a contrary opinion from the unconscious. Again you are demonstrating how to precipitate a contradiction or conflict between conscious and unconscious to keep patients off balance, in a state of creative flux, where they are more able to shake free of their limiting sets to do more creative work with themselves. Your suggestions that she be "puzzled" introduces a set for ***confusion*** that also will help her break through her conscious limitations.

MHE: I would like to have you
watch her grow up.
[Pause]
And really watch that child grow up
[Pause]
and notice the changes in her.
There are going to be many changes,
many conflicting ideas,
believing,
unbelieving,
some things that can't be shared with strangers,
and I want that little girl to grow up,
and after a while you will notice
that that little girl is really Mrs. L.
So be interested in watching Mrs. L.
[Pause]
Look at her with interest and appreciation,
and you can know anything
you wish about her,
but you will only tell those things
to me that you can share with strangers.

ER: You now embark on a series of very general suggestions that could apply to anyone, yet they evoke highly specific and personal memories.

MHE: In real life, as one grows up through puberty, one naturally goes through periods of great uncertainty: believing and unbelieving. "Some things that can't be shared with strangers," guides her into very personal feelings and experiences without my telling her to have a personal experience.

MHE: Notice at times
you forget
that girl is Mrs. L
[Pause]
and then you suddenly realize
yes, it is.
[Pause]

ER: This type of forgetting is a means of depotentiating consciousness further in trance. She is encouraged to drift along on more autonomous and unconscious fantasy currents until she again catches herself, until the observer function of the ego again checks in, as it inevitably will. I wonder if this natural alternation between unconscious drifting versus observing and in part controlling is responsible for the alternation in trance depth that takes place spontaneously in hypnosis?

MHE: Notice that she
is getting a different feeling
about her body.
[Pause]
Notice that at times
that girl thinks to herself,
Is this really me?
Notice that at times you look at that girl
you can see yourself,
that really isn't me,
but yes, it is, but it isn't, but it is.
Have a very delightful time
[Pause]

MHE: When a girl begins to develop breasts or pubic hair, she goes through such feeling: It is me but it isn't.

ER: So, without her being aware of it, you're guiding her into a re-experiencing of puberty feelings.

MHE: and time is so long,
[Pause]
no matter how short the watch says time is,
it is really long.
[Pause]
And since
you are going to share
some of that knowledge with me,
and pick out certain
definite things
that you can share with strangers,
but only those
that can be shared with strangers.
[Pause]
You have seen movies
of flowers opening
and in the same way you look at that little girl
growing up
from a little bud till full-bloom rose.

ER: This is an example of your routine use of *Time Distortion* interpolated in a place where it will obviously facilitate the work at hand. You then protect her by emphasizing that she will share only certain things she can share with strangers.

MHE: There is another indirect association to puberty: Womanhood opening up like a flower.

MHE: And when you have completed, really
looking at her, you will awaken
and tell us only those things that you are willing to share.

[After a minute or so, Mrs. L awakens and stretches her arms.]

MHE: Hi, Mrs. L.

Mrs. L: Hi.

ER: It's interesting how you make awakening contingent upon completing that inner task., which also reinforces the inner work. That's a form of the ***implied directive*** that includes a posthypnotic suggestion to tell only what she is willing to share.

MHE: That's right.

ER: You know she's going to have to awaken sometime, and she might even be eager to awake . She will thus do the inner work so she can wake up. When she finally does actually awaken, that tends to reinforce the fact that inner work has been done.

MHE: Yes, it's her admission that the inner work has been done. Awakening her in this manner compels her to do it, but I haven't verbally said, "Now you do that!" She does not recognize that I have compelled her.

[As Mrs. L awakens, Erickson greets her with a cheery "Hi" and then encourages her to recount some of her early experiences that she recovered while in the trance state. After about 10 minutes of this casual recounting, Dr. S, who had been in a trance of her own, spontaneously awakens herself. On questioning, it is learned that Dr. S felt a little bit bored, perhaps a bit resentful that Mrs. L had been getting all the attention, and she just felt like awakening to join us. She had awakened herself by saying silently to herself, "I am going to count to three and then awaken feeling refreshed and alert," and she did exactly that. She is much too polite to complain to Erickson, but she is in a quietly doubtful and questioning mood about the whole procedure.]

MHE: This cheery "Hi" on awakening is because "Hi" belongs to the world of consciousness. I'm thereby telling her to be wide awake and forget all about that unconscious activity.

ER: By so dismissing it, you're effecting an amnesia except for those things you said she could share.

MHE: Yes, I'm causing an amnesia by implying "that's all over and done with. Now let's go on to something else."

Chapter Fourteen

The Implied Directive

The "implied directive" is a label we are proposing for a fairly common type of indirect suggestion that is in current use in clinical hypnosis (Cheek and LeCron, 1968). The implied directive usually has three parts: (1) a time-binding introduction, (2) the implied (or assumed) suggestion, and (3) a behavioral response to signal when the implied suggestion has been accomplished. We may thus analyze an implied directive from this session as follows:

As soon as you know

1. A time binding introduction that focuses the patient on the suggestion to follow

only you or I, or only you and my voice are here

2. The implied (or assumed) suggestion

your right hand will descend to your thigh.

3. The behavioral response signaling that the suggestion has been accomplished.

An implied directive frequently used by Rossi to end a hypnotherapeutic session is as follows:

As soon as your unconscious knows

1. A time-binding introduction that facilitates dissociation and reliance on the unconscious.

it can again return to this state comfortably and easily to do constructive work the next time we are together,

2. The implied suggestion for easy reentry to trance phrased in a therapeutically motivating manner.

you will find yourself awakening feeling refreshed and alert

3. The behavioral response signaling that the above suggestion has been accomplished.

When the behavioral response signaling the accomplishment is an inevitable response that the patient wants to happen (as in the above examples), we have a situation where the behavioral response also has motivating properties for the accomplishment of the suggestion. The behavioral response signaling the accomplishment of the suggestion takes place on an involuntary or unconscious level. Thus, the unconscious that carries out the suggestion also signals when it is accomplished.

The implied directive engenders a covert state of internal learning. It is covert because no one can tell it is occurring since it is a series of responses taking place entirely within the subject, frequently without conscious awareness and usually not remembered after trance. Therapist and patient only know it is completed when the requested automatic response (e.g., finger signaling, head nodding, awakening from trance) takes place, signaling the end of the internal state of learning.

The implied directive is thus a way of facilitating an intense state of internal learning or problem solving. We may suppose that all of a subject's available mental resources (e.g., stored memories, sensory and verbal associational patterns, various forms of previous learning, etc.) are marshalled toward a creative state of learning and problem solving. Since recent experiments in the neurophysiology of learning suggest that new proteins are actually synthesized in the appropriate brain cells during learning (Rossi, 1973a), we may speculate that the implied directive facilitates the internal synthesis of new protein structures that could function as the biological basis of new behavior and phenomenological experience in the patient.

The implied directive is particularly interesting because of its similarity to the technique of biofeedback. In most forms of biofeedback, an electronic device is used to signal when an internal response has been accomplished. With the implied directive, the patient's own overt and autonomous behavioral response is used to signal when the internal response has been accomplished. The formal similarities between them may be listed as follows:

1. Consciousness is given a task it does not know how to accomplish by itself.

Raise (or lower) your blood pressure 10 points.
Warm your right hand and cool your left.
Increase the alpha of your right cortex.
Decrease the muscle tension in your forehead.

2. Consciousness is given a signal enabling it to recognize when any behavior changes are being made in the desired direction of response. In biofeedback, this is accomplished by an electronic transducer that measures the response (blood pressure, body temperature, alpha waves, or muscle tension in the above examples) and makes any change in this response evident on a meter that allows the subjects to monitor their own behavior.

3. In the implied directive, by contrast, the patient's own unconscious system serves as the transducer indicating when the desired internal response (blood pressure change, body temperature, etc.) has been made and translates it into an overt behavior signal that consciousness can recognize.

The advantages of the implied directive over biofeedback are obvious. The latter is a fairly cumbersome technique that requires sophisticated and expensive electronic equipment. It is limited to those responses that can actually be measured. By contrast, the implied directive requires no equipment and is limited only by the ingenuity and imagination of both therapist and patient. Although no comparative studies have been made as yet, one might expect that the electronic equipment of biofeedback might ensure a greater reliability of control than is possible with the implied directive. For this, indeed, is the major problem in ***Utilizing*** any method of hypnosis: The relative reliability of response between different individuals and within the same individual on different occasions. It may well be that this reliability problem can be dealt with in part by ***Utilizing*** this analogy with biofeedback. The reliability of biofeedback is due to the reliability of the signaling system provided by the electronic instrumentation. Hypnotic procedures can be made more reliable by having patients remember and report experiential and behavioral changes that initiate or accompany the desired hypnotic response. These changes may then function as signals to reinstate the hypnotic response on another occasion. In this case hypnosis and biofeedback share another common aim: To establish a connection between a conscious thought or behavior and a previously nonvoluntary response.

Exercises with the Implied Directive

1. The implied directive has evolved in clinical practice, but there is no research data that has experimentally validated its usefulness. Can the reader devise implied directives that can be validated experimentally in a controlled and objectively repeatable manner?

2. Devise implied directives that will facilitate the experience of all the major hypnotic phenomenon.

3. Devise implied directives that will facilitate the internal learning of therapeutically useful goals (e.g., freeing the unconscious from the limitations of a particular patient's ego programming to find a new solution for a problem).

4. Since the implied directive includes an involuntary signal that a suggestion has been accomplished, it can be used in place of "challenges" to test the effectiveness of trance work. In the older, classical approaches to trance training the operators "tested" and "proved" the depth and validity of trance and the strength of their suggestions by "challenging" subjects to try to open their eyes or unclasp their hands when they had been given suggestions that they could not do so. If the subjects were not able to open their eyes, then they passed the challenge and the validity of trance was established. The implied directive accomplishes the same purposes in a much more constructive and permissive manner. It leaves the locus of control within the patient, where it belongs, rather than fostering the illusion of the therapist's control. It is thus a valuable indicator for both subject and therapist that a desired response is indeed taking place. The therapist can now learn to devise implied directives as indicators of any stage in the development and accomplishment of suggestions requiring internal responses (memories, feelings, sensations, etc.) not otherwise open to the therapist's observation.

Questions that Focus, Suggest and Reinforce

One of the most surprising aspects of approach is his use of questions to focus attention, to suggest indirectly, and to reinforce all at the same time. Questions seem so innocent in everyday life. When other people question us, it is frequently from their own need, and the question implies that we know something and are quite fine to be helping them. Questions asking for help, directions, advice, and so on are all of this category and are most useful for focusing attention.

Another useful category of questions concerns abilities: Can we do such and such? This ability question frequently has strongly motivating properties from many years of effort in childhood, adolescence, and young adulthood to meet a developmental challenge successfully: "I'll try, and I bet I can!" These ability questions are therefore useful in motivating patients provided they are not overwhelming in their demand. We must take care because questions can also be piercing and destructive, as when they are experienced as the merciless stings of an examination situation or inquisition.

Recent research (Sternberg, 1975; Shevrin, 1975) indicates that when questioned, the human brain continues an exhaustive search throughout its entire memory system on an unconscious level even after it has found an answer that is satisfactory on a conscious level. The mind apparently scans 30 items per second even when the person is unaware that the search is continuing to take place. The results of such searches on an unconscious level are evident from many familiar experiences of everyday life. How often do we forget a name or an item only to have it pop up all by itself only a few moments later, after our conscious mind has gone onto something else? How often are we consciously satisfied with a solution only to have fresh doubts and perhaps a better answer come up autonomously a short while later?

The fact that such unconscious search and cognition are carried out in response to questions even after the conscious mind is apparently satisfied and otherwise occupied is a verification of Erickson's early research supporting the then controversial view that the mind could be simultaneously active on two entirely separate and independent tasks—one on a conscious level and another on an unconscious level (Erickson & Kubie, 1939/2010; Erickson & Erickson, 1941). This activation of unconscious resources is the very essence of the indirect approach, wherein we seek to activate and ***Utilize*** a patient's unrecognized potentials to evoke hypnotic phenomena and therapeutic responses.

As usual demonstrates and indirect approach even in his use of questions, which typically structure the patient's internal associations by implication. Questions are frequently implied directives. They are often used to depotentiate conscious sets so the patient will be more open to new response possibilities. Let us analyze a few examples of Erickson's questions.

It will be found that it is almost impossible to neatly classify these questions because even the simplest are very complex in their implications and effects.

Which hand is lighter?

Focuses attention on hands. Indirectly suggests one will be lighter and may levitate. Reinforces lightness and possible levitation as an adequate response. It is an implied directive insofar as it requires a hypnotic response to be answered adequately. Illusory choice and ***Double Bind*** are also operative because one is being bound into making a hypnotic response whichever hand feels lightest. This question indirectly depotentiates consciousness because it is no unusual that the "normal" and habitual frameworks of ego consciousness cannot cope with it, so the patient must wait for an unconscious or autonomous response.

Why did John just leave?

This question in the context of this session where Mrs. L was hallucinating John serves primarily as an indirect suggestion to cease hallucinating. It works by implication and refocuses attention.

Do you want Dr. Rossi to look at you?

In the context of this session where Mrs. L is hallucinating herself as naked from the waist up, this question strongly ratifies the hallucinatory experience with an implied directive that she show some response to being naked in front of a relative stranger (she covered her breasts with her arms).

Do you enjoy
[pause]
not knowing where you are?

This is an indirect, compound suggestion that gains its potency from many sources. It is compound because it asks two questions at the same time: Do you enjoy? You do not know where you are? It is so difficult to answer such a double question that the patient would frequently rather just go along with it and "enjoy not knowing where he is." The use of the negative "not knowing," is a further source of confusion that is frequently too difficult to figure out, so the patient goes along. "Do you enjoy," indirectly suggests pleasure and is thus reinforcing.

It is evident from these analyses that we are only beginning to make a beginning in our understanding of language in general and questions in particular. The hypnotherapist would do well to make as thorough as possible a study of that branch of semiotics known as pragmatics, the relation between signs and the users of signs (Morris, 1938; Watzlawick et al., 1967 and Watzlawick et al., 1974).

Exercises with Questions for Analysis

Perform a similar analysis on the following questions as well as all others you find interesting in the inductions of this volume.

Would you like to enter trance now or later?

Where does your body experience its greatest comfort?

Can you say, "Something?" (Note the use of this question as a test of literalism.)

Do you really understand? (The vocal emphasis is on "really.")

Can you enjoy relaxing and not having to remember?

Can your unconscious deal with that problem?

Do you feel comfortable not knowing who I am?

Questions for Indirect Trance Induction

One of the most useful forms of suggestion is the question that fixes and focuses attention while helping subjects to reach into their own associative matrix to uncover useful responses that can be structured into new behavior patterns. Erickson frequently induces trance and carries out an entire hypnotherapeutic session with a series of questions.

1. What kind of trance would you like to experience?

2. How long will it take you to go into that trance?

3. How will you know you are beginning to experience trance?

4. Now do you really think you are still fully awake?

5. How much of a trance do you feel you are in already?

6. How soon will your trance deepen?

7. You will let me know when it is deep enough, will you not?

8. What would you now like to experience in this trance as it continues to deepen? Or would you like it as a surprise? Sooner or later?

9. Will you let your hand (finger, head) move when it feels warm (cold, numb, etc.)?

10. And you don't know how much of that numbness you would like to maintain after you awaken, do you?

Each of these questions evokes associative responses to different aspects of trance experience within the patient. The effect of the first three is to reintegrate previous trance experiences as well as heightening patients' motivation for their current experience. Questions 4 and 5 help patients assess their current status and help make the transition from awakedness to trance. Questions 6 and 7 complete this transition and set up a signaling system so that patients can let the therapist know when a trance of sufficient depth has been achieved. Questions 8, 9 and 10 are all variations that can be used to explore the evocation of virtually any hypnotic phenomena or posthypnotic response. Questions are thus a fail-safe approach to trance experience. The question, more than any other hypnotic form, appears automatically to evoke partial aspects of the phenomena in question so that they may be expresses as a possible hypnotic response.

The Fragmentary Development of Trance

We feel it is better to induce a trance by fragments than by demanding the whole all at once. The questioning approach allows patients to experience trance by degrees. It also allows the therapist to continually monitor the process and know where the patient is all the time. It is similar, but not identical with Vogt's fractionation technique (Weitzenhoffer, 1957; Kroger, 1963) and the process "heteroactive hyper-suggestibility" (Hull, 1933) whereby following one suggestion tends to increase the probability of following another.

ER: Why is it better to induce a trance by fragments?

MHE: You induce a small fragment of the trance and then another. Then you can connect those two.

ER: Different fragments of trance are developed by questions that function as waking suggestions? Each waking suggestion that is accepted adds another fragment of trance?

MHE: Yes, and then you relate them together. First, you develop a catalepsy of the arm. Then you add: "And the numbness, do you notice that? And you can't move your eyes from your hand? All you can see is your hand? And all unimportant sounds have dropped out?"

ER: These questions successively build the trance by adding a possible experience of analgesia or anesthesia, immobility of the eyes and head and a negative visual and auditory hallucination for unimportant background details.

EXERCISES *UTILIZING* QUESTIONS AS SUGGESTIONS

1. Write out a complete induction using only question for the following approaches to trance:

   a. ***Hand Levitation***
   b. Eye fixation
   c. Relaxation
   d. Any other favorite approach such as visualization, etc.

2. Formulate series of questions that will focus a subject's attention and associative processes in such a manner that an experience of each of the classical hypnotic phenomena will be facilitated.

3. Formulate a series of questions that will focus a patient's memories and associations in a manner that will facilitate a therapeutic response.

4. The question approach to trance induction is very similar to the introspective approaches that are ***Utilized*** in many diverse schools of psychotherapy. The active imagination of C. G. Jung (1963; Rossi, 1972), the meditation methods of Assagioli's psychosynthe-

sis (1965), and the dialogues of the gestalt approach (Perles, 1969) all focus the individual's attention on inner realities. Thus, they are trance inducing, even though their originators usually do not recognize it. Such methods may be considered indirect approaches to trance even though they are not labeled as hypnosis. The essential identity between periods of introspection and trance was demonstrated by Erickson in his early research with Clark L. Hull (Erickson, 1964), when he found that groups of subjects asked to perform a task in introspection underwent behavioral and subjective experiences that were similar to those they had when they went through a classical hypnotic induction.

It would be instructive to the beginner in hypnosis to give subjects tasks in introspection and imagination and then ask for their subjective comparisons of these inner experiences with those of a classical hypnotic induction. What similarities are noted in their outer behavior? The relation between such introspection-imagination approaches to trance and imagination (Sheehan, 1972) are the subject of much current research (Hilgard, 1970).

Depotentiating Conscious Mental Sets: Confusion, Mental Flux, and Creativity

ER: You keep patients constantly in flux, slightly off balance, so they will continually grasp onto whatever orientation you provide?

MHE: Yes.

ER: That is one of the creative states within hypnosis; that state of constant flux wherein the patient grasps the orientations you provide.

MHE: That's right.

ER: This is in contrast to the situation where you allow patients to remain quiet by themselves in a trance (Erickson, 1955) to work out their own solution to a problem in their own way.

MHE: When a person goes into a trance, you bounce him around and keep him whirling and then you tell him to work quietly on that problem. You have first detached him from his conscious mental sets. You have broken the connections that might have been stopping him from working on his problem. That is a very important thing.

ER: You break their habitual mental sets and the conscious biases that prevented them from solving a problem and then orient them toward creative inner work.

MHE: People always have that tendency to put off working on a problem to tomorrow. But you make tomorrow today by breaking those conscious sets and keeping them in a state of flux.

ER: That is part and parcel of the confusion and the ***Surprise Techniques*** as well. All these approaches depotentiate the limitations of conscious sets.

In this conversation, Erickson clearly expresses a major aspect of his work in facilitating problem solving and creativity. Earlier in the third session, we saw that a flow diagram of trance induction went as follows:

DIMMING OF OUTER REALITY

↓

CONFUSION

↓

RECEPTIVITY TO CLARIFYING SUGGESTIONS

↓

TRANCE WORK PROPER

In this section, Erickson elaborates further on the significance of confusion. ***Confusion*** ("You bounce him around and keep him whirling") is used to detach people from their "conscious mental sets." You have broken the connections that might have been stopping them from working on their problem. A patient is a patient because of erroneous mental sets and limited frames of reference. Erickson continually seeks to break through these rigid limitations to initiate a state of mental flux that may release the patient's creative potential.

Thus, confusion becomes a major tool for breaking rigid mental sets and initiating a creative process. An entirely spontaneous example of this process occurred in the commentary of this session, where Rossi admits to feeling "woozy" trying to break through his own mental limitations to understand what Erickson was trying to teach. This feeling actually occurred many times. The breaking of Rossi's habitual frames of reference together with the complexity which which Erickson expresses himself was sometimes enough to induce a hypnotic atmosphere. The complexity of Erickson's thought, it should be noted, was not due to its abstract nature, but to his habitual use of indirection, questions, and implications that continually turn over a listener's associative processes in ways that are experienced as unusual and perhaps not self-directed (and therefore hypnotic).

Many of the verbal forms that Erickson uses to initiate confusion to break through a patient's erroneous conscious sets are already familiar to us: the use of provocative questions, implications, ***Double Binds***, ***Surprise***, not doing and not knowing.

At the simplest level, Erickson softly and insistently reiterates all the things a patient does not need to do or know. He is actually telling the patient's consciousness that it can relinquish its usual control and direction and permit unconscious and autonomous processes to take over. The whole process of trance induction is designed to relax these habitual sets of consciousness. The trance deepens, and patients are able to break out of the learned limitations of their usual mode of consciousness to the degree that they give up what they know.

Not Knowing or Not Doing

You don't need to listen, your unconscious can respond on its own.

You don't need to know consciously for when the occasion arises, your unconscious will supply that knowledge.

You don't know when you are going to change your rate of breathing [or any other behavior].

[To a restless patient] You don't know exactly when you will feel a need to move again.

You don't need to know where your hands [or feet] are.

I would like you to learn that no matter what any person believes your belief,

your unconscious belief, your unconscious knowledge, is all that counts.

In the course of living from infancy on,
you acquired knowledge,

but you could not keep all that knowledge in the foreground of your mind.

Note from the induction transcript how these last two suggestions lead up to Erickson's suggestion for forgetting.

Closely related to not doing and not knowing are the related hypnotic forms of losing abilities, the negative, doubt, contradictions, and the apposition of opposites. We will now take up each of these in turn.

Losing Abilities

Erickson likes to phrase suggestions in the form of losing abilities because it is easy to experience, it is compatible with the basic nature of trance, and it is a rather impressive demonstration of trance as an altered state. Losing abilities tends to depotentiate one's usual everyday reality orientation and thus make one more receptive to altered modes of experiencing.

It will be interesting to experience that moment when you can no longer hold your eyelids open.

You can lose the ability to lift your right hand from your thigh.

And will it be surprising when you find you cannot stand up?

The Negative

Erickson has studied the use of the negative in great detail. He admired an actor who could say "No" in 16 different ways to express 16 different shades of meaning from "absolute no" to agreeable acquiescence. A few examples are as follows:

Won't you?

When expressed with a doubting tone of voice, this has a negative meaning—"You won't." It is used only when you don't want a subject to do something.

You will, will you not?

This is a use of a negative word: "not?" is turned into a positive by being enunciated with a questioning inflection. Erickson feels this phrase meets a subject's need for a negative to balance the positive "you will" that comes just before it; this sentence is thus example of his apposition of opposites.

Research has indicated that it is much more difficult to comprehend negative formulations (Donaldson, 1959). The use of the negative, therefore, tends to depotentiate consciousness. In trance, when one would rather "not do" it is easier just to go along with a suggestion than try to figure out all its implications.

Erickson also believes that the use of the negative is another way of maintaining psychological balance and compensation as we will discuss later in the apposition of opposites. The use of the negative also enables the therapist to proffer a negative onto which a patient's resistance may be discharged and displaced. The use of negatives may thus be regarded as another approach to dealing with the "resistant" patient. The use of negation with such patients actually ***Utilizes*** their own negativity in a manner that can discharge its destructive aspects and redirect it into constructive channels.

The Negative for Reverse Suggestion

Another basic use of the negative is for indirect or reverse suggestion. On one occasion a patient insisted that he would not awaken. Erickson accepted that, while admitting it would be inconvenient since he had other patients to see that day. Then, with utter sincerity, Erickson mentioned that he hoped the patient would not have to go to the bathroom, since that would awaken him. Of course, the patient soon found that he did have an inexplicable need to use the bathroom and thus, had to awaken. Another reverse suggestion might have been, "Fine, you can try to stay in trance and do not awaken." The word "try," said with a subtly doubting tone together with the implied effort it will require not to awaken, has the net effect of actually awakening the subject.

In the reverse situation, when we want to enhance the possibility of trance, we might say, "Try to stay awake, just try and do not go into trance." The subject usually resists trance heroically for a few minutes till he is exhausted from the implied effort and falls by default into trance. These effects of negative suggestion were early described by Baudouin (1920) as the Law of Reverse Effort: the more one tries to resist a suggestion, the stronger he feels compelled to carry it out. Weitzenhoffer (1957) has described this law of reverse effort as a pseudo-law. There is actually no clinical or experimental data that indicates there is an intrinsic and necessary relation between "trying to resist" and a "compulsion to carry it out." Weitzenhoffer (1975) believes the effectiveness of such formulations is due to their containing an implied suggestion to do the exact opposite of what is purportedly suggested.

Doubt

The use of doubt is a subtle process that Erickson frequently conveys with a doubting tone of voice on key words. Erickson usually capitalizes on the minimal and perhaps unrecognized doubt already experienced by a patient. His statement about this doubt is thus as much a truism as a suggestion. Whatever the doubt, it does place the person in a less stable position, and thus, propels one into a search for more structure and certainty. Erickson, of course, then provides therapeutic suggestions that will help restructure the patient in a satisfactory manner.

Do you really understand?

means, "distrust your conscious understanding."

And you will really understand

means the same as, "You don't really understand."

Do you think you are wide awake?

implies, "You are not awake."

You are quite certain of yourself now, are you?

implies, "You are not."

Contradictions

Revealing contradictions within patients' minds demonstrates the inadequacy of their usual beliefs and prepares the way for a positive attitude toward an experience with therapeutic trance. Erickson makes something of a game of this as he helps a patient to realize contradictions between thought and feeling and, of course, between the conscious and unconscious. He frequently uses ideomotor movements as a proof of these contradictions. Thus, when a patient protests that an important memory is not available, Erickson may establish a convincing contradiction, as follows:

> **If your unconscious thinks you have a better memory** [feeling, thoughts, or whatever the patient has doubts about]**, your hand will lift.**

When the hand does lift autonomously, it tends to convince the patient that with further hypnotic work the memory may soon become available. When a patient doubts whether trance has been experienced, Erickson will use ideomotor movements to establish it.

> **Your conscious mind may doubt, but if your unconscious knows you have experienced trance, it will let your head nod slowly in the affirmative.**

Erickson can thus frequently ***Utilize*** the obsessive, ambivalent, and doubting aspects of a patient's ideation in a creative manner. The obsessive-compulsive personality can be understood as one laden with contradictions between the conscious and unconscious. These contradictions can be explored to establish rapport and cooperation between the various tendencies within the personality.

Apposition of Opposites

Another of Erickson's indirect forms of hypnotic suggestion is his penchant for the close juxtaposition, or apposition of opposites. This seems to be a basic element in his ***Confusion Technique***, but it also may be a means of ***Utilizing*** another natural mental mechanism to facilitate hypnotic responsiveness.

In the second session, Erickson illustrated the careful balancing, or apposition, of the opposite processes of remembering and forgetting. Kinsbourne & Smith (1974) have discussed how the "balance between opponent systems" is a basic neurological mechanism that is built in the very structure of the nervous system. What we are labeling as the "apposition of opposites" may be a means of ***Utilizing*** this fundamental neurological process to facilitate hypnotic responsiveness. In this case, Erickson was apparently balancing the opponent systems of remembering and forgetting without the patient making a conscious effort to do either. Another apparent balancing of these opposites that is actually a ***Double Bind*** is as follows:

You can forget to remember or remember to forget.

Other modalities for the apposition of opposites are in lightness and heaviness, warmth and coolness, relaxation and tension, etc.

As your hand lifts, your eyelids will feel heavy.

This juxtaposition of lifting and lightness with heaviness ***Utilizes*** the balance between opponent systems in another way. If we emphasize lightness and levitation, then we are shifting the subject out of equilibrium, so there will develop within the subject a countertendency to balance and oppose the lightness with heaviness. This natural countertendency could eventually defeat the levitation suggestions. If we ***Utilize*** this natural countertendency to heaviness by suggesting another response where it can be useful (eyelids heavy), however, we are actually *Utilizing* the balance between opponent processes in a way that will facilitate two hypnotic suggestions. It is a way of offering multiple tasks that can reinforce each other. Other examples of the planned use of such apposition is as follows:

> **You can remain comfortable immobile until the urge to move takes your hand across the page writing automatically.**
>
> **You may either see an unexpected image in the crystal ball or not see the ball at all.**
>
> **As your hand becomes warmer, your forehead can become cooler.**
>
> **As you make that tight fist, the lower part of your body can relax.**

Exercises with the Apposition of Opposites

1. Formulate suggestions *Utilizing* the apposition of opposites warmth and coolness, tension and relaxation, anesthesia and hypersensitivity to touch. An interesting use of the latter for a refractory case of dental anesthesia is described by Erickson (1958/2021). After a number of unsuccessful efforts by others Erickson was able to facilitate an effective oral anesthesia for dental work by first suggesting that the patient's left hand would become hypersensitive to all stimuli and needed to be carefully protected at all times. This was in keeping with the patient's fixed belief that dental work was always associated with hypersensitivity. Erickson simply displaced that hypersensitivity from the mouth to the hand, Erickson comments, "When this rigid understanding was met, dental anesthesia could be achieved, in a fashion analogous to the relaxation of one muscle permitting the contraction of another."

2. Conceptualize other opponent processes in the sensory, perceptual, and cognitive realms that can be used to facilitate hypnotic responsiveness.

3. Formulate apposition of opposites that could be ***Utilized*** to facilitate all the classical hypnotic phenomena.

Chapter Fifteen

Facilitating Hypnotic Learning

The relations between the conscious and unconscious and Erickson's means of dealing with them are explored in this session. It is apparent that Erickson, like most pioneers in depth psychology, really believes in the value of the unconscious as a useful concept in his daily work with people. He carefully points out how the conscious and unconscious each have their own interests and how successful hypnotic work frequently depends upon appealing to both. As usual, he has an indirect approach for dealing with this problem. Erickson believes that analogies are a means of simultaneously appealing to the conscious and unconscious. As such, analogies are a basic tool for facilitating hypnotic learning.

Because of this, Erickson employs a rich repertory of analogies drawn from everyday life. It will be seen that many of these analogies are about the perceptions and experiences of childhood; the child's ways of functioning are closer to unconscious, which Erickson is trying to facilitate in trance work. He likes to use examples from his own experience because he knows them best, and his sense of conviction helps mobilize similar experiences within the patient. His analogies always fixate (or bore) the attention of consciousness while simultaneously instructing the unconscious. The conscious mind does not know how to do certain things. That is why the person is in therapy. The individual's unconscious does have the resources for doing what is necessary. Analogies are frequently an effective approach for mobilizing these unconscious resources.

Session 6: Unconscious Learning with Dr. S

MHE: Do you have any questions?

Dr. S: I had a couple of questions, but I can ask them later.

MHE: Ask them now.

Dr. S: I still wasn't clear yesterday why you didn't follow through when you put me in a trance. It wasn't clear. You said you wanted me to experience it or something? I understand that a hypnotherapist should experience a trance, but I wasn't quite clear in my mind what you were doing, but maybe it isn't important for me to know.

MHE: You never completely satisfy your audience. You leave them wishing for more. That's what is happening here. She is asking, "Why didn't you do more with me?" That impresses upon them that they really do want more.

ER: You have induced a situation wherein she is asking you for more and may thus break through some of her limiting preconceptions. The fact that she finally admits that "maybe it isn't important for me to know" suggests she may be giving up some of her reliance on consciousness.

MHE: I wanted your unconscious mind to have the liberty of doing something while your conscious mind was filled with other things. You wouldn't know your unconscious was active because you are being so interested in conscious activity.
Dr. S: Yes, what was going on here. I was curious about what I did with Mrs. L. Couldn't that be considered a kind of hypno-

sis having her relaxed and concentrated on being in a different place?

MHE: Yes.

Dr. S: I think that can only be done by a good subject.

MHE: A good subject or a sophisticated one? What other questions have you?

Dr. S: That's all.

MHE: I'm making it apparent here that there are two sets of interests, and the unconscious is going to have its interests.

ER: You're carefully pointing out the separation of conscious and unconscious interests.

MHE: You can't make that too obvious or too plain. You have to rely on the unconscious.

[Dr. S gets ready to enter trance, but her hands are neatly folded together in her lap.]

MHE: One of the things that I found very important is,
don't let the hands remain in contact with each other.
Just how the contact of the hands interferes,
I don't know.
[Pause]
Now go all the way.
[Pause]

MHE: In folk language, "You have to hang together." When your hands touch each other, they tend to hang together. But you want an openness to stimuli—not something that is hanging together and excluding.

MHE: Your unconscious learned a lot yesterday.

[Pause]
It also learned
that
we could learn a lot
without
intruding upon the personality.
[Pause]
All subjects,
whatever their degree of sophistication,
are uncertain that they can do
everything,
and yet
in their personal history
they can.
[Pause]
I have hunted for a book in a bookcase
under the impression,
within the frame of reference,
that it was bound in red.
I was unable to find it.
I could resort to reading all the titles of every book
and still not be able to find it
even though I read all the titles.
The title had no meaning
because my reference was red
instead of blue, which was the correct color.

MHE: "Your unconscious learned a lot yesterday."

[MHE and ER here discuss the case of Mrs. K, whose active and conscious mind derogatorized her unconscious' very acute "literalism" while in the trance state. So acute was her literalism that it even surprised MHE. That literalism was an "accomplishment" of the unconscious, but Mrs. K's conscious mind regarded it as error.]

MHE: The conscious mind downgrades unconscious accomplishments, and you can't allow that downgrading to continue because conscious emotions filter down to the unconscious.

ER: You mean the negative sets of consciousness can inhibit unconscious potentials?

MHE: The unconscious is going to be protective of consciousness.

ER: You mean it will go along with the conscious bias?

MHE: It's going to try to reassure the conscious mind with, "You don't have to be depressed if you didn't do things." The unconscious won't say, "You did something even though you didn't know it" (e.g., Mrs. K's acute literalism). It doesn't function that way. It just says, "You don't have to worry because you failed."

ER: That is how the unconscious protects the conscious mind?

MHE: The unconscious mind, with all due respect, does not tell the conscious mind, "You're wrong?"

ER: It says instead?

MHE: "You don't have to feel bad about it." So, you must see to it that the conscious mind gets the impression, "I only think I've failed."

ER: That's how you correct the conscious mind.

MHE: Yes. With Mrs. K we had to assure her that I, Dr. Erickson, failed in my instructions to her and that her acutely literal response was a success as a hypnotic response on the part of the unconscious.

MHE: That has happened to me many times.

It seems true to others.
Others who haven't been in a trance.
[Pause]
Now, why wouldn't I have seen
a book covered with blue
when I read its title?
[Pause]
Because we all have
the ability
not to see
when we are wide awake,
and in trance state
that ability can be called upon
at any time.
[Pause]

MHE: This illustrates the biasing influence of a conscious set on true knowledge.

ER: You're trying to tell Dr. S with all these examples, "Give up conscious biases and sets."

MHE: Don't let conscious frames of reference occlude your vision.

[MHE here gives many everyday examples of how conscious sets, e.g., rose-colored glasses, continually interfere with an objective perception of things. What is an objective perception? Seeing from many points of view to get a rounded picture.]

MHE: There are many times
in the past
when you haven't seen something
that was there;
you haven't felt

things that could be felt.

ER: Now, you're shifting into suggestions that may lead to an experience of negative visual hallucinations: not seeing, hearing, or feeling.

MHE: It is a very common experience
to develop
a hypnagogic state
and arouse in the morning
from your sleep
and not know where you are.
Everybody has the experiences
of deja vu.
[Pause]
Those who have seen something before
think they have
as if it really happened to them.
Hearing something before
that you really haven't,
of being someplace where
you haven't been
but still think you have been there.
Everybody has those experiences.
Transforming a familiar experience
into an alien one,
not recognizing
that which is familiar,
not recognizing a place,
a sound,
feelings.
In hypnosis,
you utilize
those past learnings.

ER: You now review a number of fairly common everyday experiences to make certain hypnotic phenomenon seem plausible. The experience of deja vu is a nice analogy that may evoke associative pathways leading to positive hallucinatory experience. So you are carefully apposing the possibility of either a negative or positive hallucination in whatever sense modality it may occur. It is all very open-ended; you will accept and applaud whatever hypnotic experience she is ready to have.

MHE: Yes.

> **MHE: One of the most charming experiences**
> **that children can demonstrate—**
> **and they all do—**
> **they bend over and**
> **look at the world from between their legs,**
> **[Pause]**
> **because the world is so strange.**
> **Some people remember doing that.**
> **[Pause]**
> **Most do not remember.**
> **[Pause]**
> **Memories are so many times**
> **discovered to be false**
> **when they are true memories.**
> **It is due to a change**
> **in the person**
> **that's not been recognized.**

MHE: This is a terribly important experience. In psychotherapy, you have to look at a problem upside down and sidewise.

ER: To break out of your conscious sets.

MHE: You have to look at your patient as if you were sitting on a seat higher than his. You also have to look at him from a much lower seat. You need to look at him from the other side of the room. Because you always get a totally different picture from different points of view. Only by such a total look at the patient can you gain some objectivity.

ER: All these different views add up to a more total objectivity.

MHE: That's one of the drawbacks of conventional psychoanalysis: You get just one view, 18 inches behind and to the left of the patient. That is a very stereotyped thing.

MHE: As examples
I can cite personal incidences.
[Pause]
When I went back
to the farm
after being in college,
I found that the stove was
unusually small.
[Pause]
I remembered how I had
to stand on my toes
to reach up to the warming oven.
My son Allan returned from Washington, D.C.,
walked through all the rooms of the house,
and remarked,
"I know it is impossible
that these rooms have all shrunk.
They are much smaller,
very much smaller."
[Pause]

[MHE cites another example wherein one of his daughters as a baby looking up from her crib learned to associate his head as close to the ceiling. The confusion this association came up on a later occasion when she saw him closer to his true proportions.]

MHE: In hypnotic experiences

you do not try
to correct your memories.
You receive them
without automatic correction.
I have watched babies' perception develop.
They start out
by seeing one person
standing by the crib
until one day,
without verbalizing it,
they now realize there are two.
It takes some length of time
to differentiate between
mother and father.
It takes still more time
to differentiate between
big brother or mother
and to recognize three.

MHE: Pointing out here the child's frame of reference.

ER: All of this is to train Dr. S to give up her conscious sets, to break down her conscious frameworks in preparation for change.

MHE: I want to make her aware that she has many, many rigid sets. Everybody has.

ER: So, this is a general understanding you try to give every patient in the beginning. You try to soften up their rigidities by talking of the plasticity of perception and behavior, etc.

MHE: That's right. You try to make the person aware. There is nothing wrong with having rigid sets. But if you want to alter yourself in some way, you must be unashamedly aware that you do have sets and it's better to have a greater variety of sets.

ER: So, you will have a much wider range in your behavior.

[Erickson here gives several clinical examples of how he gently broke through the inhibiting conscious sets of patients so they gradually began fuller self-exploration of their body, etc. (Haley, 1973; Rossi, 1973a)]

MHE: You have those learnings
in adult life, you can correct them,
[Pause]
but there is no real need to correct them.
They should be appreciated.
A child sees a walking
stick
[Pause]
As an adult she still shows
her wonderment
at the walking stick
that is actually a snake.
Psychotherapy using hypnosis,
taking note of past memories
in their purity
without any need to correct them.
As you should want to know what they are.
[Pause]
We learn to recognize
those individual memories
without correcting them.
You then have an opportunity to assess, evaluate
the components of a total understanding.
You meet a person,
and for no reason at all
you dislike that person,
but you do have a reason.
You have a walking-stick reason,
you have a head-between-legs-looking-at-the-world reason,

because you have seen something new in that person
in terms
of memories, of learnings.
But as an adult
you usually correct these memories,
and you simply say
you don't like that person
for no reason at all.
[Pause]
I'll cite personal incidences,
as I know them better than other instances.
When I walked into the house
and my son Lance,
then a small boy
had a problem.
He knew he could not see through a brick wall.
He could see only through windows.
Yet, Daddy walked into the house
and said, "You were told not to play
with that doily on the table."
He had played with it,
and he happened to be over by a window.
and saw me approaching.
So, he carefully replaced the doily
except he didn't center it on the table.
That was what he didn't know.
He then attributed my knowledge
that he was playing with the doily
to my being able to see through a brick wall.
[Pause]
So far as the patient
is concerned
you do not remind yourself
of adult understandings.
Nor do you look at behavior
with adult understandings.
[Pause]

ER: Here you suggest a hypnotic phenomenon (early memory) by ***not doing*** (no need to correct early memories and childhood distortions) so that it appeals as being effortlessly easy to one in a placid state of trance. This is actually an indirect approach to age regression. You don't directly tell her to age regress. By simply mentioning the ways in which a child sees the world differently, you are hoping to actually evoke her early modes of perception and thereby facilitate the possibility of a genuine age regression.

MHE: That's right.

> **MHE: How soon**
> **do you think**
> **you will be willing**
> **to open your eyes**
> **and not see your hands?**

MHE: What does this question really do? Put it into separate sentences:
You will open your eyes.
You will see.
You will not see certain things.
Those are actually commands.

ER: But they are stated in a question as a ***fait accompli.***

MHE: Yes. It's stated as a question, but the only real question it asks is, "At what time will it be done?" You are displacing all doubt onto the question of the time. That is the only thing that needs to be doubted. All the rest is actuality.

ER: You've done that with a question I would call an implied directive.

MHE: Yes. The common mistake in psychotherapy is to give a patient directions without recognizing there have to be doubts.

ER: In our society, we invariably doubt and test any suggestion that is made to us. This may be the social basis of the so called resistance. Perhaps that is why the Freudians talk so much about resistances. The typical therapist does not know how to present directives in a way that would discharge resistances automatically as you have here illustrated. You are always discharging resistances and doubts by the way you express things.

> **MHE: You have not seen**
> **your hands many times in the past**
> **when they were in direct line of vision.**
> **[Pause]**
> **An adult can learn to see things**
> **in direct line of vision.**
> **And you also learned**
> **not to see your hands**
> **when they were in a direct line of vision.**
> **[Pause]**

MHE: Now, I tied that question to an actual thing: "You have not seen your hands many times in the past."

ER: You validate the suggestion by juxtaposing it with a common perceptual experience of the past.

MHE: How many times have we not seen "the impossible not to see?"

ER: As I'm looking at this microphone I'm holding in front of you right now I realize that I was not seeing my hand that's holding it.

MHE: That's right! A magician makes his living out of that. He *Utilizes* your ability not to see what he is doing.

[Here Erickson gives another fairly complex example of how adult and child memories of the same phenomenon can be different because of their different points of view. Because of this, we find that there are frequently two sets of memories, which sometimes gives rise to confusion in patients.]

MHE: In psychotherapy,
you learn to recognize
how things can be different things.
[Pause]
I am going to suggest that you open your eyes
and keep them open,
and be aware
not to see.

[Pause. Dr. S opens her eyes and reorients to her body.]

ER: So, it is a good approach to tie your suggestions to an undeniable experience they have had. That tends to validate your suggestions. What are you trying to convince with these validating analogies from everyday life? The conscious or the unconscious?

MHE: The unconscious knows all about these things!

ER: You're telling the unconscious what mental mechanisms to use by analogy.

MHE: Yes.

ER: At the same time, the logic of the analogy impresses the conscious mind. Would you say that?

MHE: The logic appeals to the conscious mind, and the unconscious has the conviction of actual knowledge (experiential knowing.)

ER: So, you're speaking to both the logic of the conscious mind and the experience of the unconscious.

MHE: The conscious mind understands the logic of it, and the unconscious understands the reality.

ER: What do you mean by reality here?

MHE: You just demonstrated it by seeing the microphone but not your hand.

ER: The unconscious knows reality from concrete experiences.

MHE: Yes.

ER: When Dr. S opened her eyes and came out of trance, she rubbed her hands together as one of her typical acts of reorientation to her body, but she did not comment on whether or not she was actually seeing them. By implication, we can assume that she was not seeing her hands since she was so absorbed in recounting her early memories. You did not tell her to awaken, but in her case the association between opening eyes and ending trance was stronger than your implication that she could open her eyes and remain in trance and not see.

> **Dr. S: I had an experience where I was actually a year old and looking up from a crib. There was an experience from three years old when I was drinking from cups and getting splashed on my left hand. I was thinking about the feeling that I had. It's like the song about Alice, "She was ten feet tall," and I had the fear of getting a glass of water and having to bend over**

her because I was so tall.

MHE: And even that
you could do without
terrifying emotions.

Dr. S: Yes, it was like untrue, like I had been eating some magic mushrooms. I guess you look at things different. That flashed through my mind when I tried to walk on stilts as a child. It took all afternoon, and they finally did work.

MHE: And you saw things
very high?

Dr. S: They were! Those stilts were over my head.

[This session terminates with a recounting of the many memories that returned to Dr. S during her trance experience.]

Dr. S later wrote the following about her inner experience at this point:

"As I later read my remarks, I was confused because I could recall only the first part where I described myself as ***being*** in a crib. I remember that experience as though I actually were small and looking up at a big world (genuine age regression). I have amnesia now for the three year-old incident, and the last one is not as I recall it. My recollection here is that I was thirsty after the trance work and wanted to go into the next room for a drink of water. However, I could not seem to mobilize myself. I could not pick up the glass of water by my chair. I was somehow still Alice in Wonderland, ten feet tall, so I was afraid that I would have to bend to get through the doorway and that might make me dizzy.

My explanation is that I must have gone into a trance again as I began to describe the trance events. I recall that I was wearing a dress with long butterfly sleeves. My wrists were bent over the end of the arm of the chair and covered by my sleeves. This is in contrast to my usual habit of keeping them in my lap. Apparently, since I had the impression that I could not pick up a glass, I had (in a complex fashion) followed the suggestion (unrecalled by me) of not seeing my hands.

There is an unconscious!"

ER: This was a fantastically successful trance experience for Dr. S. She managed to give up some of the limiting sets of her conscious mind, so she had an apparently genuine experience of age regression wherein she experienced herself in a crib and actually saw the world the way a child would. She experienced hypermenesia (the extensive recall of early memories) and, paradoxically, she also experienced an amnesia (she forgot some trance events). She acknowledges how she managed not to see her hands to comply in her own individual fashion with your suggestion and how this immobilized her so, she could not even pick up a glass of water. You attempted to evoke a negative visual hallucination for her hands "when they were in direct line of vision." But apparently her unconscious could only manage not seeing her hands by immobilizing them out of her view at this time. It's really charming to witness her individuality: to immobilize is easier for her at this point than not seeing. And, most significantly for future hypnotic work, she really acknowledges the reality of the unconscious!

Chapter Sixteen

Displacing and Discharging Resistance

In practical clinical work, we find that "resistance" frequently means that the patient is stuck with a few patterns of association and experience that are interfering with opportunities for new learning. We thus tend to view resistance as an erroneous mental set that gets in the way of new experience. Resistance need not always be understood in the psychoanalytic sense as something that is continually maintained by deep and unconscious forces. Rather, resistance can be a relatively simple stubborn attitude that prevents people from Utilizing their own abilities.

Erickson has developed a number of approaches for displacing and discharging resistance that seem merely humorous, clever, and superficial. These approaches can help patients dodge free of their own "mental blocks" in relatively short order, however.

In a typical case, an aggressive patient may enter the situation blustering, "I need hypnotherapy and I'm sure I can't be hypnotized." On one such occasion, Erickson happened to have three other empty chairs in the office and proceeded as follows:

MHE: There is, of course, a possibility that you can be hypnotized.

[Pause]

Erickson opens the door by mentioning the "possibility" of trance.

There is more possibility that you can't be hypnotized.

He then reinforces or gains acceptance of that "positive possibility" by his open acknowledgment and acceptance of the patient's negative attitude. The patient immediately feels respected, and a positive rapport is established.

Now let's try this chair.

Implying that the question of going into trance has something to do with which chair is being used. This begins the process of displacing the resistance from the patient to the chair.

If you fail in this one, there is still the possibility that you can go into trance.

This gives the patient an opportunity to fail and thus, prove his point that he "can't be hypnotized." This initial failure allows the patient to "use up" and discharge his resistance.

> [The patient failed to enter trance in three of the chairs. He finally experiences a satisfactory trance in the fourth chair. Each time, he failed he "used up" another increment of resistance until trance became inevitable because of the way the above implication displaced the resistance from the patient to the details of seating arrangements, etc.]

Erickson will typically vary the procedure slightly with each effort (e.g., shifting direction of the chairs, shifting his chair, altering the induction procedure to find the one most satisfactory to the patient.

Another means of displacing and discharging resistance is through games and seemingly irrelevant, but humorous challenges whereby the therapist actively evokes and then discharges the resistance by way of a predictable denouement.

As an example, say that you have a bunch of marbles only one of which is a solid color. You tell a child that you are going to write down on paper which marble he is going to choose. You take the position that you are going to predict and force the child to accept your choice. The child accepts the challenge and maintains that you cannot predict his choice. You then begin describing the various marbles as his possibilities: the blue one with white stripes, the brown and white, and so on. He hears you describing all the marbles in a seemingly random manner. He does not notice that you always pick a color combination. He can escape by picking a marble with no color combination—the solid color marble that you previously wrote down as his eventual choice.

In this case, you create the resistance by saying, "I can predict your choice." You insisted that he was going to choose one of the color combinations you mentioned, but he puts an end to your speculations by choosing the solid color you had previously predicted when you wrote it down. The child does not know how you did it, yet there was a genuine rationale for predicting his choice. The child is now intrigued and open to other things you have to say to him.

The same procedure can work with a resistant adult. You look at the bookcase in your office and say that you can predict which book the patient will choose. You then mention all the various possibilities of choice: the dark books with light printing and those that are the reverse, the multicolored bindings, the odd-sized books, and others. You carefully avoid mentioning just one book. Patients invariably resist all the possibilities you mention and pick the one you did not. Patients experience a ***Surprise*** upon finding out that you had written down their choice before the game started. Their resistance tends to remain in the bookcase, and they are now simply open and curious about what you are up to. When the whole procedure is carried out in a low key, fun manner rapport is enhanced. Any serious challenge, of course, is to be avoided with an adult. Should the therapist fail to predict the book that the patient chooses, all is not lost. The patient is now "one up" and feels more relaxed; he now owes it to the therapist to be obliging by entering trance, etc. Resistance has been discharged in the play, and the patient is now available for therapeutic work.

Erickson's efforts to displace doubt and discharge resistance are a unique contribution to psychotherapy. It is clear that this approach can be useful in any form of therapy where careful consideration is taken to help the patient circumvent his own learned limitations in order to achieve something new.

Erickson provided another example of a very common situation in therapy where he regularly displaces doubt and discharges resistance as follows:

MHE: A woman patient came to me with a great many doubts about how much she could tell me. So I said, "All right, hold back everything that you could possibly have some doubt about telling me."

ER: So that immediately mobilized in her mind all the possible things she could say.

MHE: Yes, by the end of the hour she told me everything because once she told me one thing it led to the next. She finally found she had nothing she had any doubts about telling me. An analyst could have dealt with those resistances for several years.

ER: Whenever you give important directives, you try to provide a lightning rod to discharge their resistances.

MHE: Without bringing an awareness of that resistance into the foreground. You don't want your patient to think about resistances.

ER: You discharge resistances without their even being aware that it is happening.

MHE: To discredit this as manipulation is as faulty as it is to describe food as being manipulated because you have seasoned it properly.

We use "resistant" here to mean a lack of understanding. One usually resists when, through lack of understanding they anticipate harm. Further insight into Erickson's approach to discharging negativity and resistance is in the way he gets a patient's "No" away from the therapy situation and gradually replaces it with "Yes." With a resistant patient he sometimes begins by saying, "You don't like all that smog out there t you?" Of course, the patient answers with "No." Erickson then continues with a series of questions that elicit a "No" response about things far removed from the therapy situation. This process gives patients an opportunity to displace and discharge their resistance away from the therapy situation. Erickson then proceeds to ask questions that will elicit a "Yes" about the therapy situation (e.g., Are you as comfortable in that chair as you can be?")

The "Yes" responses then generalize to a greater extent than the patient realizes. One question about comfort, for example, does not convince patients that the therapist is concerned about their comfort and welfare. But a series of questions about comfort begins to generalize through the patient's associative process. The possibility of comfort, for example, now becomes associated with the difficult or traumatic material the patient is struggling to express.

It is apparent that Erickson is using a process orientation to shift ***resistance and "No"*** out of the therapy situation and to bring ***comfort and "Yes"*** into the therapy situation. That is, the actual content of the "No" or "Yes" is irrelevant. Any expressed "No" will help discharge negativity regardless of its particular content. Any expressed "Yes" will generalize further cooperation regardless of the subject matter.

On careful reflection, it will be found that this orientation to ***process*** is more frequently prominent in Erickson's approach than his concern about ***content***. In inducing trance, for example, he ***Utilizes*** the ***process*** of confusion to depotentiate consciousness; the actual subject matter or content of the confusion is irrelevant. In training, a hypnotic subject, it is the process of experiencing one and then a series of hypnotic phenomena that is important, not the content of the particular phenomena. In facilitating therapy, it is the process of getting any noticeable improvement that is important, even if it is initially far removed from the content of the patient's most pressing problem. Content, to be sure, is important, but its importance is usually as a vehicle to gain entry to the patient's attention and associative structures where the process of therapy can be facilitated.

Exercises in Displacing Doubt and Resistance

1. ***Discharging resistance in everyday life.*** Think of occasions in which you were firmly against something and to your surprise found yourself going along with it nonetheless. You may later criticize yourself for "compromising," "giving in," or having "weak willpower." But actually you were probably caught in a situation where your resistance was intentionally or accidentally discharged by another person or circumstances. Can you recall your feelings at the moment when you "gave in?" Can you trace out the psychodynamics of how your resistance was discharged? Can you formulate how you could utilize this example of discharging resistance in a psychotherapeutic situation?

2. Keep a record of all your examples of displacing doubt and discharging resistance in everyday life and psychotherapy. When you have enough examples, try to formulate some general hypotheses about the psychodynamics of displacing doubt and discharging resistance. Can you now design psychological experiments that could test the validity of your hypotheses? Publish your results!

Multiple Levels of Communication: Analogy, Puns, Metaphor, Jokes, and Folk Language

Erickson's penchant for communication by analogy is herein explained as communication on two levels: the conscious and the unconscious. The logic of an analogy can appeal to the conscious mind and break through some of its limiting sets. When the analogy also refers to deeply engrained (automatic and therefore functionally unconscious) associations, mental mechanisms, and learned patterns of behavior, it tends to activate these internal responses and make them available for problem solving. Suggestions made by analogy are thus a powerful and indirect twofold approach that mediates between the conscious and unconscious. Appropriate analogies appeal to the conscious mind because of their inherent interest while mobilizing the resources of the unconscious by many processes of association.

The authors (Erickson and Rossi, 1976) have discussed multilevel communication in terms of Jenkins' contextual theory of verbal associations (Erickson & Rossi, 1974/2010). Analogy, puns, metaphor, paradox, and folk language can all be understood as presenting a general context on the surface level that is first assimilated by consciousness. The individual words and phrases used to articulate that general context, however, all have their own individual and literal associations that do not belong to the context. These individual and literal associations are, of course, usually suppressed and excluded from consciousness in its effort to grasp the general context. These suppressed associations do remain in the unconscious, however, and under the special circumstances of trance, where dissociation and literalness are heightened, they can play a significant role in facilitating responsive behavior that is surprising to consciousness.

This situation can be made clear by analogy. The adult reader is usually searching for an author's meaning. Within certain limits it really doesn't matter what particular sentences or words are used. Many different sentences and combinations of words could be used to express the same meaning. It is the meaning or the general context of the sentences that registered in consciousness, while the particular sentences and words used fall into the unconscious and are "forgotten." In the same way, one reads the meaning of a whole word rather than the individual letters used to make up the word. The general context of the letters registers as the conscious meaning of a word rather than the individual associations of each letter. Jenkins (1974) has summarized the data of recent experimental work in the area of verbal association, event recognition, information integration, and memory that places a similar emphasis on the significance of context to understand these phenomena. In any discourse or phenomena using words, it is usually the general context that establishes meaning rather than the structural units that create the discourse.

The obvious exceptions to this, of course, are in puns, allusions, and all sorts of verbal jokes where the punch line depends on literal or individual verbal associations to words and phrases that originally escaped the attention of consciousness. Verbal jokes depend on literal or individual associations that are usually suppressed.

In the same way, Erickson's two-level communication ***Utilizes*** a general context to fixate the attention of consciousness while the individual associations of words, phrases, or sentences within that context are registered in the unconscious, where they can work their effects. From this point of view, Erickson's ***Interspersal Technique*** (1966b) is the clearest example of two-level communication wherein subject matter of interest to a particular patient is ***Utilized*** as a general context to fixate conscious attention while ***Interspersed*** suggestions are received for their effects on an unconscious level.

Erickson has devised a number of other techniques to activate the individual, literal, and unconscious associations to words, phrases, or sentences buried within a more general context. Turns of phrase that are shocking, surprising, mystifying, non sequiturs, too difficult or incomprehensible for the general conscious context, for example, all tend momentarily to depotentiate the patient's conscious sets and to activate a search on the unconscious level that will turn up the literal and individual associations that were previously suppressed. When Erickson overloads the general context with many words, phrases, or sentences that have common individual associations, those associations (the interspersed suggestion) gain ascendency in the unconscious until they finally spill over into responsive behavior that the conscious mind now registers with a sense of surprise. The conscious mind is surprised because it is presented with a response within itself that it cannot account for. The response is then described as having occurred "all by itself" without the intervention of the subject's conscious intention; the response appears to be autonomous or hypnotic.

Analogy and metaphor as well as jokes can be understood as exerting their powerful effects through the same mechanism of activating unconscious association patterns and response tendencies that suddenly summate to present consciousness with an apparently "new" datum or behavioral response.

The Microdynamics of Suggestion

Once Erickson has fixated and focused a patient's attention with a question or general context of interest (e.g., ideally, the possibility of dealing with the patient's problem), he then introduces a number of approaches designed to depotentiate conscious sets. By this, we do not mean there is a loss of awareness in the sense of going to sleep; we are not confusing trance with the condition of sleep. In trance, there is a reduction of the patient's foci of attention to a few inner realities; consciousness has been fixated and focused to a relatively narrow frame of attention rather than being diffused over a broad area, as in the more typical general reality orientation (Shor, 1959) of our usual everyday awareness. When fixated and focused in such a narrow frame, consciousness is in a state of unstable equilibrium; it can be depotentiated by being shifted, transformed, or bypassed with relative ease.

Erickson believes that the purpose of clinical induction is to focus attention inward and to alter some of the individual's habitual patterns of functioning. Because of the limitations of patients' habitual frames of reference, their usual everyday consciousness cannot cope with certain inner and/or outer realities, and they recognize that they have a "problem." Depotentiating patients' usual everyday consciousness is thus a way of depotentiating facets of their personal limitations; it is a way of deautomatizing (Deikman, 1972) an individual's habitual modes of functioning so that dissociation and many of its attendant classical hypnotic phenomena (e.g., age regression, amnesia, sensory-perceptual distortions, catalepsies, etc.) are frequently manifest in an entirely spontaneous manner (Erickson and Rossi, 1975.) Depotentiating the limitations of the individual's usual patterns of awareness thus opens up the possibility that new combinations of associations and mental skills may be evolved for creative problem solving within that individual.

Erickson's approaches to depotentiating conscious sets are so subtle and pervasive in the manner with which they are interwoven with the actual process of induction and suggestion that they are usually unrecognized even when one studies a written transcript of his words. In order to place them in perspective, we have outlined the microdynamics of induction and suggestion in Table 2 as:

1) Fixation of Attention

2) Depotentiating Conscious Sets

3) Unconscious Search

4) Unconscious Processes

5) Hypnotic Response

We have also listed a number of Erickson's approaches to facilitating each stage. Most of these approaches are illustrated in this volume and are discussed in more detail elsewhere (Erickson and Rossi, 1974/2010; Erickson and Rossi, 1975; Haley, 1963; Rossi, 1973a). Although we may outline these processes as stages of a sequence in Table 2 for the purpose of analysis, they usually function as one simultaneous process. Because of this, and in order to distinguish these processes from the broader dynamics of induction and mediating variables previously outlined (Barber and De Moor, 1972) we designate ours as "microdynamics." When we succeed in fixating attention, we automatically narrow the focus of attention to the point where one's usual frames of reference are vulnerable to being depotentiated. At such moments there is an automatic search on the unconscious level for new associations that can restructure a more stable frame of reference through the summation of unconscious processes. There is thus a certain arbitrariness to the order and the headings under which we assign some of the approaches Erickson used in Table 2. He could equally well begin with an interesting story or pun as with a shock, ***Surprise***, or a formal induction of trance. Once the conditions in the first three columns have been set in motion by the therapist, however, the patient's own individual unconscious dynamics automatically carries out the processes of the last two columns.

A number of Erickson's most interesting approaches to facilitate hypnotic response are the hypnotic forms listed in column 3 of Table 2. All these approaches are designed to evoke a search on the unconscious level. Allusions, puns, metaphors, implications and so on, are usually not grasped immediately by consciousness. There is a momentary delay before one "gets" a joke, and in part, that is what is funny about it. In that delay period, there obviously is a search and processes on an unconscious level (column 4) that finally summate to present a new datum to consciousness so that it gets the joke. All the approaches listed in column 3 are communication devices that initiate a search for new combinations of associations and mental processes that can present consciousness with useful results in everyday life as well as in hypnosis. The hypnotic forms listed in columns 2 and 3 are also the essence of Erickson's indirect approach to suggestion. The study of these approaches may be regarded as a contribution to the science of pragmatics: the relation between signs and the users of signs (Watzlawick et al., 1967). Erickson relies upon the skillful ***Utilization*** of such forms of communication, rather than hyper-suggestibility per se, to evoke hypnotic behavior.

As noted previously, it is important to recognize that while Erickson thinks of therapeutic trance as a special state (of reduced foci of attention), he does not believe hype-suggestibility is a necessary characteristic of such trance (Erickson, 1932/2010). That is, just because patients are experiencing trance, it does not mean they are going to accept and act upon the therapist's direct suggestions. This is a major misconception that accounts for many of the failures of hypnotherapy; it has frustrated and discouraged many clinical workers in the past and may have impeded the scientific exploration of hypnosis in the laboratory. Therapeutic trance is a special state that intensifies the patient-therapist relationship and focuses the patient's attention on a few inner realities; ***trance does not ensure the acceptance of suggestions***. Erickson depends upon certain communication devices such as those listed in column 3 to evoke, mobilize, and move a patient's associative processes and mental skills in certain directions to ***sometimes*** achieve certain therapeutic goals. He believes that hypnotic suggestion is actually this process of evoking and *Utilizing* a patient's own mental processes in ways that are outside his

Table 2 (10.12.T.2) The Microdynamics of Trance Induction and Suggestion				
Fixation of Attention	*Depotentiating Conscious Sets*	*Unconscious Search*	*Uncon- scious Processes*	*Hypnotic Response*
1. Sto- ries that motivate, interest, fascination, etc.	1. Shock, ***Surprise***, the unrealistic and unusual	1. Allusions, puns, jokes	1. Summa- tion of: a. Inter- spersed suggestions b. Literal associa- tions c. Individ- ual associa- tions d. Multiple meaning of words	New datum or behavioral response experi- enced as hypnotic or happen- ing all by itself
2. Standard eye fixation	2. Shifting frames of ref- erence; dis- placing doubt, resistance, and failure	2. Metaphor, analogy, folk language	2. Autono- mous, sen- sory, and perceptual processes	
3. Pan- tomime approaches	3. Distraction	3. Implica- tion	3. Freud- ian primary processes	
4. Imagina- tion and vi- sualization approaches	4. Dissociation and disequilib- rium	4. Implied directive	4. Person- ality mech- anisms of defense	

5. ***Hand Levitation***	5. Cognitive overloading	5. Ideomotor signaling	5. Ziegarnik Effect Etc.	
6. Relaxation and all forms of inner sensory, perceptual or emotional experience Etc.	6. Confusion & non sequiturs	6. Words initiating exploratory sets		
	7. Paradox	7. Questions and tasks requiring unconscious search		
	8. Binds and ***Double Binds***	8. Pause with therapist attitude of expectancy		
	9. Conditioning via voice dynamics, etc.	9. Open-ended suggestions		
	10. Structured amnesia	10. Covering all possibilities of response		
	11. Not doing, not knowing	11. Compound statements		
	12. Losing abilities; the negative; doubt Etc.	12. Intercontextual cues and suggestions Etc.		

usual range of ego control. This ***Utilization*** theory of hypnotic suggestion can be validated if it is found that other therapists and researchers can also effect more reliable results by carefully ***Utilizing*** whatever associations and mental skills a particular patient already has that can be mobilized, extended, displaced, or transformed to achieve specific "hypnotic" phenomena and therapeutic goals.

In the therapeutic trance situation, the successful ***Utilization*** of unconscious processes leads to an autonomous response; patients are surprised to find themselves confronted with a new datum or behavior (column 5.) The same situation is in evidence in everyday life, however, whenever attention is fixated with a question or an experience of the amazing, the unusual, or anything that holds a person's interest. At such moments, people experience the common everyday trance; they tend to gaze off (to the right or left, depending upon which cerebral hemisphere is most dominant, (Baken, 1969; Hilgard and Hilgard, 1975) and get that "faraway" or "blank" look; their eyes may actually close, their body tends to become immobile (a form of catalepsy), certain reflexes (e.g., swallowing, respiration) may be suppressed, and they seem momentarily oblivious to their surroundings until they have completed their inner search on the unconscious level for the new idea, response, or frames of reference that will restabilize their general reality orientation. We hypothesize that in everyday life consciousness is in a continual state of flux between the general reality orientation and the momentary microdynamics of trance as outlined in Table 2. The well-trained hypnotherapist is acutely aware of these dynamics and their behavioral manifestations. Trance experience and hypnotherapy are simply the extension and ***Utilization*** of these normal psychodynamic processes. Altered states of consciousness—wherein attention is fixated and the resulting narrow frame of reference is shattered, shifted, and/or transformed with the help of drugs, sensory deprivation, meditation, biofeedback, or whatever—follow essentially the same pattern but with varying emphasis on the different stages. We may thus understand Table 2 as a general paradigm for understanding the genesis and microdynamics of altered states and their effects upon behavior.

Exercises with Analogies Puns, and Metaphors

1. Create analogies and metaphors that are interesting and arresting to the conscious mind while also activating habitual modes of unconscious functioning that can be used to facilitate all the standard hypnotic phenomena.

2. When planning a therapeutic approach to a particular patient's problem, ***Utilize*** puns, analogies, metaphors, and folk language that will have the following:

a. A direct appeal for that individual in terms of his lifetime interests.

b. Directly activate by association habitual modes of functioning in the patient that can facilitate a therapeutic goal.

Note that such analogies can be effective with or without trance. In trance, however, analogies can be considered as specific tools for facilitating desired responses.

Chapter Seventeen

Indirectly Conditioned Eye Closure Induction

Erickson continues in this session to deal with Dr. S's major problem in learning to experience trance: allowing and trusting unconscious modes of functioning. This is the most typical problem the modern hypnotherapist must learn to cope with in our western culture where the rational aspect of mind is valued above all others. It is the bias and hubris of the rational and intellectualized mind to downgrade the accomplishments and possibilities of the unconscious. The conscious mind likes to believe in its autonomy and power. In actuality, consciousness is always focal and thus limited to what is within its momentary focus. It cannot possibly deal with everything all at once; at every moment in our lives we are dependent on unconscious processes to regulate everything from our blood chemistry to our next verbal association. Consciousness is a relatively recent evolutionary acquisition. Although we like to believe that consciousness is a high form of evolutionary development, it is in fact extremely labile and limited in its abilities.

A major problem of consciousness as it is presently constructed is that it frequently excludes everything outside of its immediate focus and it tends to believe only in its own momentary mood and truth. No wonder there are so many lethal conflicts within us as individuals and between us as people. Because of these limitations it is important that consciousness be expanded (awareness heightened) by learning to relate optimally to the unconscious. For Erickson, this would mean allowing the unconscious an opportunity to do its own work. Therapeutic trance can be understood as a state in which unconscious work is to some extent freed from the limiting foci and sets of consciousness. Once the unconscious has done its work, the conscious mind can receive and focus it appropriately in the various moments and sets (circumstances) of life. The unconscious is a manufacturer and consciousness is a consumer; trance is a mediator between them.

Erickson begins the session with remarks that tend to confuse and depotentiate consciousness. He then demonstrates another indirect approach to induction by conditioning eye closure. He emphasizes the need for careful observation of trance induction by a scaling procedure. Of particular value in the commentaries of this session are examples of Erickson's unusual perceptiveness in dealing with a number of difficult issues in trance work, including sources of psychological confusion in trance, alternating rhythms of suggestibility in trance, posthypnotic suggestion, dealing with spontaneous awakening, and ways of protecting the subject in trance.

Session 7: Confusion in Trance Induction with Dr. S

Erickson begins the session by asking Dr. S what she would like to accomplish today. Dr. S mentions a wart she would like to have go away but does not volunteer any personal problems she might want to deal with. A desultory conversation takes place for a few minutes. Then Erickson quietly remarks, "Probably Dr. Rossi is noticing something." This was a hint to ER to notice that Dr. S's eye blink reflex was spontaneously beginning to slow down. ER isn't sure just what is happening, but he is aware Erickson is telling him to observe Dr. S carefully. Dr. S laughs self-consciously and asks what is going on. Erickson assures her that she will know soon enough. After a moment's pause Erickson continues.

MHE: How soon do you think you will know?

Dr. S: I don't even know what I'm supposed to know. What I'm ready for?
[Pause]
What am I supposed to know?
[Pause]

ER: You frequently use this approach of hinting that something is happening that the patient's consciousness is not tuned into. It tends to confuse the patient, it depotentiates the ego's subjective sense of control, and it builds up a high expectancy that something unusual and significant will happen. Her questions clearly indicate the great confusion that has been induced by your simple remark, "Probably Dr. Rossi is noticing something."

MHE: Now I'll say odd and even for a specific purpose.

Dr. S: Will you tell me?

MHE: At the end.
Even.
Odd.
[Pause]
Odd.
Odd.
Odd
Even.
[Pause]

[Dr. S is obviously puzzled by Erickson's odd-even statements. He is talking in a way that is apparently meaningful, yet she cannot grasp his meaning. After a moment of concentrated attention she apparently gives up and lapses into herself]

MHE: You say "odd" when the eye blink is slow and "even" when it is fast.

ER: You just say that without her being aware of what you were doing?

MHE: Yes.

ER: What does that do to her?

MHE: She makes the connection unconsciously. She begins with two blinks, one fast and one slow. Unconsciously she noticed that I said "odd" after the slow blink. So then she pauses and then blinks slow three times. She gives a more rapid blink and pauses again.

ER: This is an induction procedure or what?

MHE: It is an induction procedure because you're closing the eyelids. It is a technique to close the eyelids.

ER: Why will the eyelids close?

MHE: Because it becomes a conditioned response. "Odd" becomes associated with a sensation of slowness if you say it each time there is a slow blink.

ER: Once you've established that association, you need only say "odd" and the eyelids will get slower and slower and finally close. Is this another subtle or indirect way of inducing trance? Is it an unconsciously conditioned response for induction?

MHE: Yes. It's an unconsciously conditioned response. She is going back and forth on a scale of 1 to 100.

Dr. S: I usually don't blink so much.

MHE: Now she is up to about 15.
[Pause]
50
35, 40
15, close
[To ER] Now I let that be prolonged. I interrupted it so it could be
demonstrated thoroughly. Ordinarily you wouldn't make prolonged use of
this. This is a chance for you to see it in operation.

MHE: On a scale of 1 to 100 where a 100 is deep trance. When the eyes close when you say "close," the subject is perhaps at 10.

ER: You are using your own subjective scale when you say she is up to 15, 50, etc. When she was up to 15, I noticed her face beginning to iron out. At 40, I noticed more quietness.

MHE: I said "close" here when the eyes were closing on a slow blink, and that served to close them.

MHE: Now I know that Dr. S wants to drift.
[Pause]
Now there you saw the conscious mind recognizing a word of significance.
After a while she will let the drifting remain unconscious.
[Pause]
[To Dr. S] Now searching through things you really want
for many different reasons,
not only for an understanding of them
but for an experience of them.
[Pause]

ER: At the word "drift" there was a visible relaxing of Dr. S that was apparently mediated by ego consciousness, since it was obvious and quick. When relaxation is mediated by the unconscious, it is somehow more subtle. Her conscious mind recognized the work "drift" as her own description of deepening trance.

MHE: Now Dr. S has been trying to get some rational understanding of hypnosis. She doesn't realize that to learn to swim you have to get in the water to actually experience it. Intellectual book knowledge about swimming won't do it. She has been trying to get in the trance and understand. But she should just get in the water first.

ER: When the patient tries to observe and understand, it interferes with the process of learning by the experience of just letting things happen. In trance, it is necessary to learn by experiencing rather than intellectualizing.

> **MHE: As you know enough**
> **about phenomena**
> **so you can let your own unconscious mind**
> **elaborate**
> **whatever phenomena you wish.**
> **And in any direction.**
> **And you should do that as an experience for yourself**
> **as a discovery of what your unconscious mind can do.**

MHE: "Elaborate" is separated off as a separate word to make it a command.

ER: What's the command?

MHE: "So you can let your own unconscious mind" is a permissive statement that the conscious mind hears. "Elaborate" makes it a command which the unconscious hears. It's an interspersal technique. It's not noticeable that a command has been given.

ER: What's the interspersed message here?

MHE: The word "elaborate." The emphasis on this word changes it from just another word in the sentence to a specific word.

ER: A specific direction and command the unconscious is given with the emphasis on that word "elaborate." This is an indirect message to further separate the conscious from the unconscious.

> **MHE: Your unconscious mind can decide what part**
> **or what aspects**
> **of the experience should be shared by Dr. Rossi and me.**
> **By others in general.**
> **By patients with whom you work.**
> **[Pause]**
> **With others within you.**
> **Also, your understandings belong to you.**
> **But it is possible**
> **for you to share with others**
> **in ways you never thought of before.**

MHE: She thinks, "Should I share this with Dr. Rossi, knowing that I know Dr. Rossi only to such and such a degree? Is this something he can tolerate? Is this something he can be interested in?"

ER: These statements are a series of psychological truisms wherein you mention all possibilities of response and thereby bring whatever she does into association with you and your words. It is easy for her to accept and follow any one of these truisms, but whatever she chooses will actually place her in the situation of following your words and thus reinforce her rapport with you and her tendency to follow other suggestions. This is a way of covering all possible responses.

Depotentiating Consciousness with Boredom: An Example of Indirect Suggestion

MHE: I'll give you a personal example.
In learning the multiplication tables at school, my teacher said, "I do not
know what you are doing, but you have all the answers right."
I had to wait until I got to college to explain to my teacher what it was I had done.
[Pause]
I have a son whose teacher said, "Now I don't know what you are doing in
your arithmetic lessons, but you do have the right answers, so keep right on with whatever you are doing."
The reason he didn't know
was that my sixth grade son was using algorithms.
This baffled the teacher.
This bewildered my son,
and he reached the conclusion that a slide rule was a child's plaything.
I sent him to a library to find some books there that might interest him.
He found a book of logarithms
and began a formal study of logarithms
and tried to teach them to his teacher.
But he really couldn't explain logarithms to his teacher,
and he later found that to teach logarithms to college students is quite a job.
I told him how I did my math.
He said,

"Well I tried that long ago, but it's too simple."
When you use multiplication tables, there is a mathematical relationship
among the answers. If you know the mathematical relationship, you know all the answers.

Take the 7 times table:
7 x 1 = 7
7 x 2 = 14
7 x 3 = 21
7 x 4 = 28
7 x 5 = 35
7 x 6 = 42
7 x 7 = 49
7 x 8 = 56
7 x 9 = 63

If you know this relationship of progression in the algorithm, it is easy to remember the whole table.

ER: Dr. S is in a light trance at this point, so what is the purpose of giving such a complex and detailed mathematical example in such a disjointed manner? Won't this activate her conscious mind and defeat the process of deepening the trance and unconscious learning?

MHE: *Often* with highly sophisticated subjects, you resort to uninteresting detail to bore the hell out of them.

ER: That's what you're doing here? You're boring the hell out of her? That's why you used this mathematical example! Well, you were succeeding because at that point I was also going into a trance myself.

MHE: They don't know what you are doing. They try to be polite, and this, past experience has taught them, can be awfully fatiguing.

ER: So this is a way of making her tired.

MHE: Yes. ***Without telling her to be tired!***

ER: I see. You're taking all the spunk and fire and energy out of her intellect. You're discharging it with this boredom. You're fizzling it out with boredom.

MHE: That's right.

ER: I see! I was bored too! I was wondering, "Is this supposed to be brilliant hypnotherapy? What is this?" But now that I can see what it was used for, I can realize it's marvelous. You were depotentiating consciousness by boring it out of existence.

MHE: Yes. That's right.

ER: This is an excellent example of your indirect approach to suggestion. You did not directly suggest she would be relaxed or tired. Rather, you had recourse to evoking a certain psychological situation or stimulus (boring arithmetic) that will arouse an internal response (acting polite) that will in turn evoke an experience of mental fatigue by associations and processes that already exist within her. She is not able to recognize the relation between what you are saying and what she is actually experiencing. Because of this the indirect suggestion escapes her conscious attention. She is responding in a certain way but may not know exactly why. This ***not knowing*** is compatible with the essence of trance, which is to allow more autonomous or spontaneous responses take place without the habitual sets of consciousness structuring, directing, and controlling them.

For the benefit of the reader, I'll point out that there are a number of different ways to identify patterns in math. Of course, it would be hopeless for someone trying to go into trance to figure that out, so their consciousness just gives up. And that is trance when the normal ego consciousness is no longer directing and controlling things as usual. The distraction results in boredom.

MHE: Now personal meanings
to you
are yours.
The application
of all those meanings
to others
is an entirely different thing.
I could know
mathematical relationships
and couldn't explain them
to my teacher.
My son could not explain to his teacher.
But we get the same answers as they get.
We could not explain why we preferred our way.
[Pause]

MHE: I'm trying to get her to understand: what may be pleasant and agreeable to one may not be pleasant and agreeable to others.

ER: Why do you put that in here?

MHE: How many times has a patient said to you, "But you wouldn't be interested in hearing this." That's a very inhibiting thing in them. They are inhibiting themselves. You've got the task of telling them, "You are interesting."

ER: You're breaking through a negative attitude of consciousness. Again you're telling Dr. S that she does not have to understand trance intellectually, she just needs to experience it.

MHE: Now the matter of hallucination,
of regression,
of Time Distortion,
the selection of memories,
the achieving of understandings,
the isolation of the self from a situation.
[Pause]
I exist in the office.
[Pause]

MHE: She might be intellectually interested in any of these phenomena, but she doesn't know if her unconscious wants them.

ER: We have to be humble enough to let our unconscious direct and experience whichever of these possibilities it needs.

MHE: Yes. We let the unconscious direct. Whenever subjects try to do what they understand, [try to direct their unconscious with their conscious], they run into confusion.

ER: I wonder if that throws light on the general significance of confusion when we deal with personality and inner problems? Confusion is the result of trying to impose our conscious and more limited understanding on the broader patterns of unconscious functioning?

MHE: Confusion results from trying to impose some form of regimentation upon natural processes.

ER: I see. That's how you would define psychological confusion.

MHE: A centipede can be walking along happily until some son of a gun asks him which leg comes after which. Then he falls into confusion trying to figure that out. As long as the centipede does not try to rationalize, he is okay.

ER: From a neuropsychological point of view, I wonder if psychological confusion and error can result from trying to impose the rational programs of the left hemisphere on the gestalt patterns of the right?

MHE: You can learn to hear my voice
as only meaningful sound.
Meaningful sound
to which you give the interpretation.
And it isn't necessary
for you to
waste mental energy
on the realities,
the external realities.
Now I will illustrate that.
[Pause]
When I was demonstrating in a
hospital, I had some subjects on a stage with me.
They were not in a trance.
I told the audience that the people on stage were going to go
into a trance.
While I was doing that, I noticed some people in the audience
that were going in a trance.
They were very still.
I told the people in the audience they could look around and
see which of
them had gone in a trance. Some might have to stand up to
look around.
[Pause]

MHE: I want her to hear my voice as something which evokes memories and associations meaningful to her.

ER: You're trying to associate your voice with meaningful dimensions within her. She can even reinterpret your words in terms of her own mental sets and personal contexts into which she places your words.

MHE: My words are not limited to the words themselves. They will just naturally trigger off many different associations in her.

ER: So you're actually describing another natural mental mechanism here: the process of association. At the same time, you're associating your voice with whatever personal associations are evoked.

MHE: That's right, to elaborate their associations at the unconscious level. You've already told them they don't have to share it all with you, but you do want them to elaborate.

ER: You're activating the unconscious, you're getting them moving here?

MHE: You're getting them moving because there is a lot of territory they can cover.

ER: In other words, you want patients to be active in the inner world, not just sitting there passively.

MHE: That's right.

> **MHE: One girl in the audience stood up and looked around.**
> **I told her she could do something she liked to do.**
> **[Pause]**
> **She nodded her head agreeably.**

**She would do so.
I worked with the other subjects on stage.
I later asked her to give me some attention.
I asked her to tell me
if she could share it with others,
to tell me what she had been doing
and to explain it.
She said she had been down to the bay and looked all around.
There was nobody in sight so she went in swimming in the nude and had a
most delightful time.
And then she heard my voice from a long distance away.
A distance of 50 miles.
It was hard to recognize my voice, because of the distance, asking her to
come back to the hospital room.
She came back and explained how she enjoyed swimming in the nude very
much
and often swam nude alone at that place.
She had enjoyed that swim
and now felt very rested,
[Pause]
refreshed.
[Pause]
You have done comparable things in your dreams at night.
[Pause]
You can do comparable things in the trance state.
[Pause]
You can read a book.
You can go swimming.
You can converse with friends.
And everything will be totally real
because the only reality
that things possess
is the reality that our senses give them.**

ER: It is not unusual for you to notice the spontaneous trances that people in the audience fall into while they are apparently listening to you. Their bodies are still, they typically have a "vacant" or "faraway" look in their eyes, and their faces may be "ironed out." This sort of trance or reverie is a natural part of everyday life, and you have developed approaches to ***Utilize*** these spontaneous trances for demonstration and therapeutic purposes. The very fact that this girl from the audience did stand up indicated she was in rapport with you, and your simple suggestion that she could "do something she liked to do" was sufficient to ***Utilize*** her spontaneous trance for demonstration purposes.

MHE: When she stood up, I could tell she was in a trance by the economy of effort in her movements: a slow and highly coordinated way of moving.

ER: So you ***Utilized*** her spontaneous trance for demonstration purposes.

MHE: At an invitation by her.

ER: I see. Since she did go into a spontaneous trance and followed your suggestion to stand and look around, you concluded that her unconscious was asking for a trance experience directed by you.

> [Erickson here gives several other examples of how he detected the unconscious wishes of experimental subjects and patients and then Utilized these wishes in deep trance to help them achieve them.]

ER: This accounts for much of your success in helping subjects achieve significant objectives in deep trance. By being sensitive to what they want and need and "giving them permission" to achieve these things, they go into intense periods of inner absorption (deep trance) focused on their needs and thereby achieve their inner realization. That accounts for the potency of your clinical, patient-centered approach; you go along with the natural currents that are there striving for expression. You simply ***Utilized*** what is there.

MHE: And when a patient says, "I don't want to do this," I say, "Okay, then I'll take care of it while you do this other." So they can dissociate.

ER: You help them dissociate their negative affect from something that needs to be done.

MHE: A blind person
hears and feels
and smells someone else.
He cannot see that person,
but he can hear how tall a person is.
He can tell,
talking with the person,
just by his own speech to the person
he can tell if the body is male or female,
because there is a different sound bouncing off that person's body back to
his ears.
He can tell if a person is facing him or has his back to him.
We all have so much knowledge.
of which we are unaware.
[Pause]
Will you stop to think about it?
We do not know
[Pausc]
which use
of your awareness
of things
you will use.

MHE: Most people do not know of their total capacities for response to stimuli. They place mystical meanings on much of the information they get by subtle cues.

[Erickson goes on to explain that the ability to make a subject turn around by looking at their back, for example, is achieved because the person who turns around has actually picked up minimal cues from others in the audience who have noticed the looker. If two people are alone, the same effect is achieved by detecting subtle smells or sounds of the presence of the other without even being aware that these subtle smells or sounds were Utilized. On numerous occasions, people have asked Erickson about the existence of ESP and other psi phenomena in hypnosis. Erickson simply replies that he has never personally encountered a situation where such "parapsychological" events could not be accounted for by minimal sensory cues which people were unaware they were capable of using.]

ER: Yes, many of the mind-reading, thought-reading, and muscle-reading experiments of the early days in hypnosis (Hull, 1933) can be explained as forms of ideomotor or ideosensory cues that most people do not ordinarily recognize.

MHE: You can drive straight west
and pass
a distant mountainside.
The landscape impresses you
very
warmly.
Ten years later
in driving east
you recognize that landscape.
One can think
of a situation
without using a single muscle.
Or one can think of a situation
and use only the memories
of muscle action.
Or one can very slightly
use the muscles.
One can remember

a long past fear
and be completely passive
but feel all the memories of that fear.

[Erickson here gives a personal example of memories associated with muscle action.]

And you can make my voice
just a meaningful sound
that you can interpret
in any way that you please.
[Pause]
And you have no occasion to be
frightened
or excited
or confused
except for your own
desires
and your own
understandings.
You can look at anything
you wish
to see it.
You use your memories
to construct it.
If opening the eyes aids the construction, that's all right.
But you can construct with the eyes closed.
In brief,
there is a wide field of
exploration
for you.

[To ER] Now when a patient has this opportunity to explore themselves,
you are careful not to place any interpretation on anything they do.

MHE: This is another example of the same thing: you don't know which cues you are using, but you do remember the landscape. The whole effect is registered.

ER: The whole, the gestalt?

MHE: Yes, the gestalt.

ER: So you're telling Dr. S by this example to be sensitive to gestalts?

MHE: I'm telling her, "Don't assume it must be just one cue or fact that you can name in recognizing things."

ER: Why are you telling her this? What are you getting at?

MHE: You don't know what the cues are that you are using, but you can recognize things.

ER: So your unconscious is automatically identifying all those cues and ends up by telling the conscious mind, "It's so and so," without telling the conscious mind all the details of how it came to that perception. So you're telling her unconscious to ***Utilize*** all its cues.

MHE: It doesn't have to have a cue that is nameable. The conscious mind tends to think it has to have identifiable cues, but you don't need specific cues to do things.

ER: But why are you giving her this lesson here?

MHE: Because she's been trained as a psychologist, and one of the defects in teaching psychologists is they try to make you aware of all the cues to different things.

ER: They train you to consciously label everything rather than learning to utilize your intuition (unconscious perception.) With Dr. S you must undo some of this over rational training to force the unconscious to work on its own. This is necessary if she is to experience hypnotic phenomena wherein the unconscious operates autonomously. You are thus trying to activate her unconscious by emphasizing all the things it does well all by itself and depotentiate her over rational conscious orientation by emphasizing that it is not needed.

MHE: She has learned in college that you use words and numbers to express everything.

ER: That rational approach is good for certain intellectual things, but for total human functioning it is not good.

MHE: It's ***not*** good!

ER: It freezes you up. It limits you to your conscious awareness. It locks out unconscious perception and mentation. You don't trust your unconscious perception.

> [Erickson here tells a charming story of how he and several of his male colleagues at a convention happened to be standing together watching a young female child hovering in obvious difficulty in

front of a men's room. Dr. Erickson immediately wagered that she would pick the married man with the most children from among them to take her into the men's room. With unerring unconscious perception she did. The child did not stop to think, "Now the ablest man to help me would be the one who had the most children and is therefore used to this sort of thing."]

ER: So you want Dr. S to learn to trust that unconscious knowing and doing in her trance work. This experience will then help her eventually achieve a better balance between rational and irrational processes in her daily life.

MHE: Yes! You don't actually have to look for a wedding ring to spot a married man or woman.

MHE: [Turning to Dr. S] We learn early that to see things we have to have eyes open. But in reconstruction of a visual scene you only need the memories.

[To ER] There is that lifetime of learning that you have to open the eyes, and
so you tell them they can open their eyes since it may help them.
You give them the opportunity
to open their eyes.
They also know they can
use their nose to smell
and ears to hear,
their fingers to feel.

ER: They get all that by implication.

MHE: Yes, by implication. One can learn by reading,
by seeing,
by feeling,
by being told,

by experiencing,
and the best way of learning, to use folk language,
is by getting the feel of it.

ER: To encourage a person to go into trance you must encourage them to trust their unconscious because trance is a natural form of unconscious functioning.

MHE: That's right.

ER: Our view is that trance is an altered state. Do you go along with the idea that it is concrete mental functioning—more on the paleocortex rather than the neocortex?

MHE: Trance is a simpler and uncomplicated way of functioning.

[Erickson here gives examples of how a child learns food preferences, etc., by watching the parents and siblings reactions to food. These early learnings are based on the simpler and more direct processes of observation rather than the more complicated forms of learning involving the mediated use of words and logical thought processes that come later. Erickson does not believe, however, that trance is an atavistic state.]

MHE: You get the feel of a poem,
the feeling of a picture,
the feeling of a statue.
Feeling is a very meaningful word.
We do not just feel with the fingers,
but with the heart,
the mind.
You feel with the learnings of the past.
You feel with the hopes for the future.

You feel the present.

[Dr. S is making slight "Yes" head nodding motions. So slight and slow were the movements that Erickson had to silently point them out and Rossi had to carefully study Dr. S for a minute or two before he was convinced that they were really taking place. These slight "Yes" responses are apparently Dr. S's expression of agreement with what Erickson was saying.]

ER: You like to use pantomime and nonverbal approaches to trance because they activate and reach in more deeply to the simpler levels of functioning.

MHE: Yes. You thereby bypass the enforced rigid forms of later conscious acquisitions. You don't have to have things put into words.

[Erickson gives examples in courtship. A girl may tilt her head for a kiss, but it would spoil the situation for her to verbalize her wish.]

You just ruin things with your later learnings. A tilt of the head is far more meaningful than words.

ER: How can we generalize this to trance behavior as a whole? Trance is not so much regressed behavior as a simpler form of behavior—behavior that is not necessarily dependent on words and adult patterns of understanding?

MHE: Yes, it's awfully simple behavior.

[Erickson gives examples of the economy of body movement in trance. Nodding the head "Yes" in trance is very slight and slow;

this is in marked contrast to the rapid and large nodding movements to signify "Yes" when we are awake.]

ER: You can differentiate conscious from unconscious movements because the latter are always slower and more abbreviated.

MHE: If something is very important, then the movement [e.g., head nodding] will be continuous rather than just once—still slow and abbreviated but continuous so you ***really*** understand. They will continue the head nodding until you give some acknowledgment that you understand. Repetitive movements in trance mean a thing is more important.

MHE: Now I would leave
instruction in neurosis primarily to your unconscious.
[Pause]
And I want you to know
that in each person's life
there are things
we like and don't want to know about.
It would spoil the magicians art if you knew
how he did that trick.
How did he get that rabbit out of a hat?
Of course, there is some kind of an explanation,
but you would rather enjoy having him perform
than know how he did it.
All magicians keep their own special secrets,
and they all respect each others' secrets.

[Erickson gives several examples of how he and others have enjoyed not knowing how magicians performed their mysterious feats.]

And another thing all patients
should keep in mind,
adults are only children grown tall.

ER: It seems strange to suddenly pop out with that didactic statement, "Now I would leave instruction in neurosis primarily to your unconscious." Why did you come out with that right here?

MHE: Because I have prepared her for it with the previous context, where I was giving many instructions for more freedom for unconscious functioning. So that statement would mean, "Leave all the instructions concerning your neurosis to your unconscious. Let us turn this problem over to the unconscious."

ER: Because your conscious mind does not know how to cope with it? You are leaving the understanding to the unconcious.

MHE: That's right. But you do not tell them they cannot deal with it consciously.

ER: Again you've taken something out of the biased, rigid sets of consciousness and given it to the more flexible system of the unconscious.

MHE: It would spoil the magician's art if you knew how he did that trick. If you want to enjoy swimming, do not analyze it. If you want to make love, don't try to analyze it.

ER: Right, Masters and Johnson even talk about getting hung up in the "spectator" role in sex, which interferes with sexual experiencing (Masters and Johnson, 1970; Rossi, 1972).

> **MHE: The unconscious is**
> **much more childlike**
> **in that it is direct**
> **and it is free.**
> **Children have asked me**

why I walk that funny way
when their parents had not even noticed that I limped.
They were appalled at the children calling attention to my limp.
The children saw something they wanted an understanding of.
They were willing to reach out for an understanding.
When you have a patient in a trance, the patient thinks like a child and
reaches for an understanding.

MHE: Patients tend to disparage themselves as being childish during trance, but don't let them disparage themselves that way. You rob them of that sort of ***neurosis shelter***.

ER: Self-disparagement is a neurosis shelter. So you emphasize the creative aspects of a child's fresh perception and curiosity about the world to loosen patients from their negative adult bias against natural free inquiry in trance. This is one of the characteristic ways you attempt to facilitate an attitude that will encourage them to take a fresh look at their problems from new points of view.

MHE: Juvenility is far superior to senility.

MHE: Your task is to protect them.

ER: To protect them?

MHE: To protect a patient so he doesn't get alarmed at what he discovers.

MHE: When patients came in to stop smoking, they may say when in trance, "I don't really want to stop smoking." The therapist then sees physical alarm; they now know the truth about themselves. So you say to them, "I don't think you should know that when you're awake ***yet***." You protect your patient. You're protecting the conscious mind by keeping that self-understanding unconscious.

ER: Because the conscious mind should not have its sets shattered too rapidly.

MHE: Yes, that can be a shattering experience unless the patient has the strength to endure it.

> **MHE: An example is in lying. Children are entitled to tell lies. They are entitled to see things as they are without being frightened.**

MHE: When a person in a trance says something you know is a lie, you better look it over because it has another meaning.

ER: It has meaning other than being a lie?

MHE: Yes, in some way the person is telling the truth. A truth as seen from a totally different point of view. And bear in mind that you as the therapist also have your own set and rigid points of view to deal with.

ER: Would lies in a trance also be an indication of regression to a more childlike state?

MHE: It's a regression to a more simple mode of functioning, less complicated. A person may tell you of going to a circus in Wisconsin, yet they have never been to Wisconsin. That may mean they are identified with somebody in Wisconsin. This is their way of telling you about an identification when they don't have a vocabulary to permit them to say, "I identify with so and so."

ER: They express an identification by attributing something about the other to themselves. This kind of psychological language accounts for many of the so-called lies and distortions expressed in trance.

> **MHE: A child will drop a glass on the floor and say with wonderment, "It broke!" And not necessarily have to react with adult understanding that it was a valued antique.**
> **[Pause]**
> **Every patient needs to know that the emotional content of something can be experienced with no knowledge of what caused the emotion.**
> **[Pause]**
> **A patient can also recall the intellectual memories of an event as if they happened to someone else.**
> **Many other things have no meaning to the self, and then later the emotions and intellectual content gets together piece by piece, like a jigsaw puzzle.**

MHE: It's well to let them experience this state of wonderment in the trance.

ER: That would mean that in the trance state their unconscious is free from the biases of the conscious mind?

MHE: Yes. It shows the unconscious can forget what the conscious mind knows, It may leave certain knowledge in the conscious mind.

ER: I see. So the conscious and unconscious really are separate systems?

MHE: Yes, they are separate systems.

ER: Do you have any therapeutic goal for the ideal mode of psychological functioning? A certain amount of interchange between the conscious and the unconscious, for example?

MHE: The ideal person would be one who had a readiness to accept the interchange between the conscious and unconscious. Children are uncluttered by rigid conscious sets, and therefore children can see things that adults cannot.

MHE: I taught my sons the best way of hoeing a garden.
You have a square yard at
the northeast corner,
a square yard at the northwest corner,
and then the southeast and the southwest.
Now that you have hoed a square yard at all corners, you hoe a square yard in the center. Then hoe a line from the middle to a corner.
Now you're making a design of the garden.
That is a very interesting way of doing a laborious piece of work. You
become so interested in the design that it's a pleasure.
In working at a problem of difficulty, you try to make an interesting design
in the handling of it.
That way you have an answer to the difficult problem.
Become interested in the design and don't notice the
back-breaking labor.
In therapy, that is often a very delightful thing to do.
[Pause]
When you do work freely and willingly,
one has a right to take a rest period at any time.
You are free to resume work at any time.
Free to alter the design and pattern in which the work is done.

[Erickson here gives a detailed clinical example of a child who wrote backwards and upside down and from right to left, but not the conventional way. Rather than attempt to correct the child by prohibiting his unusual ways of writing, Erickson pointed out to the child his superiority in being able to write in three different ways while Erickson could only write in one: the conventional way. Erickson then proceeded to try to learn to write one of the ways the child did, and the child, to maintain his superiority, now wanted to learn yet another way of writing—the conventional way. He was now learning his fourth way of writing while Erickson was still struggling to learn his second.]

MHE: Another simple technique of distracting consciousness from a laborious piece of work.

ER: So here again in this lengthy example you're telling Dr. S to let go of her conscious sets and orientation because they are so laborious. You are suggesting that she substitute a kind of creative, aesthetic play with patterns for the hard work of hoeing in laborious linear rows.

Throughout this and many previous sessions many of your efforts could be understood as distracting or depotentiating the linguistic, rational, linear, and directed modes of left hemispheric functioning in favor of the spontaneous perceptual aesthetic, kinesthetic, and synthetic modes of right hemispheric functioning. Dream, reverie, and trance have recently been characterized as right hemispheric functions. When you emphasize trusting natural or unconscious patterns of functioning in trance, you are actually emphasizing the paralogical or appositional (Bogen, 1969) characteristics of the right hemisphere. It may well be that future research will establish that much of what we have until now characterized as the dichotomy between the conscious and unconscious (secondary and primary process thinking) is neuropsychologically a dichotomy between left and right hemispheric functioning. From this point of view many psychological problems could be understood as the erroneous imposition of rational left hemispheric approaches to situations that could be better dealt with by the right hemisphere.

MHE: Now the next thing I want to say to you is this: It is never necessary when you sleep at night to remember your dreams the next day.
It's possible to dream
tonight
and wait a year before you remember
the dream.
You may remember a part of the dream
tomorrow and part of it next week.
Your remembering the dream
has to be in accord
with what you need.
You don't have to remember.
The important thing is
to have
certain experiences
recorded in your mind.
Some day their presence will be of service to you.
It is necessary for you to be aware
that you know they are there.
The important thing always is
to do the right thing at the
right time.
To know that you can rely on yourself.
To let your unconscious feed to you
the right information
that permits you
to do the right thing at the right time.
It may be this year or
next year
or two years from now.
[Pause]

ER: You are again illustrating the unimportance of consciousness relative to the unconscious in trance. With all these examples you are telling Dr. S that she can rely on her unconscious. This approach is needed with Dr. S because she is, relatively speaking, a highly intellectualized person with a Ph D. This approach of retraining the patient to rely on the unconscious is going to become more important in the future as more and more people become highly intellectualized. Direct authoritative suggestions may have been appropriate 100 years ago, when it was possible to reach the unconscious that way. But the modern hypnotherapist has to help people relearn that natural mode of functioning where they leave things to their unconscious.

MHE: An illustration is when you awaken. One of the most pleasant things you have to experience is in coming out of the trance thinking you are ready to go into a trance
for the first time.
And then becoming aware that you must have been in a trance.
Maybe the degree of light outside indicates that.
The indication is from the outside.
That can be assessed by you
as a beautiful learning experience.
[Pause]

ER: This is an example of an indirect posthypnotic suggestion. First you carefully lay the groundwork by talking about forgetting dreams until it is the right time to remember them. You thereby hope to evoke forgetting mechanisms. Just as she can forget a dream until it is important to remember it, so can she, by implication, forget she was in trance until it is important to remember it. You then administer the indirect posthypnotic suggestion. You don't directly tell her to forget she was in trance. That might only evoke the typical reaction of consciousness, "But I don't know how?" Instead, you describe the kind of pleasant experience she can have "coming out of the trance thinking she is ready to go into a trance for the first time." Instead of giving a direct suggestion to do something consciousness would find difficult, you simply motivate her for a "pleasant" experience. You talk about the degree of daylight outside as an indication of the passage of time. Perhaps that will be the only cue that will enable her to recognize she was in trance for some time. You also prepared for this earlier when you talked about the way the unconscious uses cues and the value of relying on the unconscious to do things.

Thus, during the earlier part of this session you were laying an important foundation for this seemingly casual posthypnotic suggestion. You were building an associational network and activating mental mechanisms that might be ***Utilized*** to facilitate forgetting in an entirely autonomous or dissociated manner.

MHE: Yes, you are always building one thing on another and relating what you are saying now to what you said earlier.

> **MHE: In everyday life,**
> **you overhear people saying to themselves,**
> **"Now just how did I do that?"**
> **What they mean is,**
> **they don't know how they did it.**
> **They have only an incomplete view of how they did it.**
> **They then have to recover**
> **step by step**
> **the manner in which they did it.**
>
> **ER: Experiencing and learning come before understanding.**
>
> [Erickson here gives several clinical examples of how he recognized minimal cues of hand, eye, and lip behavior that indicated that certain patients did not really want to give up smoking even though they presented themselves in therapy for that purpose. These examples illustrated the difference between conscious purpose and a deeper understanding of motivation.]

ER: Here you're giving examples of lapses in consciousness in everyday life. By simply mentioning these possibilities, you hope to facilitate their occurrence in Dr. S as a means of depotentiating her consciousness so she can learn to rely more on her unconscious.

> [Much of the above actually appeared to be a conversation between Erickson and Rossi. Dr. S and began spontaneously to awaken, as was indicated by minimal movements of her lips, nose,

forehead wrinkling, and some finger movements. Erickson notes this and remarks that she is awakening and getting ready to talk to us.]

Dr. S: What do you want to know?

MHE: Only what you want to tell us.

Dr. S: Well, I was jumping around a lot. When you were saying I was trying to wake up, I actually had already abandoned the idea because my hands were so heavy I couldn't move them. But when you said I was waking up, I tried to wake up again. But I'm kind of curious why you don't follow through with someone who is in trance. Like when I do hypnotherapy, I stay right with the patient the whole time, and then when I judge it's right, I say you can count to wake up or whatever. Why don't you do something like that?

ER: [Laughing] Yes, Dr. Erickson, why don't you behave like a regular hypnotherapist should?

ER: Here you accepted her spontaneous awakening and *Utilized* it as part of a hypnotic suggestion by simply remarking on it and helping it happen further. People are continually going in and out of trance, so when they are coming out you may as well *Utilize* that behavior to strengthen the hypnotic relationship rather than contesting it and setting up a battle of wills between therapist and patient. You can be with them whether they are in or out of trance.

MHE: You may as well join them when they come out, and later they will join you in following your suggestions more easily. You always give the patient approval for what she is doing.

ER: There is no need for the beginning hypnotherapist to panic when a patient spontaneously comes awake. That's just their natural mode of functioning and is to be accepted as a way of strengthening the hypnotic relationship.

MHE: If it is their way of functioning, you'd better go along with it.

ER: The therapist is not really in control of anyone.

MHE: That's right!

ER: There are only moments when the therapist can effectively direct something the patient wants to experience. But it is "touch and go—touch and go." Moments when a suggestion can be accepted alternate with moments when they cannot.

MHE: And the therapist can remain comfortable in that situation.

ER: Yes, this is very important for the beginning therapist to learn: there is a natural rhythm in patients that the therapist learns to recognize and go along with. I used to get all tense in working with patients by thinking, "Oh, this is not working, that doesn't work either, the whole thing's not happening." Such an attitude I now see is ridiculous.

MHE: It is so ridiculous! You never give the patient the impression that you must be constantly alert. You give them the impression that they are always sharing in the responsibility for the success of the work. Dr. S had expressed her belief that when she did hypnotherapy she had to stay right with the patient all the time. Therefore when I appeared to be distracted, that gave her reason to wake up.

> **Dr. S: What is the logic of what you do?**
>
> **MHE: In a learning situation, you have to do your own learning. I want you to learn a lot faster than I did. It took me about 30 years to learn, and there is no sense in that. Now if I were**

treating you for a problem, I'd stay with you and give you support at different points. But you are in a learning process, getting the feel of everything.

Dr. S: But this way I just trip around 'till I'm bored and then come out of it.

MHE: Are you sure you come out of it because you are bored?

Dr. S: It's almost as if I fell asleep because I caught myself nodding a few
times. What was happening on your left side, some distance off to the left? Were you looking for something?

[Erickson now puts a detailed series of questions to Dr. S regarding the subjective experiences that were associated with her behavior in trance, such as eye and head movements to the left and right, minute movements of the face, breathing alternations, etc. In an amazing way Erickson revealed he had actually observed many more details of S's trance behavior than she could recall.]

ER: With this question Dr. S reveals her highly rational approach. That is why you've spent most of this session telling her to give up consciousness control. Could you elaborate here on just what you want her to learn on her own? This appears almost like self-hypnosis, where the person has to do it all on their own. You're telling her to learn to let things happen?

MHE: That's right.

ER: If an itch happens, fine, go along with it. If heaviness happens, fine, go along with it. If memories happen, fine! If you flash and trip around in your head, fine!

[Erickson here tells an amusing anecdote about a husband and wife trying to outdo each other in growing tomatoes. A few days after planting them the wife decided they needed more sun, so she transplanted them. Later, it seemed to her they needed more shade, so she transplanted them again—and so on. She was still transplanting them when her husband was harvesting his tomatoes.]

ER: So what's the relevance of that story for what we are discussing?

MHE: You let the subject grow!

ER: Oh, they learn to do their own thing at their own pace. You let them grow and not interfere with their natural growth process.

MHE: My learning over the years was that I tried to direct the patient too much. It took me a long time to let things develop and make use of things as they developed.

ER: That accounts for your development of *Utilization Techniques*—one of your basic contributions to modern hypnosis. You *Utilize* the patient's own behavior to initiate trance, self-exploration, and the like.

Dr. S: When I tried to lift my arms toward the end in an effort to awaken, I got dizzy.

MHE: Why do you think you got dizzy?

Dr. S: It was like when you first wake up in the morning and you are very groggy. It was a disorientation, as if I could be tipping all sorts of ways. It was a strange body sensation. I was myself enjoying the trance in the beginning; then I became the therapist, wondering why the heck you weren't telling me what to do.

ER: I think Dr. S has been getting impatient with us.

MHE: Impatient in a curious way, and that is always a barrier.

Dr. S: Well, I guess I want to know the practical things about hypnosis: what it is, how you deal with problems, how you deal with smoking, weight problems, etc.

ER: Dr. S used to intellectual learning rather than the experiential learning of trance.

ER: You attempted to extend her trance training in this session by giving her an interesting posthypnotic suggestion to forget she was in trance. To carry out that suggestion successfully, she would have to rely on her own unconscious, as she did in her last session when she experienced that marvelous age regression, hypermenesia. But in this session, she was irritated because you did not meet her preconceived expectations of how closely attentive you should be to her during trance. Because these more personal emotional needs were not met, your indirect posthypnotic suggestion paled into insignificance and was not received. That she was experiencing trance is indicated by the heaviness of her hands, but then the therapist observer within her may have gotten in the way of further experiential learning in this session. This is a clear indication of how important it is to recognize and meet in some way the patient's emotional needs before we can expect them to relax to the point where they can rely upon their unconscious to carry out suggestions.

[Erickson terminates this session by giving several examples of experiential learning and knowing versus intellectual learning.]

Chapter Eighteen

Trance Training and *Utilization*

Erickson makes a highly significant statement in this commentary:

"My learning over the years was that I tried to direct the patient too much. It took me a long time to let things develop and make use of things as they developed."

This entire session with Dr. S was an effort on Erickson's part to train her to allow things to happen spontaneously, unconsciously. The most basic learning in hypnotic work is to let things to happen of themselves, to let the unconscious function as free as possible from the learned habits and programs of consciousness.

It took Erickson a long time to learn that this is the first essential in all sound hypnotherapeutic work. Patients are patients because they are out of rapport with their own unconscious. Trance allows the patient to experience his own unconscious free, to some extent, from the limitations of his conscious sets. Once this unconscious mode of functioning becomes manifest, then Erickson feels free to help the patient ***Utilize*** it for therapeutic purposes.

Therapeutic hypnosis is not just another technique for programming patients. Patients are people who have had too much programming—so much outside programming that they have lost touch with their inner selves. Therapeutic trance is an experience wherein patients receive something from within themselves. The astute hypnotherapist is one who arranges circumstances to permit such receptivity to inner experience. He helps the patient to recognize the value of his unique inner experience and provides suggestions about how it may be ***Utilized*** therapeutically.

We may note that this way of defining therapeutic trance is very similar to the classical use of meditation. The word "meditation" comes from the Latin ***meditari***, a passive form of the verb that means literally "being moved to the center." Consciousness remains passive as it is moved to the center (the unconscious), where it can achieve wholeness: a reunion with contents and tendencies that have been excluded from consciousness (Jung, 1960).

The Dynamics of Indirect and Direct Suggestion

Erickson's use of a boring explanation of arithmetic to fatigue Dr. S in this session reveals some basic principles of his use of indirect suggestion in a particularly clear manner. Erickson did not directly suggestion that she would be relaxed, tired, or fatigued.

Rather he used an arithmetic explanation as a stimulus (^{S}arithmetic) for evoking an external response of being polite (^{R}polite),which in turn evoked within Dr. S an internal response of boredom (^{r}boredom), which led her to feel fatigued (^{R}fatigue).

There is little or no identity between the suggestion (^{S}arithmetic) and the final response (^{R}fatigue) that the subject can recognize or influence in any way. This process of outer stimulus, internal mediation, and behavioral response can be outlined as shown in Figure 2.

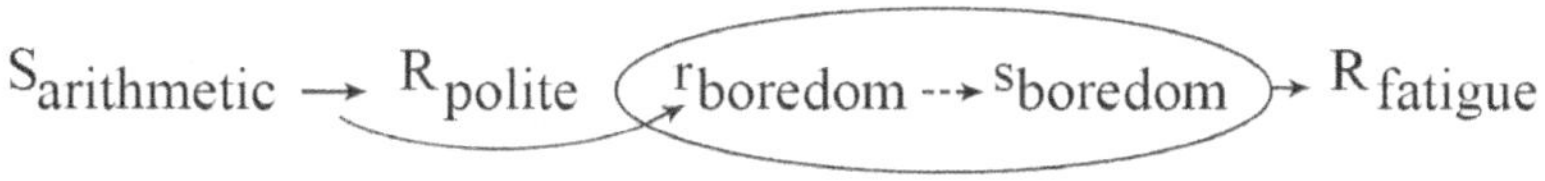

Figure 2 (10.18.F.2) The Process of Indirect Suggestion with No Obvious Relation Between the Suggestion and Response

The process of indirect suggestion with no obvious relation between the suggestion (^{S}arithmetic) and response (^{R}fatigue). The large letters represent overt, external, objective events, while the small letters (r and s) represent covert, internal, subjective events that are usually not understood or even recognized by the subject.

Direct suggestion, by contrast, presents subjects with a stimulus that identifies what the response should be. Frequently the therapist offering direct suggestions will actually tell subjects exactly what internal processes they should use to mediate the response. In giving a direct suggestion, the therapist can only hope the subject will cooperate with this exact suggestion or find other internal processes by which the response can be mediated. How the response is mediated within is sometimes understood at least in part by the subject. When they are successful, subjects usually report that they imagined themselves in a fatiguing situation, for example, and then by association they managed to evoke a response of fatigue they could actually feel. Some investigators (Barber, et al., 1974) actually train their subjects to use conscious ideation in this way. Direct suggestion could be diagrammed as shown in Figure 2, where there is a clear identity between the initial suggestion, the internally mediated responses, and the outer response that the subject can recognize and influence.

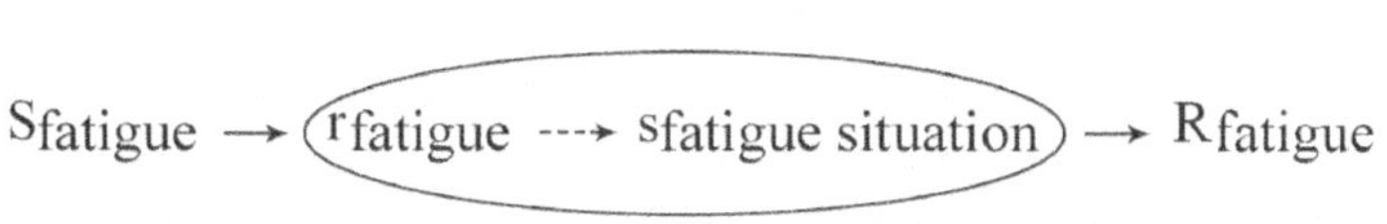

Figure 3 (10.18.F.3) The Process of Direct Suggestion with an Obvious Relation Between the Suggestion and the Response

The process of direct suggestion with an obvious relation between the suggestion (^{S}fatigue) and the response (^{R}fatigue). The internal mediating responses (rfatigue - - -> Sfatigue situation) are in part recognized and understood by the patient.

Direct and indirect suggestions can both achieve effective results, but they are mediated in different ways such that their relations to consciousness and volition are different. Direct suggestion is mediated by internal processes that the subjects usually have some awareness of. The subjects recognize that they made the response happen. The response is more or less under voluntary control. Indirect suggestion, by contrast, is usually mediated by internal processes that remain unknown to the subjects. The response, when it is noticed, is usually acknowledged by the subjects with a sense of surprise. The response appeared to occur in an involuntary and spontaneous manner. It has a curiously dissociated or autonomous aspect that is usually acknowledged as hypnotic.

A problem with direct suggestion is that the responses obtained may simply be voluntary compliance on the part of the subjects. They may simply be trying to please the therapist in a fully conscious way. Thus, theorists who have identified hypnosis and trance with suggestibility (compliance with direct suggestions) have been led to a downgrading of the autonomous or involuntary aspects of hypnotic experience. Thus, we have theories of trance as voluntary roleplaying (Sarbin and Coe, 1972) or a form of voluntary conscious cooperation in thinking and imagining along with the theorist's suggestions (Barber, et al., 1974). These are all actually theories of direct suggestion. An unconscious or involuntary component is not necessarily evident when a subject accepts and acts on a direct suggestion.

With indirect suggestion, however, subjects usually do not recognize the relation between the suggestion and their own response. There thus can be no question of voluntary compliance with the therapist's suggestion. If a response does take place, then it has been mediated by involuntary processes outside of a subject's immediate range of awareness. This involuntary mediation of responses is what we use to define the genuineness of trance behavior. The involuntary or autonomous response that surprises consciousness is what differentiates hypnotic from ordinary awake behavior. Such autonomous responses can be elicited by direct suggestions—e.g., all the suggestions of the Stanford (Hilgard, 1965 and the Barber et al. 1974) hypnotic suggestibility scales—but with direct suggestion there is always the problem of simulation: Did the response take place in a voluntary or involuntary manner? With indirect suggestion, however, the very appearance of a response can be a satisfactory criterion of its involuntary nature, since the subject is unaware of why or how it happens.

Weitzenhoffer (1957, 1974, 1975) has emphasized that the defining feature of hypnotic suggestion is the absence of conscious volition in the production of the hypnotic response. We agree with this basic formulation. In order to take a preliminary step in making a distinction between direct and indirect suggestion, we have discussed the role of conscious awareness and intention in our formulation above. In direct suggestion, it is possible for the patient to have some conscious awareness of how the hypnotic response is mediated within and may in consequence attempt either to inhibit or to facilitate the hypnotic response with conscious intentionality. With indirect suggestion, care is taken so that the typical patient will not become aware of how the hypnotic response is mediated within; hence there is less opportunity for conscious intentionality either to facilitate or to block the response.

Indirect Conditioning of Trance

Erickson's use of indirect eyelid conditioning in this session is another prime example of his indirect approach. He labels a slow eye blink (associated with trance) with the word "odd" and a fast eye blink with the word "even." The subject did not know the connection between her eye blinks and the words. An association can be made between the rapidity of eye blink and the words "odd" and "even" without conscious awareness. Once this association is made, then saying the word "odd" will tend to evoke slow eye blinks, and since slow eye blinks are associated with the beginning of trance (by previous eye fixation induction as well as by everyday life experience wherein we do begin to blink slowly as we drift into altered states like daydreaming and sleep), subjects find themselves drifting into trance without knowing exactly why.

Erickson actually uses many forms of indirect or incidental conditioning that take place all by themselves. Often he relies on nothing more than the natural processes of associational conditioning that are formed between trance experience and the situation in which the first trance occurred. Subjects who have successful experiences with trance the first time they come into Erickson's office will have many associative connections built between trance experience and Erickson as a person, his voice, his manner, and other characteristics. There will be associative connections between trance and the subject's presence in the office and sitting in the same chair as the first time. There will be associations between the appearance of the room, the presence of the cut-glass paperweight that Erickson usually uses as a point for eye-fixation induction, etc. Indeed, for some subjects the simple behavior of going to an appointment with Erickson is enough to initiate the expectation of trance so that inner adjustments are being made to facilitate the trance experience even when the subjects are on their way to an appointment.

Erickson simply watches for these natural processes of conditioning the experience of trance. When patients enter the office, Erickson carefully observes their behavior for the subtle signs of trance. Many of these are standard signs that are fairly applicable to most people: slow eye blink, economy of movement, smoothing of facial features, response attentiveness, and so on. Some signs are characteristic of an individual: a part of the body held in an inconspicuous catalepsy (e.g., the finger of one hand bent in a characteristic way), a particular gaze or manner. When Erickson sees these signs of naturally conditioned trance behavior emerging, he simply adopts his own usual manner when inducing a trance. He will look at the patient with his characteristic attitude of expectancy. He may look meaningfully at the cut-glass paperweight. He might take a deep breath and visibly relax. He might even close his eyes for a moment. These are all nonverbal cues for patients to enter further into the trance they may already be experiencing. Patients are surprised to find how easily trance develops, and they frequently have no idea of how or why. Even when patients have some intellectual awareness of how they have been conditioned to experience trance, they find it more comfortable to go along than to resist. Yet, if patients want to resist the developing trance, they certainly can. Such indirectly conditioned trances develop to a significant degree only in an atmosphere of trust, comfort, and cooperation, where there is an expectation that something will be gained from the experience.

Exercises with Indirect or Incidental Conditioning of Trance

1. Learn to observe your patients carefully as they enter the therapy situation after having had a trance experience during the previous session. Can you discern signs of developing trance?

2. Carefully study your own physical office situation and induction procedures to discover what incidental associations are being formed between your patients' trance experience and the physical characteristics of the setting and your own behavior. Plan how you might ***Utilize*** these to facilitate later trances.

3. What nonverbal cues can you learn to ***Utilize*** to reinduce trance in your previous subjects? Many of these will be the slight alterations in your own behavior as you are facilitating trance experience in your subjects. It may help to have a trained observer present to help you recognize subtle behavior changes that you do not recognize yourself.

VOICE DYNAMICS IN TRANCE

Erickson's use of voice dynamics is another major approach to indirect suggestion. This use of voice dynamics ranges from simple direct suggestion that his voice will evoke personal associations to indirect conditioning wherein he associates the locus of his voice to different processes within the subject.

In the traditional style of direct suggestion the therapist often tells the patient to pay attention to the therapist's voice and ignore everything else. That is an effective approach with direct suggestion. For indirect suggestion, by contrast, Erickson will typically tell patients that they do not have to bother listening to his voice. When patients later report that during trance they lost track of Erickson's voice and did not always know what he was talking about, it can be taken as an indication of the typical development of trance. Initially many subjects report an alteration in hearing and not hearing or paying attention. This spontaneous alteration may correspond to the spontaneous alteration of trance depth that is a characteristic feature of hypnotic experience.

In this session, Erickson suggested that Dr. S could learn to hear his voice only as a meaningful sound to which she would give an interpretation. That is, the content of Erickson's words could be ignored. The sound of his voice could become a vehicle carrying Dr. S's own projections. Frequently Erickson will suggest or imply that what he says is not important. Only the patient's interpretation of what he says in important. Because of this he will use words with multiple meanings, puns, incomplete sentences, and dangling phrases, so that the patient's unconscious can project meanings that are important to itself.

One of Erickson's unique contributions to the use of voice locus is what we might call its spatial-perceptual associations. As he talks about associations and memories back in the past, he may tip his chair backward away from the patient, lower his voice, and even turn his head away from the patient, so that it seems as if his voice is coming from far away. Just as the voice is far away, so will the patient's memories come from far away in their dim past. As those memories stir and become available to the patient's awareness, Erickson may gradually tip his chair forward and come closer to the patient and speak more clearly and loudly. But his manner is always subtle, so that the patient does not recognize what he is doing.

The patient's unconscious, however, may utilize these differences in voice locus and volume as stimuli that evoke altered patterns of association that may make valuable memories available. In one striking demonstration with a subject who was visualizing a suggested scene with her eyes closed, Erickson would raise the pitch of his voice and actually project it upward by looking up when he wanted her to see something up in the air and vice versa when he wanted her to see something lower on her internal visual screen. The movements of her closed eyes were observed to follow the locus and pitch of his voice exactly. The patient later remarked about the peculiar alteration in the height at which the suggested images appeared to her. Erickson (1973) has reported how voice locus can be used to induce sea sickness, vertigo, and similar conditions.

One of Erickson's most interesting, but controversial uses of voice locus is his effort to direct suggestions selectively to the conscious and unconscious of the patient. As he goes through his induction talk, Erickson may shift slightly to the right every time he mentions the word "conscious" or talks about obviously conscious matters of interest. He shifts slightly to the left whenever he uses the word "unconscious" or talks about involuntary and autonomous processes that are usually mediated without voluntary conscious control. Without the patients realizing it, they are being conditioned to associate conscious voluntary processes with voice locus coming from the right and unconscious or involuntary and dissociated processes with voice locus on the left. Once these associations are established, Erickson can beam a suggestion to a conscious or unconscious level by shifting his voice in the appropriated direction. It will be a matter of future empirical research and practice to determine the effectiveness of this procedure and the degree to which others can learn to use it effectively in a systematic way.

Exercises with Voice Dynamics

1. Study tape recordings of your own voice during therapy sessions and in everyday life situations to become more familiar with your own natural voice dynamics in different circumstances, and what you are consciously and unconsciously communicating.

2. Study recordings of your voice before and during trance induction to learn what changes you usually make and how these changes may be facilitating or interfering with trance development in your patients.

3. The actual conscious ***Utilization*** of one's own voice dynamics requires some practice. The object is to use voice dynamics in a way that does not arouse the patient's conscious attention. Otherwise their purpose may be largely lost. One can begin by learning to speak a bit ***softly*** when one wants to obtain the listener's closer attention. One can then learn to speak more ***slowly*** when one wants to help a listener slow down. One can practice speaking just a bit more loudly and distinctly when one wants a patient to arouse from trance.

4. Explore the use of voice locus in conditioning subjects to receive suggestions at different levels of awareness (Erickson, 1973). Can you devise new field experiments or more controlled experimental situations to assess the effectiveness of this use of voice locus?

The lengths to which Erickson will go in *Utilizing* all sorts of intercontextual cues as indirect suggestion is indicated in the following dialogue:

MHE: I had some repetitive dreams last night about some things that should be said about this. In giving suggestions and instruction to hypnotic subjects in the trance state, it is not only what you say, but it is what they hear, that is important. I can give you an example.

Let us say there is a village named Sun*flower* in Arizona. Let us take another imaginary place we will call ***Weldon's Ditches***. You carry on a casual conversation about Arizona and you mention Suntower. Rather than Sun*flower*. You purposely say Sun*tower*. The person listening automatically and unheedingly corrects you and doesn't know that you actually said "Sun*tower*." In talking about the southern part of Arizona and strip mining, you mention ***Weldon's Britches*** (instead of ***Ditches***).

Now you have said two things outrageously wrong and the subject has consciously corrected what you said. So consciously they think you said Sun*flower* and Weldon's Ditches. But the unconscious heard you say Sun*tower* and ***Britches***. They detect and remember that. You can later use that because they don't know why they are impelled to talk about a *flower* and a Dutchman's ***britches***.

ER: They are impelled to use those associations which you placed in their unconscious.

MHE: Yes. They may then talk about that "Devil's Tower" in the Caribbean and have no idea of how you got that association across to them. But you know how you have done it. They can't consciously ever figure it out. Their consciousness corrected for their conscious mind, but their unconscious heard it.

ER: Your error remains lodged in their unconscious, striving for expression.

MHE: It is lodged there in the unconscious, and you can keep on talking and drive the conversation in such a fashion that the discussion of wildflowers brings up ***Dutchman's Britches*** and the Devil's *Tower* in theCaribbean.

This rather complex example intertwines the names of obscure locations with the names of specific flowers. The resultant confusion and correction may be characterized as one of placing associations within the patient's unconscious and then allowing the unconscious to ***Utilize*** them in its own way. A more common practice is Erickson's habitual use of pauses that break up his sentence structure into phrases, each of which can have its own meaning that can be entirely independent of the meaning the sentence has as a whole. In our transcripts of the induction section of each session we made an effort to note these important pauses. The separate and independent meaning of each phrase can be described as intercontextual cues and suggestions that are picked up and partially processed by the unconscious, while the conscious simply waits for the remainder of the sentence. These phrases buried in the context of the sentence thus function as another form of indirect suggestion.

This use of phrases as separate suggestions buried within the broader context of the whole sentence is actually another form of ***interspersal technique*** (Erickson,1966b). Erickson has illustrated the uses of ***interspersing suggestions*** within the broader context of a general conversation about a topic the patient can easily identify with (e.g., a general conversation about growing plants with a farmer, caring for children with a mother, and so on). Interspersed in this conversation is a pattern of suggestions that come at random intervals (frequently with a slightly different intonation of voice,) so they are unpredictable by the subject. The interspersed suggestion comes at an ***unexpected moment***, it is ***short***, it is usually a ***truism*** that is not arguable, and the therapist ***quickly moves on*** to the general conversation before the patients can react to the suggestion. The suggestion is received, but the patients have no opportunity to resist it with their habitual associations, limiting frames of reference, or other inhibiting factors.

The general conversation that is of interest to the patients has the following functions as a vehicle for the interspersed suggestions.

1. The general conversation facilitates the development of an accepting or ***Yes Set,*** since it is a topic of interest to the patients. The interspersed suggestion is thus received with acceptance along with the overt message that is motivating to the patients.

2. The general conversation keeps the patients "awake" at an optimal level

of receptivity rather than drifting to the border of trance and its associative receptivity.

3. The topic of interest facilitates patients' rapport with the therapist, rather than have them drift too far off into their own associative matrix, which might again result in uncertain receptivity.

4. The interspersing of suggestions within a familiar and redundant message facilitates *a* structured amnesia (Erickson and Rossi, 1974) for the interspersed suggestions and thus prevents a patient's usual associative structure from interfering with the suggestions.

The intercontextual cues and suggestions buried within the general context of a sentence would appear to function in the same way as the interspersed suggestions in the context of a general conversation as described above.

Exercises with Intercontextual Cues and Suggestions

1. Review the induction sections of all previous sessions to study the intercontextual cues and suggestions that are present in the phrases, but not in the sentence as a whole.

2. On the other hand, note how at times the separate phrases of each sentence have the same implications as the total sentence. In such cases, the phrases can summate and greatly reinforce the suggestion contained in the sentence as a whole, but without belaboring the point and possibly arousing the limiting reactions of an awakened consciousness.

3. Notice how often in previous commentary sections Erickson brings attention to this or that phrase as a separate suggestion buried within a more general context. It wasn't until this session,

however, that it finally dawns on Rossi that Erickson was trying to teach another indirect approach to suggestion, which we have now labeled "intercontextual cues and suggestions."

4. In actual practice, it is very easy to learn how to administer intercontextual cues and suggestions. Simply tape record your sessions and later study the transcripts to note what intercontextual cues and suggestions you are unwittingly giving. As you become more sensitive to your own buried suggestions, you will develop a heightened awareness of what you are saying when you actually say it in the therapy sessions. Soon you will welcome the pauses in your sentence structure to savor your intercontextual cues and bring them under greater control. As you administer a phrase and carefully watch the patient's face, you can study the patient's involuntary response (wincing, smiling, etc.) to each separate phrase. This can give you a sense of the reality of intercontextual suggestions. You will then be able to ***Utilize*** these immediate patient responses as a kind of feedback to make you more aware of the effect your words are having on the patient's associative structure. You can then learn to orchestrate your phrases and the patient's responses to more adequately effect the therapeutic harmonies you are attempting to create together.

Right and Left Hemispheric Functioning in Trance

In our efforts to conceptualize Erickson's understanding of trance and its facilitation we have used a number of different models:

1. The psychodynamic model of the conscious-unconscious system

2. The learning theory model of behavioral psychology

3. A linguistic model ***Utilizing*** multiple levels of communication.

From this session, it is finally clear that a neuropsychological model ***Utilizing*** the differences between right and left hemispheric functioning is also implicit in Erickson's work, even though he developed his views and skills long before the recent studies of hemispheric functioning (Sperry, 1968; Gazzaniga, 1967; Bogen, 1969). These studies suggest to some investigators that experiences of trance, reverie, and dream are all characteristic of right hemispheric functioning, while the rational, logical, and verbal modes of functioning are more characteristic of the left.

A summary listing of the differences in hemispheric functioning that can be related to Erickson's emphasis on the differences between awake and trance experience is as follows:

Table 3 (10.18.T.3) Left and Right Hemisphere Emphasis

Left Hemisphere (Awake)	Right Hemisphere (Trance)
Linguistic	Pantomime, Kinesthetic, Musical
Logical-Grammatical	Visuospatial
Rational	Intuitive
Abstract	Literal-Concrete
Analytical	Perceptual-Synthetic
Directed	Spontaneous
Focal	Diffuse
Effort	Comfort

From this dichotomy, it is clear that much of Erickson's efforts to facilitate trance experience are directed to depotentiating left hemispheric functioning. The hallmark of left hemispheric functioning is the linguistic and logical-grammatical organization of consciousness, which is usually related to the location of the speech center in the left cortex. Many of Erickson's nonverbal, pantomime, and indirect approaches to trance induction are obviously means of shifting consciousness away from this linguistic specialization of the left hemisphere. As we have discovered in this volume, many of Erickson's habitual forms of verbal expression are actually designed to jam or depotentiate the orderly, rational, abstract, and directing functions of a subject's usual modes of left hemispheric knowing. His use of shock, ***Surprise***, dissociation, shifting frames of reference, ***Confusion***, paradox, and ***Double Binds*** are thus all directed to depotentiating the left hemisphere. His emphasis on body language, cues from voice locus, emphasis, rhythm, etc. are all shifts away from the rational and analytic to the perceptual, kinesthetic, and synthetic of functioning so characteristic of the right hemisphere. When he uses hypnotic forms like implication, expectancy, partial remarks, and dangling phrases, analogies, metaphors' puns, and folk language, he is again shifting away from the abstract and analytical to the intuitive and synthetic modes of the right. Many of the most characteristic features of trance experience such as reverie, dream, literalism, comfort, and the autonomous or spontaneous flow of mental experience and behavior are all facilitated by hypnotic forms such as not doing and not knowing, open-ended suggestions and suggestions covering all possibilities of response.

Many investigations (Bakan, 1969; Morgan, et al., 1974) have explored the view that left hemispheric functions are diminished during trance, and then assumed that right hemispheric functioning was thereby enhanced. This does appear to be the case in those specialized trance states where there are suggestions made to enhance patients' perceptions of their own body and personality. The right hemisphere is more directly concerned with the perception of sensory and kinesthetic cues, spatial orientation, and the organization of the body schema (Luria, 1973). In the more typical trance state, however, it is precisely the disturbances of the body schema that we recognize as characteristics of the trance state. Distortions of the body image—such as feeling a part of the body (head, hand, etc.) as being unusually large or small, dissociated, or anesthetic—are frequently commented on spontaneously by subjects experiencing trance for the first time. Such distortions are also characteristic of patients with organic disturbances of the right hemisphere. Luria reports several other patterns of right hemispheric dysfunction that are similar to spontaneous phenomena of trance. Patients with deep lesions of the right hemisphere showed severe loss of spatial orientation and disturbances of the time sense. As we have seen in this volume, ***Time Distortion*** is highly characteristic of trance, and one of the most reliable signs of people awakening from trance are their efforts to reorient to their own bodies. Luria even reports "trance logic" in such patients wherein they firmly believe they can be in two places at once, just as do some hypnotic subjects when they are experiencing visual hallucinations (Orne, 1959).

These correspondences indicate that in the typical trance right hemispheric functions can be depressed just as well as those of the left. In fact, because of the more global and diffuse character of right hemispheric functioning, the right hemisphere may be more easily altered than the left. Because of this we frequently witness the disturbances of body schema, etc. without any blocking of the more focal linguistic-logical functions of the left. This is particulary characteristic of highly intellectualized subjects (Barber, 1975), who may accurately describe the sensory-perceptual distortions their right hemisphere is experiencing with the unimpaired verbal logic of the left hemisphere. Luria also comments on this situation, where patients will make an effort to mask changes in personality and consciousness due to lesions of the right hemisphere with glib verbal formulations. This sounds very similar to the mode of highly intellectualized subjects, who tend to deny that trance or an altered state was experienced. Such subjects are probably both right and wrong. They are right in denying any alteration in their left hemispheric functioning but are wrong in denying and remaining unaware of alterations in their right hemispheric functioning. This very denial of any disturbance in functioning is also characteristic of patients with organic dysfunctions of the right hemisphere.

These considerations indicate that it may be too simple to view trance as a function of the right hemisphere. The way trance is usually induced with suggestions for relaxation and comfort tends to alter the functioning of both left and right hemispheres. We can understand why right hemispheric functions are usually more obviously altered than those of the left, however. Since the left hemisphere is dominant and more focal in its functioning, the right hemisphere tends to be depotentiated more easily in the early stages of learning to experience trance. Most people have well-established habits to maintain and control their left hemispheric functions more than those of their right, so the right hemisphere tends to be more easily depontentiated or altered than the left. And since the left hemisphere is the center of verbal-logical consciousness, it can contradict or "defend" itself against the verbal-logical suggestions of the hypnotherapist. The right hemisphere, by contrast, is used to cooperating with the verbal-logical formulations of its own left hemisphere. The right hemisphere thus need only generalize this function of cooperation to go along with the verbal suggestions of the therapist.

These recent studies of the characteristics of left and right hemispheric functioning can thus greatly enhance our understanding of trance phenomena. They provide a source of interesting hypotheses for further explorations of trance experience and suggest means for refining classical procedures as well as the invention of new methods. This neuropsychological approach takes the verbal "magic" out of suggestions and provides us with a sound rationale for understanding hypnotic susceptibility as a function of both genetic and learned patterns of individual differences in behavioral response.

Chapter Nineteen

Infinite Patterns of Learning: A Two-Year Follow-up

After one final session, during which Dr. S discussed her initial efforts and problems in beginning to use hypnosis in clinical practice, Dr. S felt she had sufficient work with Erickson for the present and planned to continue her training in the workshops of the American Society of Clinical Hypnosis and under professional supervision in a work context.

Two years later, she was contacted for a follow-up. She reported that in the intervening period she had continued her training in hypnotherapy and was using it regularly in her clinical practice. When she came for the actual interview, she sat in the same chair where she had experienced her hypnotherapeutic training with Erickson. As she sat down and adjusted herself, it was immediately obvious that she was taking her habitual posture for induction, with her hands on her thighs, etc. Erickson recognized this body language and without a word simply looked at her as he usually does when inducing hypnosis. By reproducing the hypnotic situation in this way, Dr. S immediately went into a very deep trance, deeper than any she had experienced previously.

The follow-up interview thus became another step, a very profound one, in Dr, S's training. Erickson uses one of his own dream experiences to initiate a "two-stage dissociative regression" wherein Dr. S experiences a genuine state of hyperamnesia and recovers memories from a phase of her childhood that she had entirely forgotten. Erickson then initiates a series of open-ended suggestions that would set Dr. S on an infinite path of inner experiential learning. He successfully draws a curtain of amnesia over these suggestions so that Dr. S's conscious mind cannot interfere with them. But the new experiential learning would be available whenever Dr. S needed it.

Dr. S did manage to recall a bit of what her very deep experience was like in this session before Erickson initiated the process of amnesia. She wrote a few revealing paragraphs, "Reflections After Trance Induction," to describe her experience.

Of particular interest in this session is Erickson's illustration of the type of open-ended suggestions that can give rise to infinite patterns of learning that can be of life-saving value. He discusses the Pearson incident, where open-ended suggestions given to a student were *Utilized* by him years later in an emergency situation, where he was able to self-induce anesthesia and an accelerated healing of the physical body after being hit on the head with a brick (Pearson, 1966).

[**Editors' note:** ***Robert Pearson, a physician who practiced in a small town where he was the only MD, was injured when a brick fell from a construction site and hit him on the head. Instead of falling unconscious, he rallied his memories of working with Dr. Erickson to keep him alert until he had been transported to distant medical facilities. Dr. Pearson experienced minimal long term consequences from that serious injury, other than a dent on his temple where a part of his skull had been removed.***]

The infinite possibilities of learning initiated by trance work were also illustrated by Dr. S's ingenuous response to reading these transcripts two years after they occurred. She reported that in these two years she had thought of herself as particularly inventive in her approaches to initiating her patients into trance and the therapeutic uses she developed for trance in groups as well as individuals. Upon reading these transcripts, however, she realized how many of her "original" approaches had their origin in one thing or another that Erickson had said or done here or there. Her trance experiences with Erickson had obviously interacted with her own creative processes to originate new thinking and behavior patterns.

Session 8: Two-year Follow-up with Erickson, Dr. S with Rossi and Dr. Z as Observer

[After being introduced to Dr. Z, who was present as an observer, the interview proceeds as follows. Dr. S sits comfortably with her palms on her thighs, exactly as she did two years ago when she was ready to enter trance. Erickson instantly recognizes this readiness and without saying a word begins to look steadily and expectantly into Dr. S's eyes.]

Dr. S: You are staring at me again.

MHE: Describe your feelings as you sit there.

Dr. S: Oh, I feel fine. Relaxed and comfortable.

[Pause as MHE and Dr. S continue to look into each other's eyes. Dr. S then blinks slowly a few times.]

MHE: Now I thought that was very interesting the way she sat down and began to sink back into two years ago. All I did was give a look of confident expectation. Now that's the important thing. An infant learning to walk, you know he can learn to walk, but the infant doesn't know. You give the infant the confident support of your expectation.

ER: Her body language cued you into the fact that she was ready for trance work. Your expectant look silently acknowledged that readiness and permitted her to enter trance without a word being said.

Dr. S: It is getting foggy again.
[Pause]
Getting more
relaxed.

[Pause as the looking continued for a few moments longer until Dr. S finally closes her eyes, takes a deeper breath, and quite obviously enters trance with a relaxation of facial muscles and an absolute immobility of body.]

MHE: And now enjoy very much
going deeper and deeper.
[Pause]

ER: She experiences this fogging even before she closes her eyes. It's her usual way of experiencing the first stages of trance, just as she did two years ago. She also demonstrates the "trance state" when she experiences this fogging. Her eyes have an unblinking stare, a fixity of regard or a faraway or distant look. Weitzenhoffer (1971) regards the trance stare as due to a decrease in the blink rate together with an appreciable decrease in the spontaneous, random, saccadic movements of the eyeball. Other subjects report all sorts of subjective changes in the visual field during trance induction: alterations in the color background, tunnel vision, perceptual distortions, illusions, blurring, an apparent decrease in illumination, a veil before the eyes, a grayness over the visual field, and similar changes.

MHE: It is often said,
we learn to skate in the summer
and to swim in the winter.
We achieve certain
level of learning
to skate in the winter.
But the next winter

we start skating with a higher degree of excellence.
Because the random movements of skating
that complicated the first learning
have dropped out.
And the first winter
the random movements
were still fresh in mind.
[Pause]
Now you can go
much deeper
because
there are many fewer
random movements
or processes.

ER: This was a way of deepening trance after a long period of absence from experiencing an induction. You simply describe a truism of the learning process: random movements drop out during a period of rest. Therefore, this will be an even deeper trance than before.

MHE: And that is a past experience everyone has had.

ER: So you've deepened trance by *Utilizing* an innate learning process we all have experienced.

MHE: You learn to write by grimacing your face and moving your feet, but after a while these random and irrelevant movements drop out.

MHE: And now I don't know
what particular experiences
you want to sense.
I don't know if you have any conscious idea,
but always the unconscious mind has its own thoughts.
Its own desires.

[Pause]
And you can feel very pleased
in discovering
what your unconscious is going to do.
[Long Pause]
And it will be your own experience.
[Pause]
And experience can be any place,
any time,
in any situation.
[Pause]
To look at one self
doing something
is always a charming thing.
[Pause]
I can give you a personal account.
In 1930,
in the early May,
I dreamed one night
that I was on the north side of an
east and west road.
in Wisconsin.

ER: Here you begin a typical pattern of open-ended suggestions. You begin depotentiating consciousness by saying that you "don't know," and that implies that it is okay if her conscious mind does not know either. But you emphasize that the unconscious does have thoughts and desires, and you reinforce them by noting that she can be pleases to discover what her unconscious is going to do. As her "reflections" later indicate, she did use these open-ended suggestions in a manner that was uniquely her own. You emphasize the open-ended aspect of your suggestion by mentioning that it will be ***her experience*** any time, any place, any situation. This sounds like a great deal of freedom. It is freedom as far as the conscious mind in concerned, but it is being highly determined by her own unconscious.

MHE: And I stood there
knowing that I was Dr. Erickson.

And I was looking at a small boy
who was running up and down.
By the grading on the side of the road by the hills
was a maintenance crew.
A fence on the top of the grade
and barbed wire fence.
Hazel bush,
an oak tree,
a wild cherry tree.
And I saw that barefoot boy with overalls
curiously probing the freshly graded ground,
and excavating around the cut ends of the roots,
and looking at the oak tree,
and looking at the wild cherry tree,
and then examining the cut ends of the roots,
trying to determine
which roots came from the wild cherry tree
and which came from the oak tree.
The little boy was sure
none of those roots came from hazelnut bush.
I approved of that boy.
I could see him plainly.
I recognized him
as little Milton Erickson.

ER: This two-state dissociative regression wherein a person sees and sometimes even relates to himself at an earlier age level was well described in your trance work with Aldous Huxley (Erickson, 1965/2021). You hoped to trip off this state in Dr. S by giving this charming example of how it occurred to you in a dream state, where it is not uncommon (Rossi, 1972/2000, 1973). As Dr. S remarks in her "reflections" on this session, you did succeed at this point because she did see herself as a child reading a book by Louisa May Alcott. She reports the actual recovery of memories from an entirely forgotten phase of her life when she wanted to be a writer. That is, she experienced a genuine ***hypermnesia***!

MHE: But he could not see Dr. Erickson.

He didn't even know I was on the other side of that east-west bound road.
And I enjoyed watching that little boy.
And thinking
but how little appreciation he had of the fact that he was going to grow up
and become Dr. Erickson.
And then the dream terminated.
In September of that year,
I did take a vacation trip to Wisconsin.
I went to the county seat,
got out all the records
of the county road maintenance work.
And I found out where that road was.
And then I drove to that area.
I found out how it was possible for
me to have been there.
There is a gravel pit near that road.
I remember going there with my father when he got a load of gravel.
But I had no memory of ever examining that
fresh grading in the road.
But I found there was a hazelnut bush,
an oak tree,
and a wild cherry tree.
And I was still a little boy,
a barefoot boy.
I had long forgotten that,
but my unconscious mind
had remembered it.
[Pause]

ER: It is utterly fascinating how in dreams and trance states the personality can encounter itself at different age levels as if time did not exist. This was particularly clear in your work with Huxley. These are states of active and creative imagination wherein the person as an adult personality can actually relate to and help himself as a child. In this way old traumas and needs, just about any form of "unfinished business," can be resolved. This is a form of psychological healing that I believe is the essence of any form of therapy, whether it takes place in dreams, trance, free association, active imagination, meditation, or whatever. The common denominator is that something new is synthesized within the personality (Rossi, 1973a.)

MHE: I'm suggesting this to you as a possible experience.
[Long Pause]
I began work on the research service
in Worcester, Massachusetts
and was tremendously interested
in the thinking and behavior of people
at various levels.
And I knew I was going to Wisconsin on vacation in September.
And so my unconscious mind
furnished me with an opportunity
of observing myself
at a previous age.
[Pause]
And you work with patients
and you work with your understanding
and your understandings come
from your knowledge
of how you behave.
In your observations,
of the behavior of others
[Pause]
you need
to have a vivid observation
of your own past behavior.
[Long Pause]

MHE: Now it is my interpretation that she was a bit abashed by Dr. Z's presence. But I think Dr. Z isn't here now [in Dr. S's awareness. As far as I can judge, there are quite a number of mobile memories being manifested.

ER: How can you tell?

MHE: By those muscle quiverings around that elbow. And the alterations of her breathing are very suggestive of mobility. Sometimes those are suggestive of, for example, going for a walk in the woods.

ER: What is the meaning of those slight vibratory movements of the eyes?

MHE: Sometimes they are random movement, sometimes they signify a kind of relaxation. You don't know really. I think a proper thing to do is let her discover bit by bit more and more things about herself.

ER: You like to have your patients discover and tell you about these minimal movements rather than making spurious generalizations about them. This is very wise because individual differences between people are so great in trance experience it is really difficult to relate inner events to external behavior in any consistent way.

MHE: That's right.

ER: Weitzenhoffer (1971) has investigated "slow eye movements of a pendular (sinusoid) type resembling those which have been reported to accompany Stage I of natural sleep and certain other altered states of consciousness. . . . At such times the subjects have been found to be still responsive to the hypnotist." Spiegel (1972) has found eye-roll (the ability to look upward on signal while closing the eyelids) and squint during induction to be indications of clinical hypnotizability. Other investigators (Switras, 1974; Wheeler et al., 1974,) however, have found no relation between eye-roll and other measures of hypnotic susceptibility in the laboratory. Ancient images as well as modern photographs of yogi in meditation also show the upward roll of the eyeball. Even though there are great individual differences in eye behavior during trance, it can be studied for whatever clues it provides regarding altered states of consciousness.

MHE: Now it isn't important
for you
to recall
what you have achieved
here today.
Your unconscious can unfold it to you
in bits and parts
at the appropriate time,
and you will have a good understanding.
And anything not remembered today
is still recorded in your mind.
[Pause]

ER: In her later "reflections" Dr. S reported that this remark did in fact cause a dramatic and unwanted amnesia.

MHE: I'm giving Dr. S an opportunity for inner experiential learning in this trance, which she won't know about until the time is right to use it.

ER: You don't want her to know about it till the time is right, because you don't want her conscious mind to interfere with it.

MHE: I don't want her conscious programs to depotentiate it!

ER: So theoretically a patient could leave feeling you've done absolutely nothing for her?

MHE: That's right! And they often do!

ER: Until later, when they call you up with reports of the value of what you've helped them accomplish.

MHE: That's right.

> **MHE: You need not know today**
> **that perhaps you are anesthetized completely.**
> **That you are immobilized completely.**
> **[Pause]**
> **You need not even know**
> **if you have**
> **dissociated yourself from your body.**
> **At the right time, you will discover**
> **All the things that you have accomplished.**
> **you will repeat these learnings**
> **subsequently.**
> **And you are beginning to realize**
> **that you are a far better subject than you previously thought.**
> **[Long pause]**
> **And you keep right on in a trance,**
> **learning the things you need to learn.**
> **And I'm going to turn away from you and talk to Dr. Rossi.**
>
> **[Long pause during which Erickson quietly talks to Drs. Z and Rossi]**

MHE: In therapy, this is often the way you get patients to become aware of their capabilities. You are essentially giving them the freedom to use themselves. Patients come to you because they don't feel free to use themselves.

ER: Now, is this like the way you gave Dr. Robert Pearson open-ended suggestions for the anesthesia? He was suddenly able to the ability in an emergency (Pearson, 1966). You say you had never given him specific suggestions to experience anesthesia.

MHE: No.

ER: But he was able to develop an anesthesia that may well have saved his life because years before you had given him such open-ended suggestions for the possibility of anesthesia when he might need it.

MHE: I told him, "You know a lot of things you need to know, only you don't know you know them. When the appropriate situation develops, use the appropriate learning."

ER: Even though he had never experienced hypnotic anesthesia before, in an appropriate situation, in the emergency situation when a brick hit him on the head, he was able to develop a hypnotic anesthesia.

MHE: At that moment he said to himself, "If only Erickson were here." Erickson connoted hypnosis for him, and that meant he should use hypnosis.

ER: He should use hypnosis for his obvious need in that emergency situation. So this is an extremely valuable suggestion you are giving to patients. You are stimulating in them an infinate number of learnings that they will be able to apply at the appropriate time.

MHE: That Pearson incident was a beautiful example of that. His associations to me were primarily about hypnosis, anesthesia, and the ***Utilization*** of the unconscious. He added healing to that, better healing.

ER: So he was able to effect faster body healing through hypnotic suggestion?

MHE: He was back lecturing in a few days with only a bandaid. His skull had been fractured and chips of bone taken out. The surgeon had expected him to pad around in his slippers for a few weeks.

[Erickson now studies Dr. S very intently for a few minutes.]

MHE: I don't know how to understand your finger movements,
the elbow movement,
the alteration in your breathing.
But comfortable,
slowly, agreeably,
bring your trance to an end
at a time of your own choice.
And come out of it feeling rested
and comfortable
and at ease,
with a sense of having done something very well.

ER: What are you studying now?

MHE: I'm trying to determine how quickly I should awaken her.

ER: What criteria are you using?

MHE: I don't know. I do know I won't do it now while she is taking a deep breath.

ER: Why?

MHE: I don't know what is going on then. If you awaken a subject at the wrong moment, they resent it. They can then demand that you put them back in trance so they can finish.

ER: How do you know when they are finished and ready to awaken?

MHE: You look for a quiet moment when all you can see is comfort.

> **[Pause as Dr. S reorients to her body, opens her eyes, and awakens. As soon as she opens her eyes, before she is completely awakened, Erickson quickly distracts her.]**
>
> **MHE: Did Dr. Rossi ever tell you about my ironwood carvings?**
>
> **Dr. S: Wha...?**
>
> **MHE: Did Dr. Rossi tell you about my ironwood carvings?**
>
> **Dr. S; Ironwood carvings?**
>
> **MHE: And yesterday I became the proud possessor of a frog riding a tricycle.**
>
> **Dr. S: [laughs]Just what everybody needs, I guess.**
>
> **[With laughter and mirth all around Erickson continues to talk about everything under the sun except anything related to the session that has just taken place. We all then join him to look at the ironwood carvings and newly acquired whimsical clay sculpture of the frog in the living room of his home.]**

MHE: Now what I had to do was awaken her and distract her so whatever she has done can remain at the unconscious level. I don't want it shoved into a conscious frame of reference.

ER: You produced an hypnotic amnesia by distraction (Erickson and Rossi, 1974/2010), and by this means you hoped to keep the trance work effective at an unconscious level. As her later "Reflections" indicate, you were highly effective in facilitating this amnesia even though she greatly regretted it.

Reflections Written by Dr. S About Her Trance Experiences.

Some material did slip through to consciousness, and this is the essence of her reflections.

I first experienced fog and then trance, relaxed.

In response to Erickson's comments (roots, etc.,) I remember various

childhood memories including a forgotten phase where I wanted to be a writer—I see myself reading a book by Louisa May Alcott at the beach and planting a maple tree from seed which grew outside my bedroom window.

Scenes of walking on the beach, etc.

I think I must tell Dr. Erickson my wart is gone (Dr. S had removed a wart on her own finger by self hypnosis).

And that I have gotten to be a smoother therapist.

Patients comment, "She helps you and it doesn't hurt." I feel somewhat pleased.

I remember feeling my body numb and still.

I hear Dr. Erickson say something like "You won't have to remember what happens." Then, suddenly, I look and my memories become fogged up. Then I see myself in a bed reflecting to myself," You are really going into a deep sleep—you will be so relaxed you won't remember your dream."

I can't remember anything after that. But have a feeling I was in a dream-phantasy trance for some time. I wake up after a suggestion (that's the first thing I can recall) relaxed, serene, satisfied and great!

Chapter Twenty

Update: What is a Suggestion? The Neuroscience of Implicit Processing Heuristics in Therapeutic Hypnosis and Psychotherapy

Ernest L. Rossi & Kathryn L. Rossi
Reprinted with permission from the American Society of Clinical Hypnosis 49:4, April 2007

Abstract

Neuroscience and bioinformatics research on activity-dependent gene expression and brain plasticity in memory and learning are used to reconceptualize a fundamental question of therapeutic hypnosis, "What is a suggestion?" John Kihlstrom's cognitive-behavioral perspective of implicit (unconscious) and explicit (conscious) memory and Eric Kandel's Nobel Prize winning neurobiological research are integrated for a 30-year update of Milton H. Erickson's neuropsychophysiology of therapeutic hypnosis. Implicit processing heuristics are proposed as a more general framework for Erickson's concept of permissive indirect suggestions in therapeutic hypnosis and psychotherapy. These perspectives are illustrated by utilizing implicit processing heuristics to facilitate the four-stage creative process in converting implicit to explicit memory in a brain-damaged patient.

Keywords: Activity-dependent Gene Expression & brain plasticity, consciousness, implicit processing heuristics, therapeutic suggestion

INTRODUCTION: WHAT IS SUGGESTION?

"What is a suggestion?" is a fundamental and highly controversial question explored by the late André Weitzenhoffer (2000) in his critical analysis of the clinical and research literature of hypnosis. We will reconceptualize this question by first reviewing Erickson and Rossi's (1976/2021) perspective on psychological implication as a model of Erickson's indirect approach to hypnotic suggestion. We will update this perspective with new insights about the role of consciousness and attention in the formation of implicit (unconscious) and explicit (conscious) memory and learning by John Kihlstrom (2007, 2008) and Eric Kandel (2006). We will outline how such research is consistent with our hypothesis that the function of consciousness in general and the focus of attention, in particular, is to turn on activity-dependent gene expression, brain, and behavioral plasticity in the normative dynamics of adaptation, problem solving, and healing, which are highly conserved during evolution at the molecular-genomic level (Rossi, 2002b, 2004, 2005, 2007b). We apply this neuroscience and bioinformatic framework to illustrate how implicit processing heuristics may be utilized as the most general class of permissive therapeutic suggestions for facilitating memory, learning, problem solving, and healing (Erickson & Rossi, 1976).

Psychological Implication as a Model of Erickson's Therapeutic Suggestion

While Erickson used direct suggestion, particularly during the early, experimental stage of his career, he later emphasized that attempting to directly program people without understanding their individuality was "a very uninformed way of doing therapy" (Erickson & Rossi, 1979/2008). In our first collaborative effort to describe his use of indirect suggestion, we found that Erickson's "implied directive" was the most useful for conceptualizing therapeutic suggestion. Erickson believed that implication contributed to therapeutic suggestion because it is not what the therapist says that is important as much as what the patient does with what the therapist says (Erickson & Rossi, 1976/2021).

> An understanding of how Erickson uses implication will provide us with the clearest model of his indirect approach to hypnotic suggestion. Since his use of implication may involve something more than the typical dictionary definition of the term, we will assume that he may be developing a special form of "psychological implication." For Erickson, psychological implication is a key that automatically turns the tumblers of a patient's associative processes into predictable patterns without awareness of how it happened. The implied thought or response seems to come up autonomously within patients, as if it was their own inner response rather than a suggestion initiated by the therapist. Psychological implication is thus a way of structuring and directing a patient's associative processes when they cannot do it for themselves. The therapeutic use of this approach is obvious. If patients have problems because of the limitations in their ability to utilize their own resources, then implications are a way of bypassing these limitations.
>
> It is important in formulating psychological implications to realize that the therapist only provides a stimulus; the hypnotic aspect of psychological implications is created on an unconscious level by the listener. The most effective aspect of any suggestion is

> that which stirs the listener's own mental processes into automatic action. It is this autonomous activity of the listener's own associations and mental processes that creates hypnotic experience.
>
> There are, to be sure, crude and mostly ineffective uses of implication in everyday life, where the speaker in a very obvious manner attempts to cast negative implications or aspersions on the listener. In such crude usage, the implication is obviously created entirely by the speaker. In our use of psychological implication, however, we mean something quite different. In the psychological climate of the therapeutic encounter the patient is understood to be the center of focus. Every psychological truth is consciously or unconsciously received by the patient for its possible application to himself. Psychological implication thus becomes a valuable indirect approach to evoking and Utilizing a patients own associations to deal with his own problem. (pp. 59-60)

Erickson (1964/2022b) wrote that the most effective aspect of therapeutic suggestion is that which stirs the listener's own mental processes into creative activity that generates the so called "miracle" of healing as follows:

> In each instance, hypnosis was used for the specific purpose of placing the burden of responsibility for therapeutic results upon the patient himself after he himself had reached a definite conclusion that therapy would not help and that a last resort would be a hypnotic "miracle." In this author's understanding of psychotherapy, if a patient wants to believe in a "hypnotic miracle" so strongly that he will undertake the responsibility of making a recovery by virtue of his own actual behavior and continue his recovery, he is at liberty to do so under whatever guise he chooses, but neither the author nor the reader is obligated to regard the success of the therapy as a hypnotic miracle. The hypnosis was used solely as a modality by means of which to secure their cooperation in accepting what they wanted. In other words, they were induced by hypnosis to acknowledge and act upon their own personal responsibility for successfully accepting the previously futilely sought and offered but actually rejected therapy . . . a long series of similar cases are reported here to illustrate the use of hypnosis as a tech-

> nique of deliberately shifting from the therapist to the patient the entire burden of both defining the psychotherapy desired and the responsibility for accepting it." (pp. 62-65)

From our current neuroscience perspective, it is the patient's own creative activity that evokes Activity-dependent Gene Expression, brain, and behavioral plasticity, and the so-called "miracles of mind-body healing." It is the deeply meaningful and creative replaying of the listener's own mental processes that creates hypnotic experience, problem solving, and healing. The locus of healing is within the patient; the therapist has no mysterious or extraordinary powers of control or healing. Patients heal themselves when they are fortunate enough to receive appropriate "therapeutic suggestions," that function as "implicit processing heuristics." This evokes numinous experiences of novelty, enrichment, and activities that generate Activity-dependent Gene Expression, brain plasticity, and mind-body healing (Rossi, 2007b).

Many years after the concept of the implied directive and psychological implication as important keys to Erickson's successful use of therapeutic hypnosis (Erickson & Rossi, 1976/2021) were described, the central role of implication became recognized in neuroscience. Squire and Kandel (1999), for example summarized the role of categorical learning (Rossi, 1963, 1964; Rossi & Rossi, 1965) and implication in understanding the difference between conscious (explicit or declarative knowledge) and unconscious (implicate or non-declarative knowledge) in the dynamics of memory and learning.

> The question of interest is: What kind of memory underlies the ability to knowledge about categories? The surprising answer is that at least some kinds of category learning are nondeclarative. Category learning can be independent of and parallel to declarative memory, rather than simply derivative from it. People can acquire knowledge about categories implicitly even when their declarative memory for the instances that define the category is impaired (p. 188).

Recent research efforts to assess the value of Erickson's approaches to psychological implication in therapeutic suggestion remain controversial, however. Some researchers failed to find any superiority of indirect suggestion over direct suggestion (Matthews, 2000), but many clinicians dispute the validity of the research methods used (Peter & Revenstorf, 2000). Erickson's indirect approaches to therapeutic suggestion involved the patient's "experience of re-associating and reorganizing his own experiential life that eventuates in a cure, not the manifestation of responsive behavior, which can, at best, satisfy only the observer" (Erickson, 1948/2021a). The research that purports to demonstrate that indirect suggestion was not superior to direct suggestion, however, used the so-called objective measures of responsive behavior on standardized scales of hypnotic susceptibility that typically restricted the creative replay and reconstruction of the subject's subjective associations. When investigators compared the subjective perceptions of subjects to their own hypnotic experiences with the objective behavioral measures of direct and indirect suggestion, however, they came to these interesting conclusions (Matthews, et al., 1985).

> "While the behavioral data failed to show significant differences between the two methods, however, ***subjects did report feeling more deeply hypnotized during the indirect procedure than during the direct procedure. This result is in support of an Ericksonian view...of indirect suggestion in that wider latitude for responding is offered to subjects than is typically available with direct suggestion***. Thus, the subject's unique responses to indirect suggestions can be interpreted by them to be an indication of trance depth. If subjects fail to perform in accordance with a direct suggestion, however, there is some likelihood that they may perceive themselves as less deeply hypnotized" (pp. 222-223).

It is precisely this "wider latitude for responding in the subject's unique responses to indirect suggestions that Erickson wished to facilitate as a creative experience of re-associating and reorganizing their own experiential life that eventuates in a cure." While indirect suggestion can facilitate the creative replay, re-association, and re-synthesis of subjective experiences, indirect suggestion is not necessarily useful in the manipulation and control of the subject's objective behavior as it is assessed with standardized scales of hypnotic susceptibility. Even with research that demonstrates the efficacy of indirect suggestion in facilitating the subject's personal creativity, the misperception that Erickson & Rossi's (1976/2021) indirect hypnotic suggestion is a covert method of programming the patient with the therapist's goal remains an important issue in professional practice as well as public perception. Polczyk and Pasek (2006, p. 394), for example, recently clarified these difficult and easily confused issues from another perspective in the history of hypnosis research where "direct suggestions are 'outspokenly expressed,' that is, the intention to influence is overt. In contrast, indirect suggestions are masked, that is, the intention to influence is concealed."

In a more recent paper, however, Kihlstrom has clarified how this "direct-indirect dichotomy" fails to account for what is most interesting about the "explicit-implicit distinction" as follows:

> In the final analysis, both the 'direct-indirect' and 'intentional-incidental' dichotomies fail to capture the essence of the explicitimplicit distinction—which is that explicit memory is conscious recollection, and implicit memory is unconscious memory, of the past. But if implicit memory is unconscious memory, why not simply call it that? The answer is more likely to be found in sociology than psychology, as those who would make a science of unconscious mental life have sought to avoid the taint of Freudian psychoanalysis . . . Still, ***what makes implicit memory interesting is not that implicit tests provide indirect, possibly surreptitious, assessments of what a person remembers; nor that implicit expressions of memory occur involuntarily. What makes implicit memory interesting is that it represents the dynamic influence of memory in the absence of conscious recollection.*** (2007).

Because of this confusion between (1) programming and control by the therapist with direct suggestions versus (2) creative inner work by the patient via indirect suggestions, we need to make a special effort to distinguish between them. In their first book, Erickson and Rossi (1976/2021) emphasized how the classical, directive concept of hypnotic suggestion could be complemented with indirect suggestion. Because of the ambiguity of the concept of "indirect suggestion" and its possible negative connotations of surreptitious manipulation and programming of the subject, however, "indirect suggestion" is now being replaced with the concept of "implicit processing heuristics" wherever appropriate in the recent commentaries on Milton H. Erickson's Collected Works. Implicit processing heuristics designate how permissive and positive suggestion in every day life as well as therapeutic hypnosis, psychotherapy, and rehabilitation can facilitate the implicit processing of memory and learning during "offline processing" (sleep, dreaming, etc) via gene expression, brain plasticity, and mind-body healing within the subject. We now need brain imaging and DNA microarray research to document the full range and limitations of implicit processing heuristics in modulating the molecular-genomic pathways of therapeutic hypnosis and other approaches to mind-body healing and rehabilitation. Eric Kandel's (2006) recent summary of his lifetime of research on implicit and explicit memory provides an updated neuroscience database for our explorations of memory and its facilitation with implicit processing heuristics.

Kandel's Implicit and Explicit Memory, Gene Expression and Brain Plasticity

In an incisive chapter titled, "Attention must be paid!" Kandel (2006) recounts the history research on the role of attention in memory and learning that began with William James' Principles of Psychology (1890/1981). James maintained that there are two classes of attention: involuntary and voluntary. Involuntary attention is an automatic neural process activated by the external world by big things, bright things, and moving things, or blood that is evident in implicit memory. Voluntary attention such as reading this sentence, by contrast, is a characteristic of explicit memory activated by a self-directed internal need to learn and remember. Kandel (2006) describes his research in this context as follows:

James argued that voluntary attention is obviously a conscious process in people; therefore, it is likely to be initiated in the cerebral cortex. Viewed from a reductionist perspective, both kinds of attention recruit signals of salience, such as modulatory neurotransmitters, that regulate the function or configuration of a neural network.

Our molecular studies in Aplysia [a marine snail] and mice support James's contention that these two forms of attention, involuntary and voluntary, exist. One of the key differences between them is not the absence or presence of salience, but whether the signal of salience is perceived consciously . . . the determining factor in whether a memory is implicit or explicit is the manner in which the attentional signal for salience is recruited.

In both types of memory . . . conversion of short-term memory to long-term memory requires the activation of genes, and in each case modulatory transmitters appear to carry an attentional signal marking the importance of a stimulus. In response to that signal, genes are turned on and proteins are produced and sent to all the synapses. Serotonin triggers protein kinase A in Aplysia, for example, and dopamine triggers protein kinase A in the mouse [and humans]. But these signals of salience are called up in two fundamentally different ways for the implicit memory underlying sensitization in Aplysia and the explicit memory required to form the spatial map in the mouse [and humans].

In implicit memory storage, the attentional signal is recruited involuntarily (reflexively), from the bottom up: the sensory neurons of the tail, activated by a shock, act directly on the cells that release serotonin. In spatial [explicit] memory, dopamine appears to be recruited voluntarily, from the top down: the cerebral cortex activates the cells that release dopamine, and dopamine modulates activity in the hippocampus."(pp. 313-314).

Figure 4 illustrates how Kandel's contrasts the neural pathways and neurotransmitters of implicit and explicit memory on the unconscious and conscious levels respectively. Note, however, how the dynamics of both implicit and explicit memory stimulate activity or experience-dependent gene expression, which generates the growth of new synaptic connections (brain plasticity in the marine snail Aplysia, mice, and humans.)

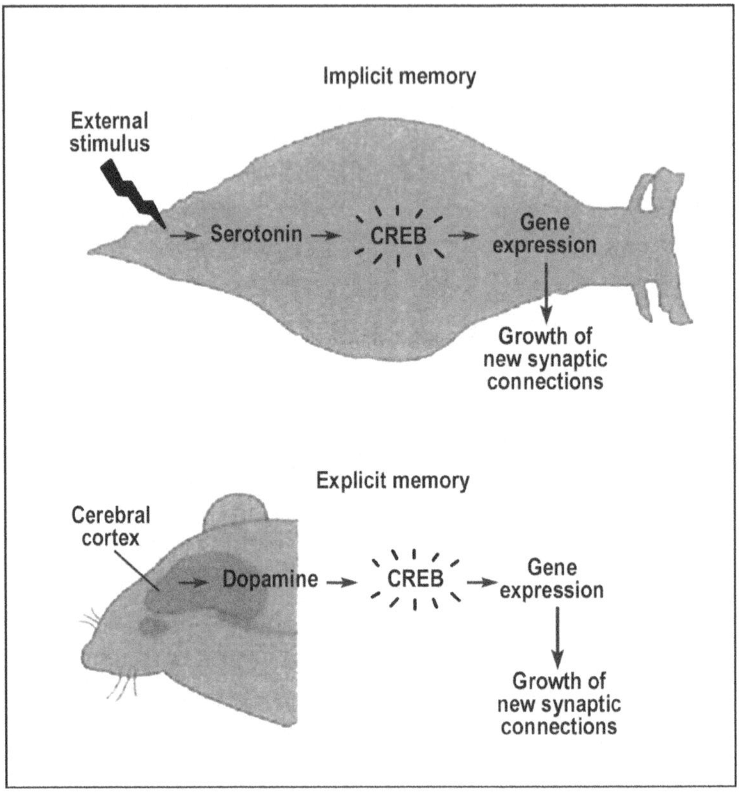

Figure 4 (10.20.F.4) How Implicit and Explicit Memory Turn on *Activity-Dependent Gene Expression* and Brain Plasticity

In implicit (unconscious) memory, an outside stimulus automatically and involuntarily triggers a salience signal (the neurotransmitter serotonin), which turns on activity-dependent gene expression and brain plasticity (growth of new synaptic connections). In explicit (conscious) memory, the cerebral cortex voluntarily recruits a salience signal (the neurotransmitter dopamine), which focuses attention modulating activity-dependent gene expression and brain plasticity in the hippocampus and eventually the cerebral cortex.

Some of the related features of attention, implication, heuristics, memory, and suggestion are listed in Table 4. To these, we would add the important contributions of Warrington & Weiskrantz (1968) and Schacter (1987) on the role of priming on episodic and implicit memory described by Kihlstrom (2007) as follows:

> In 1968, Warrington and Weiskrantz reported an experiment in which amnesic patients were asked to study a list of familiar words. Compared to control subjects, the patients performed very poorly on standard tests of recall and recognition. However, when they were presented with three-letter stems or fragments, and asked simply to complete the cues with the first word that came to mind, amnesiacs and controls were equally likely to complete the cues with items from the studied list.
>
> ***This is a priming effect, in which the processing of one item influences the processing of another item. In positive priming, the prime facilitates processing of the target; in negative priming, the prime inhibits processing of the target.*** In this instance, the priming effect indicates that the studied items were encoded in memory, retained in storage, and influenced performance on the completion test. ***The fact that equivalent levels of priming occurred in neurologically intact subjects, who remembered the priming episode normally, and amnesic patients, who had very poor memory, indicates that priming can be dissociated from conscious recollection.*** On the basis of evidence like this, Schacter distinguished between two expressions of episodic memory [autobiographical memory for events that have occurred in our personal past:] explicit and implicit (Schacter, 1987). ***Explicit memory refers to conscious recollection of a past event, as exemplified by performance on recall and recognition tests. By contrast, implicit memory refers to any effect of an event on subsequent experience, thought, or action. Priming is, of course, just such an effect. The dissociation between priming and recall in amnesic patients indicates implicit memory can persist in the absence of explicit memory.*** (p. 5-6).

We propose that while history has given these processes different names, from an evolutionary perspective they are all related on the molecular-genomic and neuropsychophysiological levels. Kandel summarizes his research on the molecular mechanisms of implicit and explicit memory and learning by emphasizing the differences in the brain dynamics of men and women as follows.

> Consistent with this idea that similar molecular mechanisms are used for top-down and bottom-up attentional processes, we have found a mechanism that may be involved in stabilizing the memory in both cases. The hippocampus of the mouse (and humans) contains at least one prion-like protein similar to the one Kausik Si discovered in Aplysia. Martin Theis, a postdoctoral student from Germany, and I found that, in much the same way that serotonin modulates the amount and state of the CPEB protein in Aplysia, dopamine modulates the amount of the prion-like CPEB

Table 4 (10.20.T.4) Related Concepts on the Unconscious and Conscious Levels

Related Concepts of Attention, Implication, Heuristics, Memory, and Suggestion on the Unconscious and Conscious Levels

Memory & Learning	Unconscious	Conscious
William James	Involuntary Attention	Voluntary Attention
Milton Erickson	Indirect Suggestion	Direct Suggestion
Ernest Rossi	Implicit Heuristics	Explicit Heuristics
Daniel Schacter	Implicit Memory	Explicit Memory
Eric Kandel	Implicit Memory	Explicit Memory

> protein (CPEB-3) in the mouse hippocampus. This discovery raised the intriguing possibility—so far just that—that spatial maps may become fixated when an animal's attention triggers the release of dopamine in the hippocampus and that dopamine initiates a self-perpetuating state also mediated by CPEB.

The importance of attention in stabilizing the spatial map raises another question: Is the spatial map, a map formed by learning, similar in all of us? Specifically, do men and women use the same strategies to find their way around an environment? This is a fascinating question and one that biologists are just beginning to explore. [There are] clear differences in the way women and men attend to and orient themselves to the space around them. ***Women use nearby cues or landmarks. . .Brain imaging shows activation of different areas in men and women as they think about space: the left hippocampus in men and the right parietal and right prefrontal cortex in women.*** These studies point out the potential benefits for group effectiveness of optimizing both strategies (pp. 314-316).

Just as Kandel found simple model organisms to differentiate between implicit and explicit memory and learning, so we need to differentiate between the implicit and explicit components of therapeutic suggestion to better facilitate problem solving and healing (Erickson & Rossi, 1976/2021). We will illustrate how implicit processing heuristics may evoke, focus, and facilitate the patient's own specific associations, life experiences, and inner resources in active, patient-centered, creative work that is sometimes so intense that the patient feels hot and actually sweats with effort (Rossi & Cheek, 1988). This is in striking contrast to the diffuse, nonspecific, and continuous singsong "hypnotic pattern" that is commonly observed in professional hypnosis training workshops when the therapist is apparently doing most of the active work by talking, which attempts to cast a "hypnotic spell" over the apparently passive patient who is merely receiving. The implicit processing heuristics illustrated in this case, by contrast, allow patients a great deal of free time for self-directed inner work during which they can find their own words, cognitions, and feelings to actively express their own creative impulses in their own way rather than attempting to passively imprint and follow the therapist's words. Implicit processing heuristics empower the patient to activate, explore, and focus their own approaches to problem solving and healing wherein they create their own metaphors, behavioral prescriptions, and neuropsychophysiological pathways.

The Hip-Nose Doctor, Brain Damage and the Hidden Tickets: Converting Implicit Memory to Explicit Consciousness

A more comprehensive presentation of this instructive illustration of the psychosocial and cultural factors involved in facilitating the conversion of implicit memory to explicit consciousness in a brain damaged patient was published previously (Rossi, 2003). In the 1970's, Rossi was first exploring new variations of Milton Erickson's ***Hand Levitation*** approaches to hypnotic induction and suggestion.

[The phone rang in Rossi's office.]

Mabel (Patient): You hip-nose doctor?

From the sound of her voice and words spoken, she sounded like a debilitated person.

Rossi: Excuse me?

Mabel: I say, you hip-nose doctor? You memory doctor?

Rossi: [Thought for a moment, trying to figure out what the woman was saying. Then it hit him.] You're wondering if I do hypnosis?

Mabel: Thas right, a hip-nose doctor to find my tickets. You dat?

Because her speech was slurred Rossi wondered whether she might be on drugs or have organic brain damage. When Mabel arrived at her appointed time, however, she was dressed appropriately, in neat, clean clothes but her hair appeared to be slightly askew and disheveled.

Rossi: So,you mentioned something on the phone about wanting hypnosis for memory loss.

[Mabel grinned and nodded her head so vigorously that her wig slipped to the floor to expose a huge scar running from the side of her head to the front. As she picked up the wig and replaced it on her head without the least embarrassment, she explained how she had recently been in a car accident and her memory just wasn't the same any more. Her problem was that she could not remember where she had hidden some very expensive tickets to a Michael Jackson concert about a month earlier after a man hand delivered the tickets to her in her home.

As a first step, Rossi tried to have her use her normal everyday consciousness to recall her steps through her house after she received the tickets to possibly recover the memory of where she may have hid them. Throughout this initial exploration, however:

Mabel: [Repeatedly comments] I only remember hiding the tickets in a safe place where nobody could find them.

The whole family had already devoted hours on a treasure hunt, practically taking the house apart to find the tickets.

Rossi was trying so hard to do a good job that he lost track of time. He kept asking her apparently futile questions about her life and family, when abruptly she sat back, shook her head sadly.

Mabel: [Asked dubiously] You not hip-nose doctor?

Rossi glanced at his watch and saw there were only ten minutes left in the session. He quickly reassured her and proceeded with the ***4-Stage Creative Process*** to activity-dependent hypnotic induction and suggestion ***Utilizing*** a series of implicit processing heuristics to facilitate her memory as follows (Rossi, 2002b, 2004).

From our current perspective, however, we can now recognize that this apparently futile preliminary period of explicit questioning—before any hypnotic induction—was actually a period of priming her implicit (unconscious) level of processing.

Application of the 4-Stage Activity-Dependent Hand Mirroring Induction with Implicit Processing Heuristics (IPH)

Stage One: Hypnotic Induction with Heightened Sensitivity & Therapeutic Dissociation

Rossi asks the patient to hold her hands up with her palms facing each other. He silently, slowly, and impressively demonstrates with his own hands to focus her attention and possibly activate her mirror neuron systems as she stares in fascination at him.

He softly and slowly suggests that she would notice when one of her hands begins to feel warmer or cooler indicating that her inner mind was starting to experience "real hypnosis."

He pauses as she mirrors the therapist's hand placement with her own and focuses her attention on them

Rossi: Or, one hand might feel heavier than the other and start to move slowly downward more or less all by itself to signal that some part of her knew where the tickets were hidden.

This is an IPH facilitating a possible therapeutic dissociation (hand "move slowly downward more or less all by itself") and ideo-dynamic signaling as she begins a memory search.

[One of her hands begins to slowly and hesitantly move down-

ward with a slightly jerky motion. Her eyes flutter spontaneously for a moment or two and then remain closed with an apparently involuntary and very fine, rapid, vibratory activity of the eyelids]

The eyelid activity has been frequently reported in the early historical literature of therapeutic hypnosis (Tinterow, 1970). We speculate that this very rapid eye activity may be associated with heightened neural activation and ***Activity-dependent Gene Expression*** and activity-dependent brain plasticity on an implicit level.

Stage Two: Incubation

[As her hand moved downward very slowly a variety of eye movements and shifts in her facial expression take place as her head hesitantly shifts from one direction to another.]

We can only speculate that she is replaying her implicit memories as one hand moves slowly downward with slight pauses now and then as she apparently searches through her house. Rossi supports the process with occasional implicit processing heuristics.

Rossi: That's right, searching carefully everyplace for these wonderful tickets.

He pauses as this IPH implies she can re-experience her memory here and now.

[After a few moments a worried look of apparent stress crosses her face.]

Rossi solicitously and sympathetically responds with a supportive IPH.

Rossi: Yes, do you have the courage to continue all by yourself for a little while longer until...?"

[Rossi pauses as this incomplete question implies further inner search with an attitude of positive expectancy.]

Since stage two is typically beset with doubts, conflicts, and uncertainties the therapeutic bond is supported further with the IPH:

Rossi: Knowing you can share with me a word or sentence or two about what your experiencing at any time, but only what I need to hear to help you further.

This is a permissive, but carefully focused and constrained IPH that limits any impulse to speak to exactly what further IPHs she may need from the therapist to facilitate her memory.

Stage Three: Illumination, Problem Solving, and Healing

[Just about the time her hand almost reaches her lap, she suddenly stiffens. Her mouth starts to open as if she wants to speak but she seems to be in conflict as if she did not want to disturb her inner focus and concentration. Facial tension now seems to drop away as a tentative and barely perceptible smile becomes very slowly evident.]

Such smiles after an experience of arousal and stress in stage two typically signal that some sort of crisis has been resolved and she may be moving into stage three of the eureka experience.

Rossi attempts to help her recognize and focus on this positive possibility with an open-ended IPH:

Rossi: You're receiving something pleasing [Pause] surprising [Pause] interesting [Pause] are you not?

Erickson believed that the close apposition of linguistic opposites with questions such as "Your are, are you not?" structured a permissive tipping point facilitating whatever the patient was engaged with. We speculate that the open-ended IHP introduces a mild confusion that could momentarily de-construct a rigid and blocking conscious (explicit) mental set so that an unconscious (implicit), fragmentary, and still nascent bit of brain plasticity and new consciousness could become manifest. (Rossi, 1972/2000)

Mabel: [Barely nodded her head to signal "Yes," very carefully, as if she didn't want to upset anything that was going on within her.]

Rossi: You are going to continue remembering it, aren't you?

Mabel: [Again nodded her head, "Yes."]

Rossi: You can really see exactly where you put those tickets.

Mabel: [Nodded, "Yes."]

[Mabel slowly opened her eyes with a fixed expression. Her body didn't move. Her hand was still in mid-air. She was apparently still in trance, staring directly into Rossi's eyes with a fixed stare.]

It is important to recognize that while she opens her eyes she does not manifest the typical nonverbal cues of reorienting to full awareness by stretching, readjusting her body orientation, etc.

Stage Four: Verification and Post Hypnotic Suggestion

Rossi: Okay, that's great. In a couple of minutes, when you are absolutely sure that you know where the tickets are, and you can tell me where they are, what is going to happen?

He pauses for these strongly directive reinforcements to consolidate her emerging explicit memory of the hidden tickets. The ambiguous open-ended question tacked on the end gives locus of control to her implicit dynamics.

[She slowly and spontaneously closes her eyes again.]

Rossi: Will your eyes remain closed when you tell me?
Or are your eyes going to open so you can fully awaken first when you tell me?

Options implying many possibilities of converting implicit to explicit memory and awakening that are satisfactory.

Mabel: Closa, Tickets in de lina closa. (Linen closet) [She said, mumbling the word indistinctly.]

[A broad grin now spreads softly across Mabel's face, she opens her eyes, stretches a bit, and pats her wig as she reorients to the room realizing she now remembers where she had put the tickets.]

These nonverbal behavioral cues indicate she is now reorienting to full awareness. She tells the story of how only she had the key to the linen closet of her home where many the important household items were kept so no one could intrude. It somehow seemed only natural to this family that everyone should avoid the linen closet during the search for the tickets. The next day, Rossi heard a message on his answering machine from one of Mabel's family members thanking him profusely for helping grandma remember where she hid the tickets.

Limitations and Scope of Implicit Processing Heuristics

The primary limitation of implicit processing heuristics is that they are not useful for the covert manipulation, programming, prediction, and control of anyone's mind or behavior. The second limitation is there are no truly adequate models for the experimental validation of implicit processing heuristics at this time. This has not been for want of trying. The entire history of the theory, research and practice of hypnosis has focused intensely on the questions and conundrums of, "What is a suggestion?" with but little critical success (Weitzenhoffer, 2000). Although Rossi (2004) proposed "64 More Research Projects" to assess permissive suggestion to supplement the previous 64 research projects proposed in David Cheek's pioneering clinical applications of finger signaling (surely another set of implicit processing heuristics) there have been but few uncontestedpublished clinical-experimental studies to date that reported modest success (Pratt, 1996; Rossi & Cheek, 1988). A third limitation is that the mouse model of Figure 4, while adequate for illustrating the highly conserved molecular-genomic basis of activity-dependent gene expression and brain plasticity that are engaged in implicit memory and learning, it does not address the full complexity of human brain neurotransmission that is now known to involve at least 1100 proteins in the postsynaptic membrane (Pennisi, 2006). This means that we are still at an early stage in unraveling the dynamics of implicit heuristics, memory, and learning.

Given these limitations it is ironic to contemplate the expanding horizon and scope of our emerging concept of the utility of implicit processing heuristics. Converting implicit into explicit processes is the essence of all consciousness studies. In the widest sense IPHs encompass the entire range of hints, crafts, and techniques in the arts and sciences of education, linguistics, philosophy, and research of all sorts (Hofstadter, 1979, 2007). It is now recognized, for example, that implication "lives at the heart of mathematics" by building upon fundamental axioms that make all higher concepts possible (King, 1992, 2000). King describes it as follows.

Table 5 (10.20.T.5) A 30-Year Update on Hyp-notic Forms of Implicit Processing

Apposition of Opposites	Multiple & Serial Tasks
Binds & ***Double Binds***	Music (Lullaby, etc)
Body Language (Mirroring Behavior)	Negating (Implicit Priming)
Compound Suggestions	Not Doing & Not Knowing
Contingent Suggestions	Open-Ended Suggestions
Covering All Possibilities of Response	Pantomime & Nonverbal Cues
Dissociation (Therapeutic)	Paradoxical Intention
Expectancy	Partial & Incomplete Suggestion
Hints (Implicit/Explicit)	Pauses
Ideomotor & Ideosensory Signaling	Poetry, Rhyme & Song
Implication	Priming Before Induction
Implied Directive	Questions Evoking Wonder
Inter-Contextual Cues	***Surprise***, Psychological Shock
Multiple Communication Levels	Truisms (Facilitating ***Yes Sets***)
Analogy, Metaphor, Saga, etc	***Utilizing*** Closure Need
Anecdotes, Myths, & Stories, etc	Vocal Locus & Dynamics
Humor & Jokes, etc	***Yes Sets***

A 30-year update of the "hypnotic forms" of implicit processing heuristics in hypnotic realities. This is a partial update of the "hypnotic forms" listed in the original hypnotic realities (Erickson & Rossi, 1976, p. 312), which we now re-conceptualize as implicit processing heuristics.

> If you want to understand pure mathematics then you must first understand this point about implications. All pure mathematicians have this understanding as part of the fiber of their being. It is as natural to them as the air they breathe. And this understanding is one of three clearly defined characteristics which separate those people who understand mathematics from thosewho do not . . .

> The development of the number system from the Peano Axioms will then consist of the formulation of statements of the form "p implies q" and the proving of each statement ... at each stage of the development, you can use only what you have specifically assumed as axiomatic ... And the understanding that it is essential is the second fundamental characteristic mathematicians possess which distinguishes them from others ... the third characteristic shared by those who truly comprehend mathematics [is] the understanding of the need for compete precision in the statement of the axioms, the definitions, and the proofs of the assertions. (King, 1992, p. 56-60).

Although it is impractical to list all possible IPHs, Table 5 is a partial 30-year update of the "hypnotic forms" listed in the original ***Hypnotic Realities*** (Erickson and Rossi, 1976, p. 312).

We now need to expand clinical and experimental research on the domain of hypnosis beyond the current constraints of the cognitive-behavioral level (Kihlstrom, 2006b). We need to document how implicit processing heuristics can focus consciousness and attention during experiences of novelty (Eriksson et al., 1998), environmental enrichment (Kempermann, et al. 1997), and exercise (mental and physical) (Van Praag et al., 1999) to facilitate gene expression and brain plasticity. Research on implicit processing heuristics needs to include the practical, clinical applications of current neuroscience and the computerized technologies of bioinformatics (Davies, 2006). IPHs are active during those momentary pauses when we stare vacantly lost in contemplation and wonder in everyday life as well as during the "offline states" sleep and dreaming when activity-dependent gene expression and brain plasticity are updating our brain and consciousness (Ribeiro, 2004; Ribeiro et al.1999, 2002, 2004). Our current and future challenge in answering the question, "What is a suggestion?" is to utilize the technologies of DNA microarrays and brain imaging to explore the utilization of implicit processing heuristics to facilitate gene expression, brain, and behavioral plasticity in therapeutic hypnosis, psychotherapy, and rehabilitation.

Chapter Twenty-One

Developing Deep Trance in Therapeutic Hypnosis

By: Jan Dyba and Kathryn L. Rossi

[**Editors' note:** *This was previously printed in The Science of Psychotherapy (SoP) Volume 12, Issue 2, Apr-June 2024. Reprinted with permission.*]

Hypnosis has been utilized in psychotherapy ever since James Braid gave its official name in 1843 almost 200 years ago (Braid, 1855/1970). The effectiveness of hypnosis in treatment of various psychological problems has been validated through many independent research studies (for example: Hammond, 2010; Langewitz et al., 2005; Patterson & Jensen, 2003; Tomé-Pires & Miró, 2012; Yapko, 2002, 2019). Although the efficacy of hypnotic interventions is well established today, clients vary in their ability to enter that "special state" of receptivity. Hypnotic responsiveness, or susceptibility, is the ability to enter hypnosis and experience different hypnotic phenomena. According to the "state" theorists (Hilgard, 1965, 1977, 1979, 1991; Hilgard, Weitzenhoffer, Landes, & Moore, 1961; Weitzenhoffer, 1997) it is a relatively stable trait of personality and remains at similar levels throughout years. On the other hand, "cognitive" oriented learning theorists advocate for a notion that hypnotic responsiveness is modifiable and requires special cognitive skills and knowledge that can be obtained through training (Bertrand, 1989; Gorassini & Spanos, 1986; Nicolas P Spanos, 1991; Nicolas P Spanos et al., 1983).

Since hypnosis is a valuable tool that can be used in treatment as one main approach (Erickson, 1948/2021; Erickson & Rossi, 1979/2014; Yapko, 2002, 2019) as well as provide additional mode enhancing non-trance interventions (Kirsch, Montgomery, & Sapirstein, 1995) an important question is: ***How can we increase the likelihood of someone entering this special receptive state deep enough to achieve satisfactory results***? The question about the possibilities to alter hypnotic suggestibility or responsiveness has been discussed and validated elsewhere in detail (for example Bertrand, 1989; Hilgard, 1965). We will focus and explore the possibilities that this ***special state*** is indeed possible. We review research on methods that have proved to be successful and analyze what actually works to provide the reader with research based tips and schemas to increase a client's hypnotic abilities.

Can Hypnosis be used to enhance more efficient utilization of brain capacities?

In our previous work (Dyba, Rossi, & Rossi, 2019; Dyba, Rossi, Żurek, & Rossi, 2021) we outlined a model of hypnosis integrating a classical two-factor theory of hypnotic experience described by Milton H. Erickson and Ernest L. Rossi (Erickson & Rossi, 1981/2014) with novel neuroscience research on attention and cognitive processes (Egner & Raz, 2007; Raz et al., 2003; Raz, Moreno-Iniguez, Martin, & Zhu, 2007; Raz, Shapiro, Fan, & Posner, 2002; Sheehan, Donovan, & MacLeod, 1988) to create a novel updated theory of hypnotic experience outlined in Figure 5.

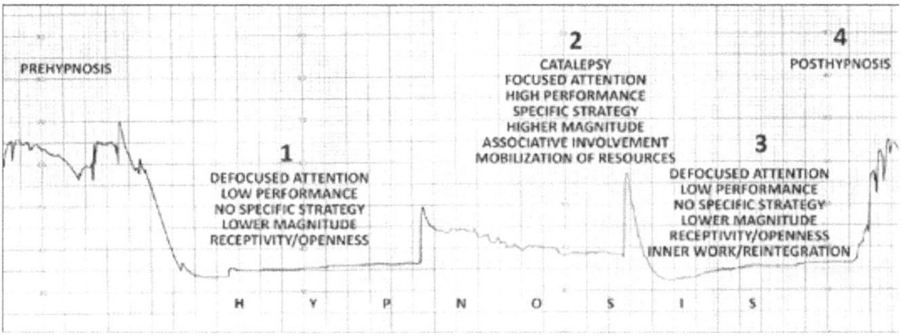

Figure 5 (10.21.F.6) A Novel Neurocognitive Model of Hypnotic Experience

According to this model (Dyba et al., 2019, 2021) hypnosis itself as a state is characterized by defocused attention, low performance, lower magnitude of electromagnetic field curve, and a state of receptivity and openness where a subject does not make any conscious effort to interfere with their own autonomous mental processes or suggestions presented by a therapist (Erickson & Rossi, 1981/2014). A client in this state does not apply any conscious cognitive strategy for dealing with a problem. However, when therapeutic work is being initiated, or any hypnotic phenomena is being elicited, then attention becomes focused, and the subject exhibits a higher performance rate as compared to being in a waking state where some specific strategy is being applied to the problem. The magnitude of electromagnetic field scores are higher, and the subject are in a process of ***associative involvement*** whereby the therapist engages and utilizes the subject's mental processes, associations, skills and resources in order to facilitate hypnotic experiences. At this moment a patient is able to better mobilize their inner resources in a goal directed manner and thus enhance or facilitate creative therapeutic change (Dyba et al., 2019; Rossi, 2002b, 2004; Rossi, Erickson-Klein, & Rossi, 2008b; Rossi & Rossi, 2013).

Multiple researchers (Crawford, Clarke, & Kitner-Triolo, 1996; De Pascalis & Palumbo, 1986; MacLeod-Morgan & Lack, 1982) demonstrated task-specific alterations of brain waves during hypnosis in highly responsive subjects as compared with low responsive ones. These results led to a formulation of a set of theories that subjects who are receptive to hypnosis demonstrate a more flexible cognitive style and therefore are more easily able to shift between different modes of functioning. This ability can be enhanced or developed with the help of hypnosis and hypnotic induction (Crawford, 1989). More recently, the main proponents of this view on hypnosis propose seeing it as a means of selectively activating different cortical and subcortical regions in accord with task-specific requirements (Crawford, 2001; Gruzelier, 1998). Based on these and additional research studies we proposed to view hypnosis as a means of more selectively, intensely, and effectively eliciting, activating and utilizing a client's resources to facilitate therapeutic change (Dyba et al., 2019, 2021).

Benefits of Deep Trance

Although much has been written on the subject of utilization of hypnosis in various clinical contexts, there are only a few papers written on its depth and what the significance of depth of trance has within a clinical practice (Barnier & Council, 2010). Campbell Perry (Perry, Gelfand, & Marcovitch, 1979), for example, provide evidence that the depth of trance, or hypnotic susceptibility, plays a role when working on problems that occur on the unconscious level, or without the client's volitional control or intent (pain, asthma or warts), as opposed to problems that occur mostly from self-initiated behavior (smoking cessation). Wadden and Anderton (1982) support this hypothesis, whereas Brown (1992) more recently adds other non-volitional problems to the list and provides evidence that hypnotic susceptibility plays a role in case of volitionally initiated problems.

If we define hypnosis as a more effective and flexible elicitation and utilization of a client's inner resources and abilities (Dyba et al., 2019, 2021; Erickson & Rossi, 1976/2010, 1979/2014; Ravitz, 2002) then the depth of hypnosis seems to be an important variable in the whole process. Generally speaking, the deeper one can enter a trance state the more readily available hypnotic abilities related with this flexibility will be. Erickson and Rossi (Erickson & Rossi, 1976/2010, 1979/2014) offered a model where they reversed the whole equation. In this model hypnosis is directly related to the client's responses to specific hypnotic suggestions. André Weitzenhoffer in an introduction to ***Experiencing Hypnosis*** (Erickson & Rossi, 1976/2010, p. xix) refers to this in the following way:

> ... there is no longer any distinction between "waking" and "hypnotic" suggestions, or if one prefers, between extra and intrahypnotic suggestions. To respond adequately to a suggestion is to be hypnotized. To put it a little differently, according to the authors, one cannot respond adequately to a suggestion without first, or at the same time, developing a hypnotic trance.

Based on these assumptions, along with additional research and conceptions, we proposed a structural model of deep trance induction and utilization (Dyba & Rossi, 2022) where the depth of trance is directly related to specific suggestion responses, and therefore depth of trance is assessed by a degree to which a subject can enact a specific hypnotic suggestion. Weitzenhoffer defines hypnotic susceptibility as a capacity to produce various hypnotic effects. In our previously described model we (Dyba & Rossi, 2022) distinguish (based on a review of previous research in hypnotic susceptibility) three different levels of hypnotic suggestion: (1) simple motor suggestions, (2) challenge suggestions, and (3) cognitive suggestions. Among other things, this model introduces a new way to estimate trance depth in clinical practice. In the past it was proposed to assess trance depth by careful observation of so called "trance indicators" (Erickson & Rossi, 1976/2010; Zeig, 2014). At the same time, however, Erickson (1952/2021) alone, as well as in his work with Ernest Rossi (1979/2014, 1981/2014) points to the individual nature of trance that can create a difficulty in assessing its depth based on some "unified" criteria. In other words, one can, but does not have to, manifest any observable behavior while being in a state of deep trance. The same observed behavior may, on the contrary, manifest itself as a light trance in other clients or on occasion within the same client. In our model the depth of trance is divided into three levels based on the difficulty of different hypnotic suggestions as described above (Dyba & Rossi, 2022). A therapist that is able to enact challenge-suggestions (for example, "You can try to lower your hand only to see that you can't") is in a deeper trance than a client who is able to achieve a simple hand catalepsy. A client who is able to demonstrate hypnotic hallucination, or amnesia, for example, is in a deeper trance state than the two described before. This view is consistent with the individuality of Erickson and Rossi's work (Erickson & Rossi, 1976/2010, 1979/2014, 1981/2014) as well as with some other perspectives described above (Crawford, 2001; Gruzelier, 1998; Weitzenhoffer, 1997).

Additionally, within this paper and in our model (Dyba & Rossi, 2022) we view a trance experience as a learning process. The same seems to be true in the view presented by Erickson and Rossi (Erickson & Rossi, 1976/2010, 1979/2014, 1981/2014). In fact, ***Hypnotic Realities*** (Erickson & Rossi, 1976/2010) consists largely of a verbatim transcript of a hypnotic training aimed at gradually developing deeper hypnotic states within a client. In Erickson's view, a trance experience is facilitated by a process of ***associative involvement***. In this way, a therapist utilizes the client's own mental processes and associations to facilitate hypnotic experiences. This hypothesis has pivotal implications. First, a client in a hypnotic trance develops hypnotic phenomena from abilities and associations that they already possesses within. Therefore, we can at many occasions witness Erickson (Erickson & Rossi, 1976/2010, 1981/2014) as he tells many anecdotes from his own life, or from the lives of others containing experiences similar to the one he would like to help develop within the trance. Such stories elicit the individual client's own associations and mental mechanisms that they can utilize to create their own hypnotic experience. In ***Experiencing Hypnosis*** (Erickson & Rossi, 1981/2014) Erickson hypnotizes a blind person to demonstrate that achieving a hand levitation will be almost impossible to her due to lack of sufficient associations and experiences with involuntary body movements. As it comes out, the hand levitation is indeed very difficult to achieve, and the client is only able to produce slight hand movements in the palm area. Erickson attributes this to the fact that blind people use their body movements very consciously to orient themselves in spatial reality, and therefore do not have a lot of experience with involuntary movements than people who base their reality orientation on visual cues have. A sighted person performs almost every movement automatically. A good example is walking. For instance, when one walks they do not analyze every muscle movement to make another step. It is an autonomous activity to such a degree that they can easily focus on other things while doing it. They can, at times, forget the path in total, and at some point in time simply realize that they reached the target. For a sighted person almost every move is automatic and does not involve conscious detailed planning. A person functioning this way possesses associations and experience that they can then utilize to create a hand levitation phenomenon. This model explains why ideomotor suggestions are one of the safest and "fail-safe" practices (Dienes & Perner, 2007; Dyba & Rossi, 2022; Nicolas P Spanos et al., 1983).

Hypnosis is an experience facilitated by a process of associative involvement through which a therapist helps a client utilize their own mental associations, abilities, and mechanisms to create hypnotic experience and construct various hypnotic phenomena. This experience is a process of learning to utilize one's own mental abilities. Therefore, developing hypnotic responsiveness may occur either by developing further associations and mechanisms, or by creating a more stimulating learning environment.

Hypnotic responsiveness

Hypnotic responsiveness is usually defined in hypnotic literature as a client's ability to carry out hypnotic suggestions. In the history of hypnosis two opposite views evolved in this regard. Mostly "***state theorists***" who believe hypnosis is an altered state of mind assume that hypnotic responsiveness is a stable characteristic of a subject and can be changed only to a certain restricted degree (Hilgard, 1965, 1979; Hilgard et al., 1961). ***Cognitively oriented*** researchers primarily associated with learning theories assume, on the other hand, that hypnotic responsiveness may be altered significantly and permanently (Bertrand, 1989; Bertrand, Stam, & Radtke, 1993; Kinney & Sachs, 1974). We focus in this paper primarily on hypnotic responsiveness modification clarifying how that can be done. We will mostly, but not exclusively, focus on the learning theorists' approaches. We will not discuss if hypnotic responsiveness is modifiable but instead will assume that it can be altered significantly.

Factors that influence hypnotic responsiveness

Below we review research literature on hypnotic responsiveness and susceptibility to discover key factors influencing a subject's hypnotic abilities.

Based on these studies we will provide our own ideas about utilizing this knowledge to help clients achieve better results in terms of their hypnotic performance.

An ability to dissociate in a special state

Many theories of hypnosis, especially in an area of "special state" theories are based on dissociation (Bowers, 1990; Dyba & Rossi, 2022; Hilgard, 1977, 1979, 1991; Kirsch & Lynn, 1998; Sadler & Woody, 2014; E Woody & Bowers, 1994; Erik Woody & Sadler, 2008), an ability to divide the experience and move part of it – a thought, an action, memory, perception, etcetera – outside of the usual range of control and conscious awareness. Although "state-dependent" theorists mostly view hypnotic susceptibility as a stable personality trait (Hilgard, 1965) dependent on a predetermined capacity for dissociation (Hilgard, 1977, 1979), quite a number of studies asked and tested if increasing a client's ability to dissociate would increased their ability to go into a hypnotic trance.

Among other methods, it was shown that meditation (Gloede, Sapp, & Susteren, 2021; Heide, Wadlington, & Lundy, 1980; McGeown, 2017; Nicholas P Spanos, Rivers, & Gottlieb, 1978), prolonged program for enhancing personal growth (Tart, 1970), and repeated hypnotic inductions (Ås, Hilgard, & Weitzenhoffer, 1963) were able to significantly increase a subjects hypnotic susceptibility. The obtained change was, however, small in magnitude. According to Bertrand (1989) such results may be an outcome of the fact that none of the above procedures addressed either directly, or indirectly, key cognitive factors that are of importance to a subjects hypnotic abilities such as utilization or development of specific cognitive strategies for carrying out hypnotic suggestions, subjects attitudes and expectations. In conclusion, techniques such as meditation, or personal growth training, produce significant but small increases in hypnotic abilities and thus they may become a part of an introductory action plan for clients willing to prepare themselves for upcoming hypnotic sessions.

Client expectations

Positive expectancy and attitude towards hypnosis is considered one of the most important factors influencing hypnotic responsiveness by many researchers (Braffman & Kirsch, 1999; Kirsch & Braffman, 2001; E. L. Rossi, 2004; E. L. Rossi et al., 2012; E. L. Rossi, Iannotti, et al., 2008).

According to research, expectancy shows the strongest correlation with hypnotic suggestibility (Braffman & Kirsch, 1999; Kirsch, Silva, Comey, & Reed, 1995). Braffman with Kirsch (Braffman & Kirsch, 1999) demonstrated in a study combined of two separate experiments that many variables, for example the "hold-back effect" (a tendency to respond to fewer non-hypnotic suggestions by subjects who have already been assessed in a hypnotic condition as opposed to those who were not) (Zamansky, Scharf, & Brightbill, 1964); motivation (Barber, 1995; Barber & Glass, 1962), absorption (Tellegen & Atkinson, 1974), and fantasy proneness are dependent on expectancy. In the case of fantasy proneness and absorption Braffman and Kirsch (1999) noted that both these valuables were correlated with expectancy, and with it controlled, neither showed significant correlation with hypnotic responsiveness. In addition, the research demonstrated a significant but relatively small effect of hypnotic induction on increase in response scores. They found that most of variability in responses during hypnosis may be attributed to differences in nonhypnotic suggestibility (Braffman & Kirsch, 1999; Kirsch & Braffman, 2001). Braffman and Kirsch (1999, pp. 585–586) summarize their research as follows:

> In this study, response expectancy was very highly associated with hypnotic responding (accounting for approximately 25% of the variance), even with prior nonhypnotic responding to the same suggestions held constant. These data indicate that the association is not merely due to observation of one's own prior responses. Instead, the data are consistent with the hypothesis of a causal role for expectancy.

In summary, the induction of hypnosis produced a modest but significant effect on responses to imaginative suggestions. This effect was unrelated to absorption or fantasy proneness but was significantly predicted by both motivation and expectancy. This data highlights the importance of nonhypnotic imaginative suggestibility, a variable that has been greatly neglected in research on suggestion and suggestibility. Nonhypnotic imaginative suggestibility was associated with absorption, fantasy proneness, and motivation, but the magnitudes of these associations were small, and the effects appeared to be mediated by the much stronger relation of expectancy to suggestibility.

The research quoted above underlines the key role of expectancy in a process of "going into trance" and increasing hypnotic responsiveness. Additionally they also support Rossi's claim that hypnosis consists mostly of focused attention and positive expectancy (E. L. Rossi, 2004; E. L. Rossi et al., 2012; E. L. Rossi, Iannotti, et al., 2008). Further in this paper we will analyze more in depth protocols that aim to increase positive expectancy and attitudes towards hypnosis.

While mentioning the effect of positive expectancy, it is also important to mention its counterpart can be boredom. It was Victor Frankl who noticed that boredom is a way of escaping reality and avoiding taking the responsibility for life (Frankl, 2009; Kondrat, 2016). According to him, it is caused by a lack of meaning in a present situation and may develop into more severe symptoms (Frankl, 1984, 2009, 2010). Frankl's claims seem to find confirmation in research on hypnotic responsiveness and susceptibility. Theodore Barber and David Smith Calverley (Barber & Calverley, 1966) noticed that scores on hypnotic suggestibility tests decrease steadily over time with each additional trial. They were the first who attributed this decrease to boredom and disinterest with the procedure. Fassler, with a research team (Fassler, Lynn, & Knox, 2008), measured the levels of boredom and demonstrated not only that it actually increases with each trial but also that the level of anger and irritation elevates accordingly, while at the same time levels of anxiety decreases and positive attitude towards hypnosis increases. These results suggest that motivation and attitude do not predict the levels of hypnotic suggestibility or responsiveness very well.

Fassler with colleges (Fassler et al., 2008), similarly to Barber and Calverley (Barber & Calverley, 1966) suggest that in order to decrease this effect it is important to reduce the similarity between sessions, or in other words, provide subjects with diverse hypnotic experiences throughout different sessions. Fassler (Fassler et al., 2008) also suggests that in a clinical practice it may be valuable to assess the clients levels of interest in a procedure, as well as previous experiences and conceptions, and modify or utilize it accordingly. While working with clients repeatedly using hypnosis it is important to work on such matters, or in such a way as to maintain their interest and, if necessary, add additional modes of treatment to make the therapy more diverse and interesting to the client (Fassler et al., 2008). Both these results, as well as conclusions, seems to be consistent with Frankl's (Frankl, 1984, 2009, 2010) claims, as well as Erickson and Rossi's theories and research (Erickson & Rossi, 1979/2014; Rossi, 1973a,

2002b, 2004). Consistent with Victor Frankl's thoughts (Frankl, 1984, 2009, 2010), meaning is a key factor in human health and healing. Lack of meaning leads to boredom and may cause progressively more severe symptoms and problems to surface. It is therefore important to provide clients with opportunities to find meaning as well as to take their current meaning and values into close consideration while building "meaningful" interventions within a therapy session. On the other hand, as Rossi (Rossi, 1973a, 2002b, 2004, 2007b; Rossi, Erickson-Klein, & Rossi, 2008a; Rossi & Rossi, 2013), and Erickson (Erickson & Rossi, 1979/2014) point out that experiences of shock or surprise as well as stimulating the numinosum – something novel, mysterious and tremendous – can focus attention to facilitate creativity and depotentiate old habitual mental frames of reference thus enabling and encouraging a deeper healing to take place within the client.

Taking all the above data and theories into consideration, we assume that it is important to provide clients with an interesting, novel, creative, and meaningful experience consistent with their goals to enhance the client's hypnotic responsiveness and suggestibility, or ability to carry out more complex hypnotic suggestions.

EEG and relaxation

Martin Batty, with a team (Batty, Bonnington, Samantha, Tang, Hawken, & Gruzelier, 2006), compared different relaxation strategies such as EEG neurofeedback, progressive muscle relaxation training, and self-hypnosis in their effects on enhancing hypnotic susceptibility. They showed that all three approaches were equally effective and were able to enhance hypnotic susceptibility in moderately susceptible subjects. The authors conclude that the common denominator of all three procedures was relaxation and that relaxation dynamics may play an important role in enhancing hypnotic susceptibility (Batty et al., 2006). Interestingly, it was only one case within the EEG neurofeedback condition that a subject demonstrated an increase from the score result of two, up three points from the others. The other subjects with low baseline hypnotic susceptibility exhibited smaller gains from the procedures (Batty et al., 2006). In the condition of EEG neurofeedback subjects underwent ten 20-minute sessions. They were instructed to close their eyes, relax, and then listen with their eyes closed to sounds contingent on theta and alpha activity. Different sounds were attached to theta and alpha activity, but the subjects were not instructed that they could control the sound to facilitate unconscious learning (Batty et al., 2006). In the relaxation training group, subjects were given one live session with the experimenter prior to home-based training with a commercially available CD anti-stress program. Those in the self-hypnosis group got one live session and were given a CD with a 20-minute hypnotic induction with visualization suggestions. Better effects might have been achieved by more frequent contact with the experimenter in the case of EEG neurofeedback or conditioning through on implicit level achieved by the sounds.

Additional research on the subject seems to support the hypothesis that training in relaxation may significantly increase the hypnotic abilities (Simon & Salzberg, 1981; Wickramasekera, 1973), although other research shows the opposite in that while such trainings produce increased levels of relaxation it does not influence hypnotic abilities in any significant manner (Nicholas P Spanos & Bertrand, 1985).

The role of structured training programs in increasing hypnotic abilities

In the past, especially with cognitively oriented theorists and researchers, attempts have been made to create training procedures aimed at increasing a subject's hypnotic abilities. Below we review and analyze the results that produced the most promising results according to research.

The Carlton Skill Training Package

The Carlton Skill Training Package is a training program that is based on an assumption that responding to suggestions and experiencing their effects are skills that can be learned (Bertrand, 1989; Bertrand et al., 1993). The training is divided into three distinct parts (Bertrand, 1989; Gorassini & Spanos, 1986):

1. Subjects are presented with positive information about hypnosis and some additional facts aimed at correcting myths and mis-

conceptions about hypnosis itself. This training seeds positive attitudes towards hypnosis and heightens expectations (Bertrand, 1989).

2. Discussion of ambiguities contained in hypnotic suggestions, as well as the importance of utilizing imaginings consistent with suggestion, produce an experience of involuntary responses. Additionally, participants are told that suggested behavior is a result of their actions and is caused by them. On this stage, participants are being presented with a movie where a female subject performs four distinct kinds of suggestions, and then follows with a detailed description of her imaginings and sensations as she experiences it. The second part of the video consists of a detailed interview with a subject where she provides a detailed description of her cognitive strategies and the activity of each of the presented suggestions.

3. The last part consists of a training during which subjects are presented with a series of suggestions that enable them to practice and utilize observed and learned cognitive strategies to develop responses to these suggestions together with a feeling of involuntariness (Bertrand, 1989).

The Carlton Skill training package is designed in such a way to: (1) heighten positive expectancies by defining hypnosis as an active (on the part of a client) process that involves "interesting and valuable cognitive skills" (Gorassini & Spanos, 1986) and removing any misconceptions, thus taking care for the client's anxieties; (2) train clients in utilizing defined cognitive strategies by way of education, modeling and (3) training of particular suggestions.

In addition to this, we assume that the following training also utilizes an idea of ideodynamic associative focusing as a mechanism facilitating a learning process. The second educational phase of training deals with the problem of ambiguities where clients are presented with detailed descriptions about how to interpret particular suggestions. For example, in hand levitation (Gorassini & Spanos, 1986, p. 1006) the subjects are provided with the following information:

> [The suggestion] will specifically tell you that your arm is like a hollow balloon being pumped up with helium... and that it's rising into the air by itself. In response... you must do everything that is required of someone who is making-believe such a thing. You must lift your arm up and you must imagine that the arm is really a hollow balloon that is being pumped full of helium, rising by itself... You must become very deeply involved in the make-believe and actually make it seem real... Rivet your attention on the hollow arm, the lightness, the fact it's going up by itself and so on. Don't imagine anything or pay attention to anything that is unrelated to the make-believe situation...

In the first part of this instruction the subject is being told that the arm will seem to feel like a "hollow balloon being pumped up with helium". This metaphor, in accord with Erickson's and Rossi's theory (Erickson & Rossi, 1976/2010, 1979/2014) as well as with other Ericksonian metaphoric communication models (Bandler & Grinder, 1975a, 1975b; Mills & Crowley, 1986) will evoke associations and processes of an inner search for meaning that could then lead to a hypnotic response. In other words, if a subject does not have enough associations connected with a hand levitation per se, such a metaphor would provide additional connections. In this way, a hypnotist provides a client with a "similar" experience that can provide information on how to enact a suggestion which asks of something that is not familiar to a client. Additionally, a subject is also encouraged to narrow their attention down to the arm and act upon it as if the whole phenomenon was real. That may launch additional associations connected with a feeling of automaticity and involuntariness. The subject is instructed to lift the arm - which suggests it is an active process - and at the same time "imagine that the arm is really a hollow balloon that is being pumped full of helium, rising by itself" - that suggests involuntariness, and at the same time to not "imagine anything or pay attention to that which is unrelated to the make-believe situation" - which by implication means to ignore the fact that they do it and focus on the idea that it is being done to them. In other words, one may also look at the whole procedure as one that builds additional associations and experiences facilitating arm levitation as well as involuntariness of the whole process itself. The balloon being pumped is also a clear example of an ***associational bridge*** (Erickson & Rossi, 1976/2010, 1979/2014, 1981/2014) between an experience of hand levitation that a client may not possess a clear representation of, and a more familiar experience of the hand being lifted up by a balloon. More familiar experiences may trigger appropriate ideomotor responses and thus facilitate the phenomenon itself.

Donald Gorassini (Gorassini, 2003) condensed the Carlton Skill Training Package down to four minutes to offer information about common misconceptions about hypnosis and to make each suggested response actively - as opposed to just waiting for it to occur, and thus to simultaneously adopt each suggestion a depiction of reality. Such a short protocol was still able to significantly increase the client's ability to respond to suggestions. Because the author did not compare it to the standard protocol we really do not know if it was equally effective. It is important, however, to note that we can significantly increase a client's hypnotic abilities in just four minutes by setting up a proper framework through which a client will perceive the whole process (hypnosis is an active endeavor on the part of the subject + correction of misconceptions) and providing them with a way of reacting to suggestions (actively make any suggested response and adopt each suggested depiction of reality).

To sum it up, we hypothesize that the following processes are involved in the development of hypnotic responsiveness: (1) education aimed at supplying a proper definition of hypnosis as well as resolving myths and anxieties that may inhibit the responsiveness; (2) education about different hypnotic phenomena, their nature, and how they are experienced; (3) a training in appropriate cognitive strategies facilitating hypnotic phenomena; (4) supply and build additional associations and bridges between hypnotic phenomena and more familiar experiences from everyday life; (5) offer a training in experiencing hypnotic phenomena and hypnosis itself.

Yet another way to build up hypnosis associations

Another training package based on ***associational bridges*** was devised by Sachs and Anderson (Kinney & Sachs, 1974; Sachs & Anderson, 1967). This training program is divided into three stages (Sachs & Anderson, 1967):

1. Present the client with a clear conception of ***sensory experiences***

associated with successful performance of any given suggestion together with an explanation that, as a result of training, will become possible to experience these involuntary sensations when appropriate cues are given.

2. Self-paced ***successive approximations***.

3. Utilization of ***double-binds***.

4. ***Verbal reinforcement*** for appropriate responses.

The first part of the training was done by using actual physical stimuli. For example, to familiarize a subject with a feeling of hand heaviness by using heavy objects (books) that were placed in the hand (Sachs & Anderson, 1967). With more abstract items - amnesia for instance - the training was based on the hypnotist's detailed descriptions of the desired sensations, stressing both subjective feelings as well as "***past experience with components in common with the item being trained***" (Sachs & Anderson, 1967, p. 174). One can view this part of a process as a training in building associations where actual physical experiences, as well as past experiences of a subject, are utilized to build more associations that can then be utilized in a process of an unconscious inner search to create and facilitate hypnotic phenomena to build up these components.

Self-paced successive approximations (Sachs & Anderson, 1967) are being achieved by repetitively introducing experiences with a subject, or a particular item, while at the same time instructing them to increase it in ***just noticeable difference*** (JND) steps. In the example of hand "heaviness," clients were told to "supply just enough additional imaginary weight to enable and experience a noticeable improvement in the degree and clarity of the subsequent sensation of "heavy" hand" (Sachs & Anderson, 1967, p. 174). This part of the training may provide client training in development of the skill to enact a particular suggestion, or to evoke designated hypnotic phenomena with an experience of ratification of trance phenomena, that facilitates the hypnotic experience by means of reinforcing it

(Erickson & Rossi, 1976/2010, 1979/2014, 1981/2014).

A double-bind situation is created in the following way (Sachs & Anderson, 1967): the client was asked to give a motor signal when they felt that the intensity of a given sensation increased by ***just noticeable differences***. After that, they were challenged on the item and tested objectively. This situation creates a double-bind because a client either discovers that their thinking is indeed correct and they achieved an increase in an objective measure, or they discover that their original thinking was incorrect. Additionally, such a situation makes clients more involved in a training procedure.

To enhance and facilitate the whole process, a verbal reinforcement was presented every step of the way for appropriate responses.

In summary, the presented trainings aim to enhance hypnotic responsiveness and susceptibility by following means:

1. Taking care of ***positive attitudes, expectancy,*** and view hypnosis by presenting it as an ***active endeavor*** on the part of a client which involves interesting and intriguing cognitive abilities.

2. Provide clients with a ***clear conception*** of what a given particular hypnotic phenomena consists of as well as how it is experienced and perceived.

3. Elicit within clients their ***own experiences*** that are similar to the defined parts of the hypnotic experience, and thus enable the client to utilize their own abilities in a process of trance phenomena elicitation and formation.

4. Provide clients with ***novel experiencestogether with detailed descriptions*** as well as additional demonstrations performed and explained by the model to create new abilities required for designated trance phenomena to be evoked.

5. Provide clients with detailed ***training opportunities*** where they can, in a ***stepwise*** fashion, exercise newly acquired abilities.

6. Supply ***verbal reinforcements*** for every successful attempt.

Suggestions – implementation and intention formation

Hypnosis is sometimes defined as a way of communicating ideas (Zeig, 2014) by means of suggestion. Hypnotic suggestion is a precise tool that enables the therapist to help a client elicit and utilize their own resources and responses in a more adaptive way (Erickson, 1948/2021; Erickson & Rossi, 1976/2010, 1979/2014, 1976/2021a, 1976/2021b; Rossi & Rossi, 2007). Michael Yapko (2019) for example, points out that in order for them to deepen or facilitate the hypnotic experience, they need to be tailored to the client and their personalities. Erickson and Rossi (Erickson, 1976/2021a; Erickson & Rossi, 1979/2014) emphasize the importance of observing and utilizing the client's individual nature in a hypnotic process.

In many theories about hypnosis an element of perceived automaticity and involuntariness of hypnotic behavior is highlighted. Zoltan Dienes (Barnier, Dienes, & Mitchell, 2008; Dienes, 2012; Dienes & Hutton, 2013; Dienes & Perner, 2007) in his ***Cold Control Theory*** of hypnosis based on Rosenthal's theory of higher order thoughts (Rosenthal, 2002, 2005, 2008) states that in hypnosis it is possible to create an intention to perform a certain defined action without second-order thoughts about intending, thus, an experience of involuntariness occurs. Based on this theory we proposed earlier, a concept of "transformative suggestion" (Dyba & Rossi, 2022) is built in such a way as to strategically alter the second-order thought about intention to facilitate any defined hypnotic phenomena.

Utilizing the same theory, Gallo with colleagues (Gallo, Pfau, & Gollwitzer, 2012) proposed an interesting way to increase hypnotic responsiveness by use of ***implementation intentions*** (Gollwitzer, 1999). Implementation intentions are a simple ***if-then plans*** about when, where, and how a particular goal will be set into action (Gallo et al., 2012; Gollwitzer,

1999). They are constructed on a simple schema - when a ***critical situation*** occurs, I will do/perform ***a particular action or response.*** Implementation intention refers to a specific goal intention (***I intend to achieve X***)(Gallo et al., 2012) and creates a commitment to react to a specific situational cue in a goal oriented manner. In Gallo's research (Gallo et al., 2012) implementation intentions were formed in such a way to block higher-order thoughts about intending (Dienes & Perner, 2007). In particular, subjects were asked to form a following goal intention: ***I will suppress any thought about my intended behavior while performing the task!*** (Gallo et al., 2012, p. 1025) and then add the following ***if-then*** plan: ***And if I receive a new task, then I will tell myself: Suppress now any thoughts about my intended behavior!*** (Gallo et al., 2012, p. 1025). The subjects were then divided into four groups: control, implementation intention, hypnotic instruction and hypnotic instruction with implementation intention. The research results demonstrated that the group that received hypnotic instruction together with implementation intention significantly outperformed all other groups. What is even more interesting is that subjects from this group improved both on measures of objective responding as well as experienced involuntary responding. They performed more suggestions and reported a higher experienced involuntariness than subjects from any other group (Gallo et al., 2012). In fact, low suggestible subjects in this group became indistinguishable from high suggestible subjects. The authors conclude that implementation intentions can create automated self-regulation of a goal striving or strategic automaticity with a single mental act of connecting a situational cue to the desired goal-directed behavior without any additional previous training.

The above research shows how important the whole process of hypnotic responsiveness enhancement is in how we structure and build suggestions. Well tailored suggestions containing implementation intention can significantly increase a client's hypnotic abilities without any previous training.

Summary

In ***Hypnotic Realities*** Erickson and Rossi (1976/2010) provide a transcript of a full hypnotic training to increase a clients hypnotic abilities. The whole process is experiential in its nature (Zeig, 2017). Erickson was constantly providing the client with experiences by either developing necessary abilities or correcting misconceptions in the thinking process. What is interesting is the theory behind the whole process was provided by Erickson and Rossi (Erickson & Rossi, 1976/2010) who assumed that trance is both an altered state of mind and a learning experience, thus building a bridge between state-dependent theories and learning theories. In Erickson's model, he understood the process of developing hypnotic abilities in subjects as one of eliciting personal associations and resources and helping a client to utilize it in a process of building trance experience together with all its features. It was, therefore, that he often used anecdotes and metaphors to facilitate this process. This was designed in such a way as to provide clients with novel ways of utilizing their own innate abilities. Clients were enhanced with countless examples of experiences of different trance phenomena to ratify the whole process complete with verbal reinforcements to deepen the experience.

Inspired by Erickson and Rossi's hypnotherapeutic work we reviewed current research in the field of hypnosis and neurocognition (Dyba & Rossi, 2022) to offer a framework for building a deep trance experience in a stepwise fashion eliciting associations and providing experiences to ratify the work being done. This paper further provides support for our structural model of deep trance induction and utilization with a special focus on techniques and technologies for deepening the experience. We reviewed research to provide useful and statistically significant techniques for increasing a client's hypnotic abilities. Much of the research also supports the work that Erickson and Rossi describe in ***Hypnotic Realities*** (Erickson & Rossi, 1976/2010) thus providing a deeper understanding of their approach. In the list below, we summarize the most prominent hints and implications to assist therapists wanting to more effectively facilitate their clients to extend and deepen hypnotic abilities.

- A form of ***meditation or personal growth training*** may be a good action plan prior to hypnotic session for clients who are willing to prepare themselves to experience hypnosis more deeply.

- ***Boredom may decrease a client's hypnotic responsiveness.*** Therefore, it is important to make sure that hypnotic sessions are diversified, interesting and meaningful to the client. It is important that the client knows why hypnosis is employed so that they can grasp the meaning of an intervention. It is also advisable to intersperse hypnotic sessions with therapeutic endeavors utilizing additional psychotherapeutic practices to increase the diversity of a treatment and thus making it more engaging. It is also a good practice to make sessions appealing and surprising to the client. Thus, one may focus their attention more intensely and facilitate the numinosum within a therapeutic experience that, in turn, enhances brain growth and brain-mind development towards an eventual cure.

- ***Relaxation*** may, to a degree, increase hypnotic susceptibility. Therefore, relaxation training incorporated within a treatment model may increase hypnotic responsiveness.

- A high level of a client's ***positive expectancy*** is of key importance. Therefore, it is important from the beginning to address this factor. Before initiating hypnosis, it is advisable to explain to the client what hypnosis is. Particularly important is understanding that hypnosis is an active process where they (the client) will need to actively carry out suggestions rather than waiting for them to occur. It is also important to describe hypnosis to the client as a process that involves interesting and valuable cognitive skills that they can master. It is crucial to correct all myths and misconceptions about hypnosis that may otherwise elicit anxiety and reluctance towards the process with a preliminary conversation.

- ***Teach clients relevant skills and strategies*** necessary to elicit hypnotic phenomena. Among the most important are active participation in the process creating and focusing on imaginings consistent with suggestions to produce an experience of involuntary responses.

- *Model examples* of other clients going into trance to elicit desired responses as well as talking about their experiences to provide clients with necessary knowledge and associations to create meaningful hypnotic phenomena.

- Provide clients ***associational bridges*** with reference experiences that are similar in nature or possesses partial components of hypnotic phenomena that enable novel experiences more familiar to them.

- Provide clients with ***stepwise opportunities*** to experience trance phenomena by themselves as well as with opportunities to exercise their own unique responses to novel suggestions based on previously learned abilities.

- Use ***verbal reinforcements*** to facilitate and ratify the process.

- ***Formulate direct and indirect suggestions*** precisely, with awareness, caution and strategic intentions in mind.

- Use ***implementation intention*** to focus attention and facilitate the hypnotic process.

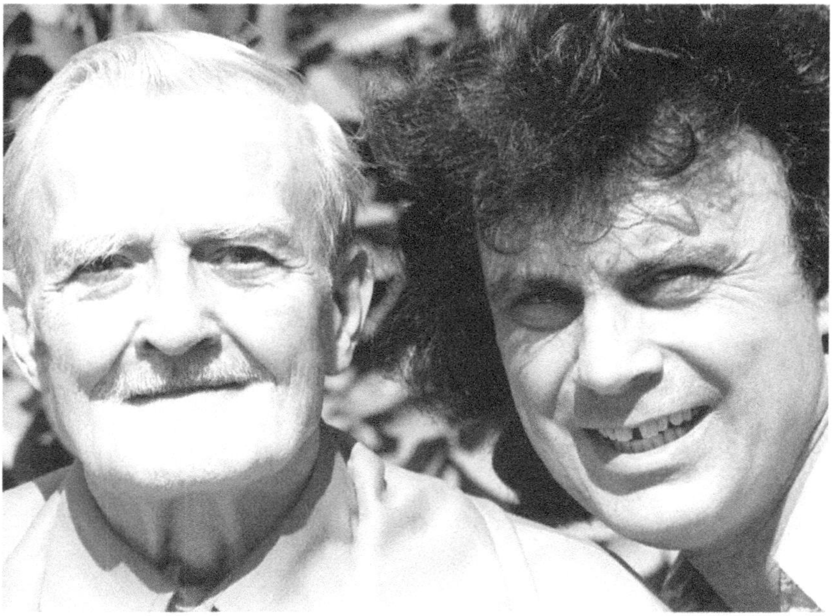

1977. Phoenix, Arizona. 1201 E. Hayward. Milton Erickson & Ernest Rossi in backyard. Photo by Rene Bergermaier.

References

Ås, A., Hilgard, E. R. & Weitzenhoffer, A. M. (1963). An attempt at experimental modification of hypnotizability through repeated individualized hypnotic experience. ***Scandinavian Journal of Psychology***, *4*(2), 81-89. https://doi.org/10.1111/j.1467-9450.1963.tb01311.x

Assagioli, R. (1965). ***Psychosynthesis: A Collection of Basic Writings***. The Viking Press.

Bakan, P. (1969). Hypnotizability, laterality of eye-movements and functional brain asymmetry. ***Perceptual and Motor Skills***, ***28***, 927-932.

Bandler, R. & Grinder, J. (1975a). ***Patterns of the Hypnotic Techniques of Milton H. Erickson, M.D. - Volume I***. Grinder & Associates.

Bandler, R. & Grinder, J. (1975b). ***The Structure of Magic Vol. 1 – A Book about Language and Therapy***. Science and Behavior Books Inc.

Barber, T. X. (1969). ***Hypnosis:A Scientific Approach***. Van Nostrand Reinhold

Barber, T. X .(1975). Responding to "hypnotic" suggestions: An introspective report. ***The American Journal of Clinical Hypnosis,18***(1), 6-22.

Barber, T. X. (1995). ***Hypnosis: A Scientific Approach.*** Van Nostrand Reinhold.

Barber, T. X. & Calverley, D. S. (1966). Towards a theory of hypnotic behavior: experimental evaluation of Hull's postulate that hypnotic susceptibility is a habit ***phenomenon. Journal of Personality***, *34*(3), 416-433.

Barber, T. X. & De Moor, W. (1972). A theory of hypnotic induction procedures. ***The***

American Journal of Clinical Hypnosis,15(2), 112-135.

Barber, T. X. & Glass, L. B. (1962). Significant factors in hypnotic behavior. ***Journal of Abnormal Psychology***, *64*, 222-228.

Barber, T. X., Spanos, N. & Chaves, J. (1974). ***Hypnosis, Imagination and Human Potentialities.*** Pergamon.

Barnier, A. J. & Council, J. R. (2010). Hypnotizability Matters: The what, why, and how of measurement. In Steven Jay Lynn, J. W. Rhue & I. Kirsch (Eds.), ***Handbook of Clinical Hypnosis*** (Second Edi, pp. 47–77). American Psychological Association.

Barnier, A. J., Dienes, Z. & Mitchell, C. J. (2008). How hypnosis happens: new cognitive theories of hypnotic responding. In A. J. Barnier & M. R. Nash (Eds.), ***The Oxford Handbook of Hypnosis: Theory, Research, and Practice The Oxford Handbook of Hypnosis: Theory, Research, and Practice*** (pp. 141-178). https://doi.org/https://doi.org/10.1093/oxfordhb/9780198570097.013.0006

Bateson, G. (1972). ***Steps to an Ecology of Mind.*** Ballantine.

Bateson, G. (1975). Personal communication. Letter of November 10, 1975.

Batty, M. J., Bonnington, Samantha, Tang, B.-K., Hawken, M. B. & Gruzelier, J. H. (2006). Relaxation strategies and enhancement of hypnotic susceptibility: EEG neurofeedback, progressive muscle relaxation and self-hypnosis. ***Brain Research Bulletin***, ***71***, 83-90.

Baudouin, C. (1920). ***Suggestion and Autosuggestion.*** Allen & Unwin.

Bernheim, H. (1895). ***Suggestive Therapeutics: A Treatise on the Nature and Uses of Hypnotism.*** Putnam.

Bertrand, L. D. (1989). The Assessment and Modification of Hypnotic Susceptibility. In Nicholas P Spanos & J. F. Chaves (Eds.), ***Hypnosis: The Cognitive-Behavioral Perspective*** (pp. 18-31). Prometheus Books.

Bertrand, L. D., Stam, H. J. & Radtke, H. L. (1993). The Carleton Skills Training Package for Modifying hypnotic susceptibility - A replication and Extension: A Brief Communication. ***International Journal of Clinical and Experimental Hypnosis***, ***41***(1), 6-14.

Birdwhistell, R. (1952). ***Introduction to Kinesics.*** University of Louisville Press.

Birdwhistell, R. (1971). ***Kinesics and Context.*** University of Pennsylvania Press.

Bogen, J. (1969). The other side of the brain: An appositional mind. ***Bulletin of the Los Angeles Neurological Societies,34***(3), 135-162.

Braid, J. (1846). ***The Power of the Mind Over the Body.*** Churchill.

Braid, J. (1855/1970). The Phisiology of Fascination and the critics criticized. In M. M. Tinterow (Ed.), ***Foundations of Hypnosis: From Mesmer to Freud*** (pp. 365-389). Charles C. Thomas.

Braffman, W. & Kirsch, I. (1999). Imaginative suggestibility and Hypnotizability: An Empirical Analysis. ***Journal of Personality and Social Psychology***, *77*(3), 578-587.

Bramwell, J. (1921). ***Hypnotism: Its History, Practice and Theory.*** Rider.

Brown, B. (1974). ***New Mind, New Body.*** Harper & Row.

Brown, D. P. (1992). Clinical Hypnosis Research since 1986. In E. Fromm & M. R. Nash (Eds.), ***Contemporary Hypnosis Research*** (pp. 427-458). The Guilford Press.

Bowers, K. (1990). Unconscious influences and hypnosis. In J. L. Singer (Ed.), ***Repression and dissociation: Implications for personality theory, psychopathology, and health*** (pp. 143–179). University of Chicago Press.

Cheek, P. & LeCron, L. (1968). ***Clinical Hypnotherapy.*** Grune & Stratton.

Crawford, H. J. (1989). Cognitive and physiological flexibility: Multiple pathways to hypnotic responsiveness. In V. A. Gheorghiu, P. Netter, H. J. Eysenck & R. Rosenthal (Eds.), ***Suggestion and Suggestibility: Theory and Research*** (pp. 155-167). Springer-Verlag.

Crawford, H. J. (2001). Neuropsychophysiology of Hypnosis: Towards an Understanding of How Hypnotic Interventions Work. In G. D. Burrows, R. O. Stanley & P. B. Bloom (Eds.), ***International Handbook of Clinical Hypnosis*** (pp. 61-82). John Wiley & Sons.

Crawford, H. J., Clarke, S. N. & Kitner-Triolo, M. (1996). Self-generated happy and sad emotions in low and highly hypnotizable persons during waking and hypnosis: Laterality and regional EEG activity differences. ***International Journal of Psychophysiology***, ***24***(3), 239-266.

Davies, K. (2006). Search and deploy. ***Bio-It World***, ***5***, 24-33.

Deese, J. & Hulse, S. (1967). ***The Psychology of Learning.*** McGraw-Hill.

De Pascalis, V. & Palumbo, G. (1986). EEG alpha asymmetry: Task difficulty and hypnotizability. ***Perceptual and Motor Skills***, ***62***, 139-150.

Deikman, A. J. (1972). Deautomatization in the mystic experience. In C. T. Tart (Ed.), ***Altered States of Consciousness***. Doubleday.

Dienes, Z. (2012). Is hypnotic responding the strategic relinquishment of metacognition? In M. J. Beran, J. L. Brandl, J. Perner & J. Proust (Eds.), ***Foundations of metacognition*** (pp. 267–278). Oxford University Press.

Dienes, Z. & Hutton, S. (2013). Understanding hypnosis metacognitively: rTMS applied to left DLPFC increases hypnotic suggestibility. ***Cortex***, *49*(2), 386-392.

Dienes, Z. & Perner, J. (2007). Executive control without conscious awareness: the cold control theory of hypnosis. In G. A. Jamieson (Ed.), ***Hypnosis and Conscious States - the cognitive neuroscience perspective*** (pp. 293–314). Oxford University Press.

Donaldson, M. (1959). Positive and negative information in matching problems. ***British Journal of Psychology, 50,*** 253-262. https://doi.org/10.1111/j.2044-8295.1959.tb00702.x

Drayton, H. S. (1899). ***Human Magnetism.*** Fowler & Wells.

Dyba, J., Rossi, E. L. & Rossi, K. L. (2019). The Neurocognitive Update of the Two-Factor Theory of a Hypnotic Experience. ***Science of Psychotherapy***, 30-45.

Dyba, J. & Rossi, K. L. (2022). A Deep Trance Phenomena Structural Model: Nature, Induction and Therapeutic Utilization. ***Science of Psychotherapy***, ***10***(10), 4-31.

Dyba, J., Rossi, K. L., Żurek, M. & Rossi, E. L. (2021). Electrodynamics of clinical hypnosis. ***American Journal of Clinical Hypnosis, 64***(2), 110-122.

Egner, T. & Raz, A. (2007). Cognitive control processes and hypnosis. In G. A. Jameson (Ed.), ***Hypnosis and Conscious States - The cognitive neuroscience perspective*** (pp. 29-50). Oxford University Press.

Erickson, M. H. (1932/2010). Possible detrimental effects of experimental hypnosis. In E. L. Rossi, R. Erickson-Klein & K. L. Rossi (Eds.) ***General and Historical Surveys of Hypnosis: Volume 8 of The Collected Works of Milton H. Erickson, MD.*** The Milton H. Erickson Foundation Press.

Erickson, M. H. (1939/2010). Induction of color blindness by a technique of hypnotic suggestion. In E. L. Rossi, R. Erickson-Klein & K. L. Rossi (Eds.), ***Classical Hypnotic Phenomena, Part 2 Memory and Hallucination: Volume 6 of The Collected Works of Milton H. Erickson, MD.*** The Milton H. Erickson Foundation Press.

Erickson, M. H. (1944). The Method Employed to Formulate a Complex Story for the Induction of an Experimental Neurosis in a Hypnotic Subject. ***Journal of General Psychology, 31***, 67-84.

Erickson, M. H. (1948/2021a). ***Basic hypnotic induction and suggestion.*** In E. L. Rossi, R. Erickson-Klein & K. L. Rossi (Eds.), ***Volume 2 of The Collected Works of Milton H. Erickson, MD.*** www.Erickson-Rossi.com

Erickson, M. H. (1948/2021b). Hypnotic Psychotherapy. In E. L. Rossi, R. Erickson-Klein & K. L. Rossi (Eds.), ***Basic Hypnotic Induction and Suggestion: Volume 2 of The Collected Works of Milton H. Erickson, MD.*** www.Erickson-Rossi.com

Erickson, M. H. (1952/2021). Deep Hypnosis and Its Induction. In E. L. Rossi, R. Erickson-Klein & K. L. Rossi (Eds.), ***The Nature of Therapeutic Hypnosis: Volume 1 of The Collected Works of Milton H. Erickson, MD.*** www.Erickson-Rossi.com

Erickson, M. H. (1954/2022). Pseudo-orientation in Time as a Hypnotherapeutic Procedure. In E. L. Rossi, R. Erickson-Klein & K. L. Rossi (Eds.), ***Opening the Mind: Volume 3 of The Collected Works of Milton H. Erickson, MD.*** www.Erickson-Rossi.com

Erickson, M. H. (1955). Self-exploration in the hypnotic state. ***Journal of Clinical and Experimental Hypnosis, 3***, 49-57, https://doi.org/10.1080/00207145508410131

Erickson, M. H. (1958/2021). The Naturalistic Techniques of Hypnosis. In E. L. Rossi, R. Erickson-Klein & K. L. Rossi (Eds.), ***The Nature of Therapeutic Hypnosis: Volume 1 of The Collected Works of Milton H. Erickson, MD.*** www.Erickson-Rossi.com

Erickson, M. H. (1959/2021). Further Clinical Techniques of hypnosis: Utilization techniques. In E. L. Rossi, R. Erickson-Klein & K. L. Rossi (Eds.), ***The Nature of Therapeutic Hypnosis: Volume 1 of The Collected Works of Milton H. Erickson, MD.*** www.Erickson-Rossi.com

Erickson, M. H. (1961/2021). Historical Note on the Hand Levitation and Other Ideomotor Techniques. In E. L. Rossi, R. Erickson-Klein & K. L. Rossi (Eds.), ***The Nature of Therapeutic Hypnosis: Volume 1 of The Collected Works of Milton H. Erickson, MD.*** www.Erickson-Rossi.com

Erickson, M. H. (1964). Pantomime techniques in hypnosis and the implications. ***American Journal of Clinical Hypnosis,*** *7*(1), 64-70. https://doi.org/10.1080/00029157.1964.10402393

Erickson, M. H. (1964/2021). Initial Experiments Investigating the Nature of Hypnosis. In E. L. Rossi, R. Erickson-Klein & K. L. Rossi (Eds.), ***The Nature of Therapeutic Hypnosis: Volume 1 of The Collected Works of Milton H. Erickson, MD.*** www.Erickson-Rossi.com

Erickson, M. H. (1964/2022a). A hypnotic technique for resistant patients: The patient, the technique, and its rationale and field experimentation. In E. L. Rossi, R. Erickson-Klein & K. L. Rossi (Eds.), ***Advanced Approaches to Therapeutic Hypnosis: Volume 4 of The Collected Works of Milton H. Erickson, MD.*** www.Erickson-Rossi.com

Erickson, M. H. (1964/2022b). The Burden of Effective Psychotherapy. In E. L. Rossi, R. Erickson-Klein & K. L. Rossi (Eds.), ***Opening the Mind: Volume 3 ofThe Collected Works of Milton H. Erickson.*** www.Erickson-Rossi.com

Erickson, M. H. (1965/2021). A Special Inquiry with Aldous Huxley into the Nature and Character of Various States of Consciousness. In E. L. Rossi, R. Erickson-Klein & K. L. Rossi (Eds.), ***The Nature of Therapeutic Hypnosis: Volume 1 of The Collected Works of Milton H. Erickson, MD.*** www.Erickson-Rossi.com

Erickson, M. H. (1965). The use of symptoms as an integral part of hypnotherapy. ***American Journal of Clinical Hypnosis, 8***, 57-65. https://doi.org/10.1080/00029157.1965.10402461

Erickson, M. H. (1966a). Experiential Knowledge of Hypnotic Phenomena Employed for Hypnotherapy. ***American Journal of Clinical Hypnosis, 8***(4), 299-309. https://doi.org/10.1080/00029157.1966.10402509

Erickson, M. H. (1966b). The interspersal hypnotic technique for symptom correction and pain control. ***American Journal of Clinical Hypnosis, 8***(3),198-209. https://doi.org/10.1080/00029157.1966.10402492

Erickson, M. H. (1967/2021). Further Experimental Investigation of Hypnotic and Nonhypnotic Realities. In E. L. Rossi, R. Erickson-Klein & K. L. Rossi (Eds.), ***The Nature of Therapeutic Hypnosis: Volume 1 of The Collected Works of Milton H. Erickson, MD.*** www.Erickson-Rossi.com

Erickson, M. H. (1973). A field investigation by hypnosis of sound loci importance in human behavior. ***The American Journal of Clinical Hypnosis, 16***(2), 92-109. https://doi.org/10.1080/00029157.1973.10403658

Erickson, M. H. & Erickson, E. M. (1941). Concerning the nature and character of post-hypnotic behavior, ***The Journal of General Psychology, 24***(1), 95-133, https://doi.org/10.1080/00221309.1941.10544362

Erickson, M. H. & Kubie, L. S. (1939/2010). Use of automatic drawing in the interpretation and relief of a state of acute obsessional depression. In E. L. Rossi, R. Erickson-Klein & K. L. Rossi (Eds.), ***Classical Hypnotic Phenomena, Part 1: Psychodynamics: Volume 5 of The Collected Works of Milton H. Erickson, MD.*** The Milton H. Erickson Foundation Press.

Erickson, M. H. & Rossi, E. L. (1974/2010). Varieties of hypnotic amnesia. In E. L. Rossi, R. Erickson-Klein & K. L. Rossi (Eds.), ***Classical Hypnotic Phenomena, Part 1: Volume 5 ofThe Collected Works of Milton H. Erickson, MD.*** The Milton H. Erickson Foundation Press.

Erickson, M. H. & Rossi, E. L. (1975). Varieties of double bind, ***American Journal of Clinical Hypnosis, 17***(3), 143-157, https://doi.org/10.1080/000 29157.1975.10403733

Erickson, M. H. & Rossi, E. L. (1976). Two-level communication and the microdynamics of trance and suggestion. ***American Journal of Clinical Hypnosis, 18***(3), 153-171. https://doi.org/10.1080/00029157.1976.10403794

Erickson, M. H. & Rossi, E. L. (1976/2010). ***Hypnotic Realities - The Induction of Clinical Hypnosis and Forms of Indirect Suggestion.*** In E. L. Rossi, R. Erickson-Klein & K. L. Rossi (Eds.), ***Volume 10 of The Collected Works of Milton H. Erickson, MD.*** www.Erickson-Rossi.com

Erickson, M. H. & Rossi, E. L. (1976/2021a). Indirect Forms of Suggestion in Hand Levitation. In E. L. Rossi, R. Erickson-Klein & K. L. Rossi (Eds.), ***Basic Hypnotic Induction and Suggestion: Volume 2 of The Collected Works of Milton H. Erickson, MD.*** www.Erickson-Rossi.com

Erickson, M. H. & Rossi, E. L. (1976/2021b). The indirect forms of suggestion. In E. L. Rossi, R. Erickson-Klein & K. L. Rossi (Eds.), ***Basic Hypnotic Induction and Suggestion: Volume 2 of The Collected Works of Milton H. Erickson, MD.*** www.Erickson-Rossi.com

Erickson, M. H. & Rossi, E. L. (1979/2014). ***Hypnotherapy: An Exploratory Casebook.*** In E. L. Rossi, R. Erickson-Klein & K. L. Rossi (Eds.), ***Volume 11 of The Collected Works of Milton H. Erickson, MD.*** The Milton H. Erickson Foundation Press.

Eriksson, P. S., Perfilieva, E., Björk-Eriksson, T., Alborn, A., Nordborg, C., Peterson, D. A. & Gage, F. H. (1998). Neurogenesis in the adult human hippocampus. ***Nature Medicine, 4***(11), 1313-1317. https://doi.org/10.1038/3305

Fassler, O., Lynn, S. J. & Knox, J. (2008). Is hypnotic suggestibility a stable trait? ***Consciousness and Cognition***, ***17***, 240-253. https://doi.org/10.1016/j.concog.2007.05.004

Fischer, R. (1971). A cartography of the ecstatic ***and*** meditative states. ***Science, 174***(4012), 897-904. https://doi.org/10.1126/science.174.4012.897

Frankl, V. (1984). ***Homo Patiens. Logoterapia i jej kliniczne zastosowanie. Pluralizm nauk a jedność człowieka. Człowiek wolny***. Instytut Wydawniczy PAX.

Frankl, V. (2009). ***Człowiek w poszukiwaniu sensu***. Wydawnictwo Czarna Owca.

Frankl, V. (2010). ***Wola sensu - założenia i zastosowanie logoterapii***. Wydawnictwo Czarna Owca.

Fromm, E. & Shor, R. (1972). ***Hypnosis: Research Developments and Perspectives***. Aldine.

Gallo, I. S., Pfau, F. & Gollwitzer, P. M. (2012). Furnishing hypnotic instructions with implementation intentions enhances hypnotic responsiveness. ***Consciousness and Cognition***, ***21***, 1023-1030. https://doi.org/10.1016/j.concog.2012.03.007

Gazzaniga, M. (1967). The split brain in man. ***Scientific American, 217(2)***, 24-29.

Geary, D. (2004). ***The origin of mind: Evolution of brain, cognition, and general intelligence.American Psychological Association***. https://doi.org/10.1037/10871-000

Ghiselin, B. (Ed.) (1952). ***The Creative Process: A Symposium.*** Mentor.

Gill, M. & Brenman, M. (1959). ***Hypnosis and Related States.*** International Universities Press.

Gloede, M. E., Sapp, M. & Susteren, W. V. (2021). Hypnosis and Mindfulness Meditation: The Power of Suggestibility. ***International Journal of Clinical and Experimental Hypnosis, 69***(4), 411-421. https://doi.org/10.1080/00207144.2021.1908830

Gollwitzer, P. M. (1999). Implementation Intentions: Strong Effects of Simple Plans. ***American Psychologist, 54***(7), 493-503. https://doi.org/10.1037/0003-066X.54.7.493

Gorassini, D. R. (2003). Brief Hypnotic Suggestibility Training: A Confirmation of its Effectiveness and a Test of Self-Report Validity. ***Imagination, Cognition and Personality, 22***(3), 291-302. https://doi.org/10.2190/L111-3X0R-W5PW-738M

Gorassini, D. R. & Spanos, N. P. (1986). A Social-Cognitive Skills Approach to the Successful Modification of Hypnotic Susceptibility. ***Journal of Personality and Social Psychology, 50***(5), 1004-1012.

Gruzelier, J. (1998). A working model of the neurophysiology of hypnosis: A review of the evidence. ***Contemporary Hypnosis, 15***(1), 3-21.

Haley, J. (1963). ***Strategies of Psychotherapy.*** Grune & Stratton.

Haley, J. (1973). ***Uncommon Therapy.*** Norton.

Hammond, D. C. (2010). Hypnosis in the treatment of anxiety- and stress-related disorders. ***Expert Review of Neurotherapeutics, 10***(2), 263-273.

Heide, F. J., Wadlington, W. L. & Lundy, R. M. (1980). Hypnotic responsivity as a predictor of outcome in meditation. ***International Journal of Clinical and Experimental Hypnosis, 28***(4), 358–366. https://doi.org/10.1080/00207148008409864

Henle, M. (1962). On the relation between logic and thinking. ***Psychological Review,***

69(4), 366-378.

Hilgard, E. R.(1965). ***Hypnotic Susceptibility.*** Harcourt.

Hilgard, E. R. (1977). ***Divided consciousness: multiple controls in human thought and action.*** Wiley Interscience.

Hilgard, E. R. (1979). Divided consciousness in hypnosis: The implications of the hidden observer. In E. Fromm & R. E. Shor (Eds.), ***Hypnosis: Developments in research and new perspectives*** (pp. 45–79). Aldine.

Hilgard, E. R. (1991). A neodissociation interpretation of hypnosis. In S. J. Lynn & J. W. Rhue (Eds.), ***Theories of hypnosis: Current models and perspectives*** (pp. 83-104). Guilford Press.

Hilgard, E. R. & Hilgard, J. (1975). ***Hypnosis in the Relief of Pain.*** Kaufmann.

Hilgard, E. R., Weitzenhoffer, A. M., Landes, J. & Moore, R. K. (1961). The Distribution of Susceptibility to Hypnosis in a Student Population: A Study using the Stanford Hypnotic Susceptibility Scale. ***Psychological Monographs: General and Applied,*** *75*(8).

Hilgard, J. (1970). ***Personality and Hypnosis.*** University of Chicago Press.

Hofstadter, D. (1979). ***Gödel, Escher, Bach: An Eternal Golden Braid.*** Basic books.

Hofstadter, D. (2007). ***I am a Strange Loop.*** Basic Books.

Honeybee Genome Sequencing Consortium. (2006). Insights into social insects from the genome of the honeybee Apis mellifera. ***Nature, 443,*** 931-949.

Hull, C. (1933). ***Hypnosis and suggestibility: An experimental approach.*** Appleton-Century.

Flanagan, O. (1993). ***Consciousness Reconsidered.*** MIT Press. ***https://doi.org/10.7551/mitpress/2112.001.0001***

James, W. (1890/1981). ***Principles of Psychology.*** Harvard University Press.

Jung, C. (1960). ***The Structure and Dynamics of the Psyche.*** Pantheon.

Jung, C. (1963). ***Mysterium Conjunctionis.*** Princeton University Press.

Kandel, E. R. (2001). The molecular biology of memory storage: A dialogue between genes and synapses. *Science, 295*(5544), 1030-1038. https://doi.org/10.1126/science.1067020

Kandel, E. R. (2006). ***In search of memory: The Emergence of a New Science of Mind.*** W. W. Norton.

Kempermann G., Kuhn, H. G. & Gage, F. H. (1997). More hippocampal neurons in adult mice living in an enriched environment. *Nature, 386*(6624), 493-5. https://doi.org/10.1038/386493a0

Kihlstrom, J. (2008). The domain of hypnosis, revisited. In M. R. Nash & A. J. Barnier (Eds.), ***The Oxford Handbook of Hypnosis: Theory, Research & Practice.*** Oxford University Press.

Kihlstrom, J., Dorfman, J. & Park, L. (2007). Implicit and explicit memory and learning. In M. Velmans & S. Schneider (Eds.) ***The Blackwell Companion to Consciousness.*** Blackwell. 525-539.

King, J. (1992). ***The Art of Mathematics.*** Springer.

King, J. (2009). ***Mathematics in 10 Lessons: The Grand Tour.*** Prometheus.

Kinsbourne, M. & Smith, W. L. (Eds.) (1974). ***Hemispheric Disconnection and Cerebral Function.*** C. C. Thomas.

Kinney, J. M. & Sachs, L. B. (1974). Increasing hypnotic susceptibility. *Journal of Abnormal Psychology, 83*(2), 145–150.

Kirsch, I. & Braffman, W. (2001). Imaginative Suggestibility and Hypnotizability. *Current Directions in Psychological Science, 10*(2), 57-61.

Kirsch, I. & Lynn, S. J. (1998). Dissociation theories of hypnosis. *Psychological Bulletin, 45*, 100-115.

Kirsch, I., Montgomery, G. H. & Sapirstein, G. (1995). Hypnosis as an adjunct to cognitive-behavioral psychotherapy: a meta-analysis. *Journal of Consulting and Clinical Psychology, 63*(2), 214-220. https://doi.org/10.1037//0022-006x.63.2.214

Kirsch, I., Silva, C. E., Comey, G. & Reed, S. (1995). A Spectral Analysis of Cognitive and Personality Variables in Hypnosis: Empirical Disconnrmation of the Two-Factor Model. *Journal of Personality and Social Psychology, 69*(1), 167-175.

Kroger, W. (1963). *Clinical and Experimental Hypnosis.* Lippincott.

Kondrat, A. (2016). Nuda egzystencjalna a sensowny wymiar człowieka. *Ruch Filozoficzny, 72*(3), 101-115.

Langewitz, W., Izakovic, J., Wyler, J., Schindler, C., Kiss, A. & Bircher, A. J. (2005). Effect of Self-Hypnosis on Hay Fever Symptoms - A Randomised Controlled Intervention Study. *Psychotherapy and Psychosomatics, 74*, 165-172.

LeCron, L. M. (1954). A hypnotic technique for uncovering unconscious material. *Journal of Clinical and Experimental Hypnosis, 2*(1), 76-79. https://doi.org/10.1080/00207145408409936

Liébeault, A. A. (1873). Ebauche De Psychologie. France.

Luria, A. (1973). ***The Working Brain.*** Basic Books.

MacLeod-Morgan, C. & Lack, L. (1982). Hemispheric Specificity: A Physiological Concomitant of Hypnotizability. ***Psychophysiology***, ***19***(6), 687-690.

Masters, W. & Johnson, V. (1970). ***Human Sexual Inadequacy.*** Little, Brown.

Matthews, W. (2000). Ericksonian approaches to hypnosis and therapy: Where are we now? ***International Journal of Clinical and Experimental Hypnosis***, ***48***, 418-426.

Matthews, W., Bennett, H., Bean, W. & Gallagher, M. (1985). Indirect versus direct suggestions - An initial investigation: A brief communication. ***International Journal of Clinical and Experimental Hypnosis***, ***33***, 219-223.

McGeown, W. J. (2017). Hypnosis, hypnotic suggestibility, and meditation: An integrative review of the associated brain regions and networks. In A. Raz & M. Lifshitz (Eds.), ***Hypnosis and meditation: Towards an integrative science of conscious planes*** (pp. 343–367). Oxford University Press.

Meares, A. (1957). A working hypothesis as to the nature of hypnosis. ***American Medical Association Archives of Neurology and Psychiatry***, ***77***(5), 549-555. https://doi.org/10.1001/archneurpsyc.1957.02330350115018

Mills, J. C. & Crowley, R. J. (1986). ***Therapeutic Metaphors for Children and the Child Within.*** Routledge Taylor and Francis Group.

Morgan, A. H., Macdonald, H. & Hilgard, E. R. (1974). EEG alpha: lateral asymmetry related to task, and hypnotizability. ***Psychophysiology, 11***(3), 275–282. https://doi.org/10.1111/j.1469-8986.1974.tb00544.x

Morris, C. W. (1938). Foundations of the theory of signs. In O. Neurath, R. Carnap & C. Morris (Eds.), ***International Encyclopedia of Unified Science, Vols. 1-2***, University of Chicago Press.

Orne, M. T. (1959). The nature of hypnosis: Artifact and essence. ***The Journal of Abnormal and Social Psychology, 58(***3), 277-299. https://doi.org/10.1037/h0046128

Patterson, D. R. & Jensen, M. P. (2003). Hypnosis and clinical pain. ***Psychological Bulletin***, *4*(129), 495–521.

Pearson, R. (1966). Communication and Motivation. Part I: A fable. Part II: The brick-A personal experience. ***The American Journal of Clinical Hypnosis***, *9*(1), 18-23.

Pennisi, E. (2006). Brain evolution on the far side. ***Science, 314***, 244-245, https://doi.org/10.1126/science.314.5797.244

Perles, F. (1969). ***Gestalt therapy verbatim.*** Real People Press.

Perry, C., Gelfand, R. & Marcovitch, P. (1979). The Relevance of Hypnotic Susceptibilityin the Clinical Context. ***Journal of Abnormal Psychology, 88***(5), 592–603.

Peter, B. & Revenstorf, D. (2000). Commentary on Matthews' "Ericksonian approaches to Hypnosis and Therapy: Where are we now?" ***International Journal of Clinical and Experiential Hypnosis, 48***, 433-437. https://doi.org/10.1080/00207140008410372

Polczyk, R. & Pasek, T. (2006). Types of suggestibility: Relationships Among Compliance, Indirect, and Direct Suggestibility. ***International Journal of Clinical and Experimental Hypnosis, 54***(4), 392-415. https://doi.org/10.1080/00207140600856764

Pratt, M. (1996). Adapting the three-step approach for use with children. ***The American Journal of Clinical Hypnosis, 39***, 48-61.

Ravitz, L. J. (1959). Application of the Electrodynamic Field Theory in Biology, Psychiatry, Medicine, and Hypnosis. ***The American Journal of Clinical Hypnosis, 1***, 135-150.

Ravitz, L. J. (1962). History, measurement, and applicability of periodic changes in the electromagnetic field in health and disease. ***Annals of the New York Academy of Sciences, 98,*** 1144-1201. https://doi.org/10.1111/j.1749-6632.1962.tb30626.x

Ravitz, L. (2002). ***Electrodynamic Man: Electromagnetic Field Measurements in Biology, Medicine, Hypnosis and Psychiatry***. Rutledge Books, Incorporated.

Raz, A., Landzberg, K. S., Schweizer, H. R., Zephrani, Z. R., Shapiro, T., Fan, J. & Posner, M. I. (2003). Posthypnotic suggestion and the modulation of Stroop interference under cycloplegia. ***Consciousness and Cognition, 3***(12), 332–346.

Raz, A., Moreno-Iniguez, M., Martin, L. & Zhu, H. (2007). Suggestion overrides the Stroop effect in highly hypnotizable individuals. ***Consciousness and Cognition, 16***(2), 331–338.

Raz, A., Shapiro, T., Fan, J. & Posner, M. I. (2002). Hypnotic suggestion and the modulation of Stroop interference. ***Archives of General Psychiatry, 59***, 1155-1161.

Ribeiro, S. (2004). Towards an evolutionary theory of sleep and dreams. ***A Mente Humana, 3***, 1-20.

Ribeiro, S., Gervasoni, D., Soares, E., Zhou, Y., Lin, S., Pantoja, J., Lavine, M. & Nicolelis, M. (2004). Long-lasting novelty-induced neuronal reverberation during slow-wave sleep in multiple forebrain areas. ***Public Library of Science (PLoS) Biology,2***(1). https://doi.org/10.1371/journal.pbio.0020024

Ribeiro, S., Goyal, V., Mello, C. V. & Pavlides, C. (1999). Brain gene expression during REM sleep depends on prior waking experience. ***Learning and Memory, 6***(5), 500-508. https://doi.org/10.1101/lm.6.5.500

Ribeiro, S., Mello, C. V., Velho, T., Gardner, T. J., Jarvis, E. D. & Pavlides, C. (2002). Induction of hippocampal long-term potentiation during waking leads to increased extrahippocampal zif-268 expression during ensuing rapid-eye-movement sleep. ***The Journal of Neuroscience: The Official Journal of the Society for Neuroscience, 22***(24), 10914-10923. https://doi.org/10.1523/JNEUROSCI.22-24-10914.2002

Rosenthal, D. M. (2002). Consciousness and Higher-Order Thought. In ***Encyclopedia of Cognitive Science*** (pp. 717-726). Basingstoke: Macmillan Publishers Ltd.

Rosenthal, D. M. (2005). ***Consciousness and mind.*** Oxford University Press.

Rosenthal, D. M. (2008). Consciousness and its function. ***Neuropsychologia***, (46), 829-840.

Rossi, E. L. (1963). Associative clustering in normal and retarded children. *American Journal of Mental Deficiency*, *67*, 691-699.

Rossi, E. L. (1964). Development of Classificatory Behavior. ***Child Development***, ***35***(1), 137-142. https://doi.org/10.2307/1126578

Rossi, E. L. (1968). The breakout heuristic: A phenomenology of growth therapy with college students. ***Journal of Humanistic Psychology***, ***8***(1), 16-28. https://doi.org/10.1177/002216786800800102

Rossi, E. L. (1972/2000). ***Dreams and the Growth of Personality: Expanding Awareness in Psychotherapy.*** In E. L. Rossi. ***Dreams, Consciousness, and Spirit.*** Zeig, Tucker, Theisen.

Rossi, E. L. (1972). Self-reflection in Dreams. ***Psychotherapy: Theory, Research, Practice***, ***9***(4), 290-298. https://doi.org/10.1037/h0086773

Rossi, E. L. (1973a). Psychological shocks and creative moments in psychotherapy. ***The American Journal of Clinical Hypnosis***, ***16***(1), 9-22. https://doi.org/10.1080/00029157.1973.10403646

Rossi, E. L. (1973b). The Dream-protein hypothesis. ***American Journal of Psychiatry***, ***130***(10), 1094-1097. https://doi.org/10.1176/ajp.130.10.1094

Rossi, E. L. (1976). The cerebral hemispheres in analytical psychology. *Journal of Analytical Psychology, 22*(1), 32-51, https://doi.org/10.1111/j.1465-5922.1977.032_1.x

Rossi, E. L. (2002a). A conceptual review of the psychosocial genomics of expectancy and surprise: Neuroscience perspectives about the deep psychobiology of therapeutic hypnosis. ***American Journal of Clinical Hypnosis***, *45*(2), 103-118.

Rossi, E. L. (2002b). ***The Psychobiology of Gene Expression: Neuroscience and Neurogenesis in Hypnosis and the Healing Arts.*** W. W. Norton Professional Books.

Rossi, E. L. (2003). The hip-nose doctor finds the Michael Jackson tickets. In Kottler, J. & Carlson, J. (Eds.) ***The Mummy at the Dining Room Table: Eminent Therapists Reveal Their Most Unusual Cases and What They Teach Us About Human Behavior.*** Wiley, 157-165.

Rossi, E. L. (2004). ***A discourse with our genes: The psychosocial and cultural genomics of therapeutic hypnosis and psychotherapy.*** (Salvador Iannotti, Translator & Editor) Editris SAS Press.

Rossi, E. L. (2005). Prospects for exploring the molecular-genomic foundations of therapeutic hypnosis with DNA microarrays. ***The American Journal of Clinical Hypnosis***, *48*(2), 165-182. https://doi.org/10.1080/00029157.2005.10401514

Rossi, E. L. (2007a). Creativity and the Nature of Numinosum: The Psychosocial Genomics of Jung's Transcendent Function in Art, Science, Spirit and Psychotherapy. In ***The Breakout Heuristic - The New Neuroscience of Mirror Neurons, Consciousness and Creativity in Human Relationships*** (pp. 415-436). Phoenix, AZ: The Milton H. Erickson Foundation Press.

Rossi, E. L. (2007b). ***The Breakout Heuristic: The New Neuroscience of Mirror Neurons, Consciousness and Creativity in Human Relationships: Selected Papers of Ernest Lawrence Rossi. Volume One.*** The Milton H. Erickson Foundation Press.

Rossi, E. L. (2008/2021). The Neuroscience of Therapeutic Hypnosis, Psychotherapy, and Rehabilitation. In E. L. Rossi, R. Erickson-Klein & K. L. Rossi (Eds.), ***The Nature of Therapeutic Hypnosis: Volume 1 of The Collected Works of Milton H. Erickson, MD.*** www.Erickson-Rossi.com

Rossi, E. L., Cozzolino, M., Mortimer, J., Atkinson, D., Iannotti, S. & Rossi, K. L. (2012). A Brief Protocol for the Creative Psychosocial Genomic Healing Experience: The 4-Stage Creative Process in Therapeutic Hypnosis and Brief Psychotherapy. In K. L. Rossi (Ed.), ***Creating Consciousness - How Therapists can Facilitate Wonder, Wisdom, Truth & Beauty - Selected Papers of Ernest Lawrence Rossi, Volume 2, 2006-2012*** (pp. 417–428). Phoenix, AZ: The Milton H. Erickson Foundation Press.

Rossi, E. L. & Cheek, D. (1988). ***Mind-Body Therapy: Methods of Ideodynamic Healing in Hypnosis.*** W. W. Norton. https://doi.org/10.1192/S0007125000006218

Rossi, E. L., Erickson-Klein, R. & Rossi, K. (2008a). Novel Activity-Dependent Approaches to Therapeutic Hypnosis and Psychotherapy: The General Waking Trance. ***American Journal of Clinical Hypnosis, 51***(2), 185-200. https://doi.org/10.1080/00029157.2008.10401664

Rossi, E. L., Erickson-Klein, R. & Rossi, K. L. (2008b). The Future Orientation of Constructive Memory: An Evolutionary Perspective on Therapeutic Hypnosis and Brief Psychotherapy. ***American Journal of Clinical Hypnosis***, ***50***(4), 341-347.

Rossi, E. L., Iannotti, S., Cozzolino, M., Castiglione, S., Cicatelli, A. & Rossi, K. L. (2008). A Pilot Study of Positive Expectations and Focused Attention via a New Protocol for Optimizing Therapeutic Hypnosis and Psychotherapy Assessed with DNA Microarrays: The Creative Psychosocial Genomic Healing Experience. ***Sleep and Hypnosis***, ***10***(2), 39-44.

Rossi, E. L. & Rossi, K. L. (2007). What is a Suggestion? The Neuroscience of Implicit Processing Heuristics in Therapeutic Hypnosis and Psychotherapy. ***American Journal of Clinical Hypnosis***, ***49***(4), 267-283.

Rossi, E. L. & Rossi, K. L. (2013). ***Creating New Consciousness in Everyday Life - The Psycho-Social Genomics of Self Creation***. Los Osos, CA: Palisades Gateway Publishing.

Rossi, E. L. & Rossi, S. (1965). Concept utilization, serial order, and recall in nursery school children. ***Child Development***, ***36***, 771-779.

Sacerdote P. (1970). An analysis of induction procedures in hypnosis. ***The American journal of clinical hypnosis***, ***12***(4), 236-253. https://doi.org/10.1080/00029157.1970.10402059

Sachs, L. B. & Anderson, W. L. (1967). Modification of Hypnotic Susceptibility. ***The International Journal of Clinical and Experimental Hypnosis***, ***15***(4), 172-180.

Sadler, P. & Woody, E. (2014). Dissociation in Hypnosis: Theoretical Frameworks and Psychotherapeutic Implications. In S. J. Lynn, J. W. Rhue & I. Kirsch (Eds.), ***Handbook of Clinical Hypnosis*** (pp. 151–178). Washington, DC: American Psychological Association.

Sandkühler, S. & Bhattacharya, J. (2008). Deconstructing Insight: EEG Correlates of Insightful Problem Solving. ***PLOS ONE, 3***(1), https://doi.org/10.1371/journal.pone.0001459

Sarbin, T. & Coe, W. (1972). ***Hypnosis: A social-psychological analysis of influence communication.*** Holt.

Schacter, D. L. (1987). Implicit memory: History and current status. ***Journal of Experimental Psychology: Learning, Memory, and Cognition, 13***(3), 501-518. https://doi.org/10.1037/0278-7393.13.3.501

Schacter, D. L. & Tulving, E. (Eds.). (1994). ***Memory systems.*** The MIT Press.

Scheflen, A. (1974). ***How behavior means.*** Aronson.

Sheehan, P. (1972). Hypnosis and manifestations of "imagination." In E. Fromm & R. Shor (Eds.) ***Hypnosis: Research Developments and Perspectives.*** Aldine-Atherton, 1972.

Sheehan, P. W., Donovan, P. & MacLeod, C. M. (1988). Strategy Manipulation and the Stroop Effect in Hypnosis. ***Journal of Abnormal Psychology, 97***(4), 455-460.

Shevrin, H. (1975). Does the averaged evoked response encode subliminal perception? Yes. A reply to Schwartz & Rem. ***Psychophysiology, 12***(4), 395-398. https://doi.org/10.1111/j.1469-8986.1975.tb00009.x

Shor, R. (1959). Hypnosis and the concept of the generalized reality-orientation. ***American Journal of Psychotherapy, 13(3)***, 582-602. https://doi.org/10.1176/appi.psychotherapy.1959.13.3.582

Simon, M. J. & Salzberg, H. C. (1981). Electromyographic Feedback and Taped Relaxation Instructions to Modify Hypnotic Susceptibility and Amnesia. ***American Journal of Clinical Hypnosis, 24***(1), 14-21. https://doi.org/10.1080/00029157.1981.10403279

Spanos, N. P. & Bertrand, L. D. (1985). EMG biofeedback, attained relaxation and hypnotic susceptibility: Is there a relationship? ***American Journal of Clinical Hypnosis, 27***(4), 219-225. https://doi.org/10.1080/00029157.1985.10402611

Spanos, N. P., Rivers, S. M. & Gottlieb, J. (1978). Hypnotic responsivity, meditation, and laterality of eye movements. ***Journal of Abnormal Psychology, 87***(5), 566-569. https://doi.org/10.1037//0021-843x.87.5.566

Spanos, N. P. (1991). A sociocognitive approach to hypnosis. In S. J. Lynn & J. W. Rhue (Eds.), ***Theories of Hypnosis: Current Models and Perspectives*** (pp. 324-361). Guilford Press.

Spanos, N. P., Radtke, H. L., Hodgins, D. C, Bertrand, L. D., Stam, H. J. & Dubreuil, D. L. (1983). The Carleton University Responsiveness to Suggestion Scale: Stability, reliability, and relationships with expectancy and "hypnotic experiences." ***Psychological Reports, 53***(2), 523-535.

Sperry, R. W. (1968). Hemisphere deconnection and unity in conscious awareness. ***American Psychologist, 23(***10), 723-733. https://doi.org/10.1037/h0026839

Spiegel, H. (1972). An Eye-Roll Test for Hypnotizability. ***American Journal of Clinical Hypnosis, 15***(1), 25-28. https://doi.org/10.1080/00029157.1972.10402206

Squire, L. & Kandel, E. (1999). ***Memory from mind to molecules.Scientific American.***

Sternberg, S. (1975). Memory scanning: New findings and current controversies. ***The Quarterly Journal of Experimental Psychology***, *27*(1), 1-32. https://doi.org/10.1080/14640747508400459

Switras, J. E. (1974). A Comparison of the Eye-Roll Test for Hypnotizability and the Stanford Hypnotic Susceptibility Scale: Form A. ***American Journal of Clinical Hypnosis***, *17*(1), 54-55. https://doi.org/10.1080/00029157.1974.10403707

Tart, C. T. (1970). Increases in hypnotizability resulting from a prolonged program for enhancing personal growth. ***Journal of Abnormal Psychology***, *75*(3), 260-266. https://doi.org/10.1037/h0029279

Tellegen, A. & Atkinson, G. (1974). Openness to absorbing and self-altering experiences ("absorption"), a trait related to hypnotic susceptibility. ***Journal of Abnormal Psychology***, *83*(3), 268-277.

Tinterow, M. M. (1970). ***Foundations of hypnosis.*** C. C. Thomas.

Tomé-Pires, C. & Miró, J. (2012). Hypnosis for the management of chronic and cancer procedure related pain in children. ***International Journal of Clinical and Experimental Hypnosis***, (60), 432-457.

van Praag, H., Kempermann, G. & Gage, F. (1999). Running increases cell proliferation and neurogenesis in the adult mouse dentate gyrus. ***Nature Neuroscience, 2***, 266-270. https://doi.org/10.1038/6368

Wadden, T. & Anderton, C. (1982). The clinical use of hypnosis. ***Psychological Bulletin, 91***(2), 215-243.

Warrington, E. & Weiskrantz, L. (1968). New Method of Testing Long-term Retention with Special Reference to Amnesic Patients. ***Nature, 217***, 972-974. https://doi.org/10.1038/217972a0

Watzlawick, P., Beavin, A. & Jackson, D. (1967). ***Pragmatics of human communication.*** Norton.

Watzlawick, P., Weakland, J. & Fisch, R. (1974). ***Change.*** Norton.

Weitzenhoffer, A. (1953). ***Hypnotism: An objective study in suggestibility.*** Wiley.

Weitzenhoffer, A. (1957). ***General techniques of hypnotism.*** Grune & Stratton.

Weitzenhoffer, A. (1960). Unconscious or Co-Conscious? Reflections upon Certain Recent Trends in Medical Hypnosis. ***American Journal of Clinical Hypnosis,*** ***2***(4), 177-196. https://doi.org/10.1080/00029157.1960.10401822

Weitzenhoffer, A. (1963). The nature of hypnosis, II. ***American Journal of Clinical Hypnosis,*** ***6***, 40-72. https://doi.org/10.1080/00029157.1963.10402321

Weitzenhoffer, A. (1971). Ocular changes associated with passive hypnotic behavior. ***American journal of clinical hypnosis,*** ***14***(2), 102-121. https://doi.org/10.1080/00029157.1971.10402158.

Weitzenhoffer, A. (1974). When is an "instruction" an "instruction"? ***International Journal of Clinical and Experimental Hypnosis,22(3)***, 258-269. https://doi.org/10.1080/00207147408413005

Weitzenhoffer, A. (1975). Personal communication.

Weitzenhoffer, A. M. (1997). Hypnotic susceptibility: A personal and historical note regarding the development and naming of the Stanford scales. ***International Journal of Clinical and Experimental Hypnosis***, ***45***, 126-143.

Weitzenhoffer, A. (2000). ***The practice of hypnotism,*** 2nd Edition. Wiley.

Weitzenhoffer, A. & Sjoberg, B. (1961). Suggestibility with & without hypnosis. ***Journal of Nervous and Mental Diseases,132***, 204-220. https://doi.org/10.1097/00005053-196103000-00002

Wetterstrand, O. (1902). ***Hypnotism and its application to practical medicine.*** Putnam.

Wheeler, L., Reis, H. T, Wolff, E., Grupsmith, E. & Mordkoff, A. M. (1974). Eye-roll & hypnotic susceptibility. ***International Journal of Clinical and Experimental Hypnosis, 22***(4), 327-334. https://doi.org/10.1080/00207147408413012

Whitehead, A. & Russell, B. (1910). ***Principia mathematica.*** Cambridge University Press.

Wickramasekera, I. (1973). Effects of electromyographic feedback on hypnotic susceptibility: more preliminary data. ***Journal of Abnormal Psychology, 82***(1), 74-77. https://doi.org/10.1037/h0034853

Wilson, E. (2006). How to make a social insect, ***Nature, 443(7114)***, 919-920. https://doi.org/10.1038/443919a

Woody, E. & Bowers, K. (1994). A frontal assault on dissociated control. In S. J. Lynn & J. W. Rhue (Eds.), ***Dissociation: clinical and theoretical perspectives*** (pp. 52-79). Guilford Press.

Woody, E. & Sadler, P. (2008). Dissociation theories of hypnosis. In M. R. Nash & A. J. Barnier (Eds.), ***Oxford handbook of hypnosis*** (pp. 81-110). Oxford University Press.

Yapko, M. (2002). ***Kiedy Życie Boli - Zalecenia w leczeniu depresji.*** Gdańsk: Gdańskie Wydawnictwo Psychologiczne.

Yapko, M. (2019). ***Trancework - An Introduction to the Practice of Clinical Hypnosis*** (5th Editio). Routledge Taylor and Francis Group.

Zamansky, H. S., Scharf, B. & Brightbill, R. (1964). The effect of expectancy for hypnosis on prehypnotic performance. ***Journal of Personality, 32***, 236-248.

Zeig, J. K. (2014). ***The Induction of Hypnosis - An Ericksonian Elicitation Approach***. Phoenix, AZ: The Milton H. Erickson Foundation Press.

Zeig, J. K. (2017). ***The Anatomy of Experiential Impact Through Ericksonian Psychotherapy: Seeing, Doing, Being***. Phoenix, AZ: The Milton H. Erickson Foundation Press.

Made in United States
Cleveland, OH
06 November 2026

47780411R00278